THE SURGICAL EXAMINATION OF CHILDREN

An Illustrated Guide

To Susan, Lin,
Kathleen, Andrew,
John, Sarah,
Rowena, Matthew
and Julia

The Surgical Examination of Children

An Illustrated Guide

John M Hutson, MB.BS (Monash), MD (Melb), FRACS
Senior Lecturer in Paediatric Surgery, Department of Paediatrics, University of Melbourne; Consultant Paediatric Surgeon, Royal Children's Hospital, Melbourne.

Spencer W Beasley, MB. ChB, FRACS
Lecturer in Paediatric Surgery, Department of Paediatrics, University of Melbourne; Consultant Paediatric Surgeon, Royal Children's Hospital and Preston and Northcote Community Hospital, Melbourne.

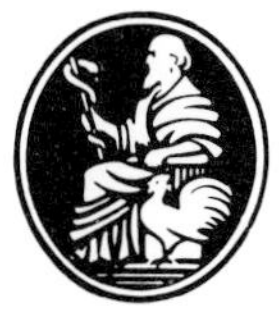

Heinemann Medical Books

Heinemann Medical Books
An imprint of Heinemann Professional Publishing Ltd
Halley Court, Jordan Hill, Oxford OX2 8EJ

OXFORD LONDON SINGAPORE NAIROBI IBADAN KINGSTON

First published 1988

Artwork by Education Resources Centre, Royal Children's
Hospital, Melbourne, Australia

A CIP catalogue record for this book is available from the British Library

ISBN 0 433 00051 1

Typeset by Tradespools Ltd, Frome and printed by Butler & Tanner Ltd, Frome.

Contents

Preface

This book aims to teach medical students and other medical and clinical personnel how to perform a clinical examination in the infant or child who has a surgical condition. Most text books of paediatric surgery focus on the pathological classification and overall management of disease, rather than on the practical details of how a diagnosis is made. In clinical practice, experienced physicians and surgeons usually use a problem-oriented approach to clinical diagnosis; yet this is rarely taught to students. This book attempts to redress this imbalance by providing a clinical approach to the patient which the student can learn with a minimum of factual information. Therefore, it should remain useful to the practitioner throughout his or her medical career. This book includes a detailed coverage of the common presentations of common diseases, and does not attempt to cover all aspects of the presentations of uncommon diseases unless their recognition is important for the well-being or survival of the child. With the increasing sophistication and specialization of children's hospitals, the exposure of medical students to rare diseases has increased in recent years. This is a counter-productive trend, since it means they obtain little experience in the range of problems that they will meet in practice subsequently. For this reason, the commonest problems are discussed in the early chapters of the book, and the last few chapters deal with uncommon or postgraduate topics.

'To study the phenomena of disease without books is to sail an uncharted sea, while to study books without patients is not to go to sea at all.'

Sir William Osler: '*Books and Men*',
Address dedicating a new building
for the Boston Medical Library, 1901

Clinical examination is a very subjective process: one should not shy away from this in a quest for objectivity, but rather one should use deliberately the subjective nature of the mind to advantage.

Acknowledgements

A large number of people have made valuable contributions to this book. We thank Miss Anne Esposito from the Royal Children's Hospital Education Resource Centre for her devotion and effort with the artwork, which is central to the success of this book. Mrs Elizabeth Vorrath, Mrs Judith Hayes and Miss Vicki Holt are thanked for their untiring help with the manuscript, despite their normal, heavy secretarial duties. We are grateful to our colleagues for support and encouragement and for their criticisms of various chapters: Mr Alex Auldist (Chapters 8, 16, 17); Dr Agnes Bankier (Chapter 2); Dr Kester Brown (Chapters 12, 20); Mr Bob Dickens (Chapter 13); Mr Justin Kelly (Chapters 7, 14, 15); Mr Max Kent (Chapters 5, 9, 21); Mr Geoffery Klug (Chapters 10, 12, 18); Dr Peter McDougall (Chapter 2); Mr Nate Myers (Chapters 1, 3); Prof. Peter Phelan (Chapters 1, 3, 6, 8); Mr Keith Stokes (Chapter 12); Mr Hock Tan (Chapters 4, 6, 11).

Dr Richard Barling of Heinemann Medical Books is thanked for his encouragement, enthusiasm and help in completing the project.

1 General principles

Clinical diagnosis in any branch of medicine requires more finesse than knowing merely how to elicit physical signs. It is often a great mystery to medical students how an experienced physician or surgeon can reach a diagnosis with the minimum of history and examination while they may have spent an hour or more with the same patient to no avail. They may despair of ever attaining the same level of expertise. The shrewd student, however, suspects that his senior colleague uses a direct approach to reach the diagnosis, avoiding the lengthy process of aimless and exhaustive history-taking and examination, much of which may be irrelevant to the patient.

It is the aim of this book to teach the student of paediatric surgery how to improve his clinical acumen, and to enable him to reach the correct diagnosis by the simplest route. This direct approach to clinical diagnosis is problem-oriented, where the diagnosis can be anticipated by the early elimination of alternatives. It is the same method that is used in 'decision trees', algorithms and flow charts. Although students may be aware already of this kind of decision-making process, its formal description in the following pages underlines the strength of the technique and demonstrates how it can be applied in clinical diagnosis. Consider the following difference in approach to the simple mathematical problem of identifying an unknown number between 1 and 1000 by asking questions with a 'yes' or 'no' answer. How many such questions are needed? There are two ways of solving this problem. One is to ask whether every number in sequence is the chosen one, beginning with 1 and continuing for up to 999 questions until the correct number is identified! An alternative approach is based on the realization that a 'yes/no' question identifies specifically a number in a two-element set. Therefore, all that is needed is to divide the 1000 choices into two and ask: 'Is the number greater than 500?' The answer will immediately eliminate half the possibilities. With this simple device, the unknown number can always be found in 10 questions! The first technique is analogous to the student who asks every conceivable question and then examines every part of the body from head to toe, before thinking about the possible diagnosis (Fig. 1.1). The latter approach echoes that of the experienced physician who reaches the diagnosis after limited questioning and physical examination.

What knowledge is needed to make a diagnosis or solve a clinical problem?

First, an understanding of the scientific foundations is required; in paediatric surgery, this involves knowledge of the embryology, anatomy and physiology of the neonate and infant, and of normal growth and development. Secondly, it is essential to be familiar with the common pathological processes to ensure a sensible differential diagnosis.

Why does a problem-oriented approach work?

The answer to this question is not obvious immediately, yet it is a fundamental principle of problem-solving by observation. In a clinical context, the clues to the diagnosis are often subtle and will be found only by someone who knows

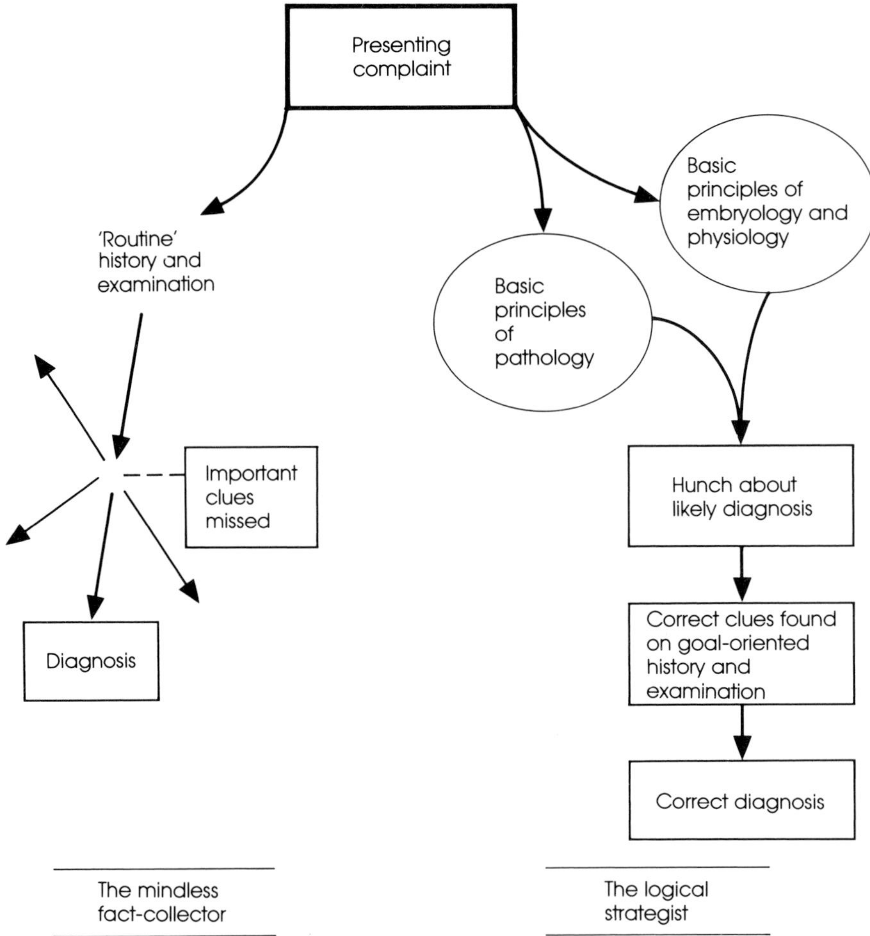

Fig. 1.1: *Unless the clinician deliberately considers the relevance of the information he obtains, he will become a mindless fact-collector, perform a meaningless examination and miss the clues vital to arriving at the correct diagnosis.*

exactly where to look and then knows how to interpret the findings. A physical sign may be detectable if the examiner is working with a hypothesis and specifically looks to see whether the sign is present, but will be missed on 'routine' examination. *It is rare that important evidence from the history or physical examination is found by accident* – the observer must be consciously prepared for it (Fig. 1.1). While it may seem improbable at first, it is a well-recognized characteristic of the brain and senses to ignore apparently irrelevant observations. Pasteur expressed the sentiment when he said: 'Fortune favours the prepared mind.' Once this limitation of the senses is appreciated, it is evident that the secret of rapid and accurate diagnosis lies in having a prepared mind at the commencement of the interview and examination. Only then can important clues be actively sought from the history and examination.

Does the problem-oriented approach work for fields of medicine other than paediatric surgery?

The approach is applicable to all branches of medicine, but the lack of degenerative diseases in paediatrics means that multiple disease processes are less likely to account for the presenting complaint; this is an example of the principle known as Ockham's razor. William of Ockham was an

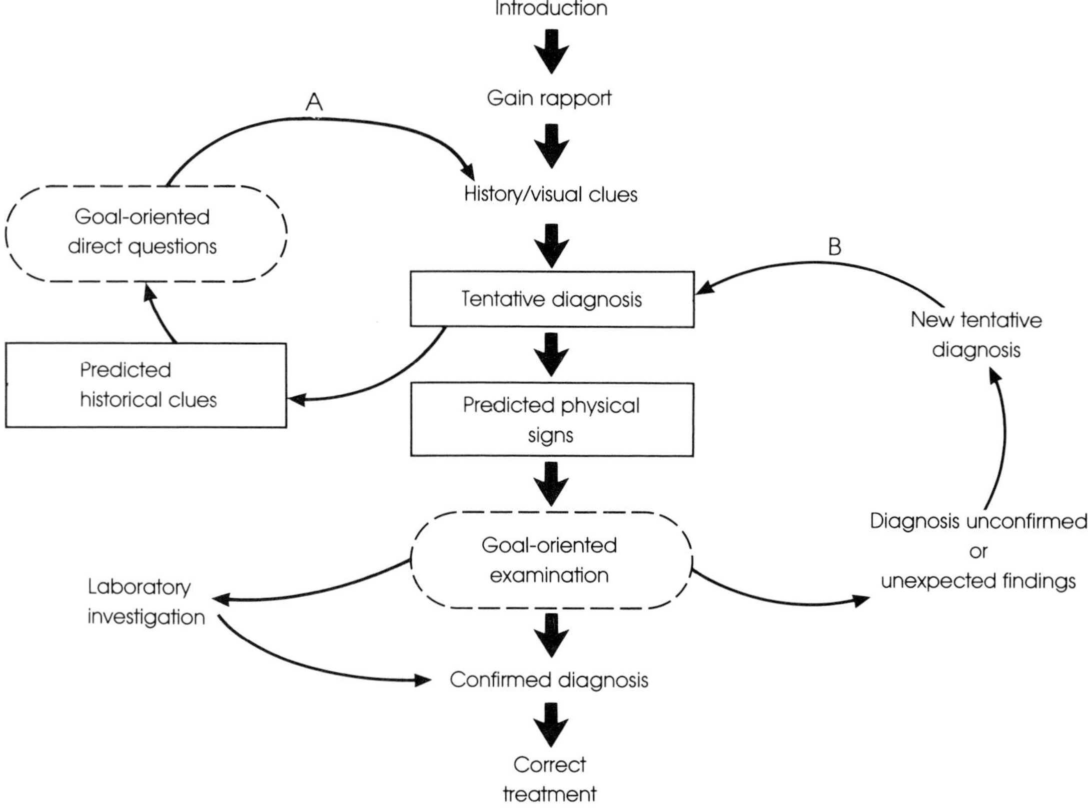

Fig. 1.2: *The process of the goal-oriented examination.*

English monk who provided scientific method with its fundamental principle seven hundred years ago when he suggested we should always favour simple explanations when trying to account for the world's mysteries.

If anticipation of the diagnosis comes with experience, how can the student hope to learn the technique while still inexperienced?

This is the 'Catch-22' of medical education. It is our belief that the technique can be learnt after limited clinical experience, subject to certain conditions.

First, the significance of each piece of evidence must be considered from the beginning of the interview, so that a simple list of differential diagnoses can be formulated. Failure to recognize the significance of information as it is provided will prejudice recognition of those clues which assist in the identification of possible diagnoses. Therefore, when first learning the method, students must ask themselves consciously what the evidence suggests and which relevant questions should be asked. Later, with experience and practice, this process occurs automatically.

Secondly, it must be understood that many problems can be solved by using basic principles, and that this can compensate in part for lack of experience. The basic principles are derived from a knowledge of the scientific foundations of surgery and paediatrics, many of which will already be known to the student. The following chapters are arranged in such a way that the most important principles are tabulated at the end of each section for easy reference as 'Golden Rules'. For many students, several years will have elapsed between the time they learned the basic sciences and their first encounter with paediatric surgery – yet their knowledge of the basic sciences is essential if their examination of children is to be effective. In the

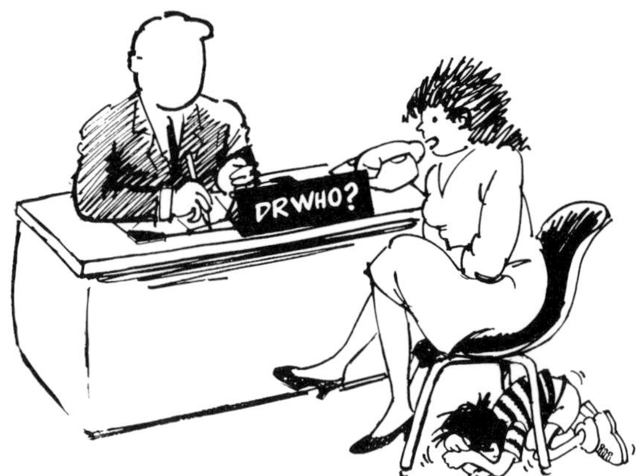

Fig. 1.3: *Beware the nameless/faceless man.*

following chapters, it will become apparent that examination in paediatric surgery demands the fusion of the preclinical sciences such as embryology, anatomy and physiology, with the clinical science of pathology. In no other branch of medicine is a knowledge of embryology more useful, but unfortunately many students will have forgotten their embryology by the time they commence their training in paediatric surgery. While no attempt has been made to provide a comprehensive description of embryology, those aspects which must be retained for clinical purposes have been highlighted.

SPECIFIC PRINCIPLES OF CLINICAL EXAMINATION

The flow chart presented here (Fig. 1.2) provides a plan of how a goal-oriented interview and physical examination can be conducted. Important points in each step are described below.

Introduction

A medical interview, like any other social interaction, needs to conform to social customs. First impressions are important and these can be used to advantage. The style adopted should be a personal one accepting that there are several minimum requirements which are necessary, regardless of your personality. It is important to introduce yourself to both the parents and the child by telling them your name and position. Many parents (and even children) will expect you to shake hands, and this may be an important step in the social interaction. It represents mutual recognition that you will be friends and not antagonists during the interview, and helps both parties to relax.

Many students and, unfortunately, many doctors in senior positions neglect to tell the parents their name and position. No one wants to be confronted by a nameless 'white coat' (Fig. 1.3): personal accountability is important even when still a student. It is not acceptable to hide behind a white coat and remain anonymous through lack of social confidence; such action will insult the child and parents and make rapport difficult to achieve.

Gain rapport

This is an extension of the introduction and is directed primarily at the child to gain his/her friendship and confidence. If the child can be spoken to in a relaxed fashion, the parents will be reassured that you are competent and comfortable with the situation. It is important not to rush this step, because once the child is happy to cooperate,

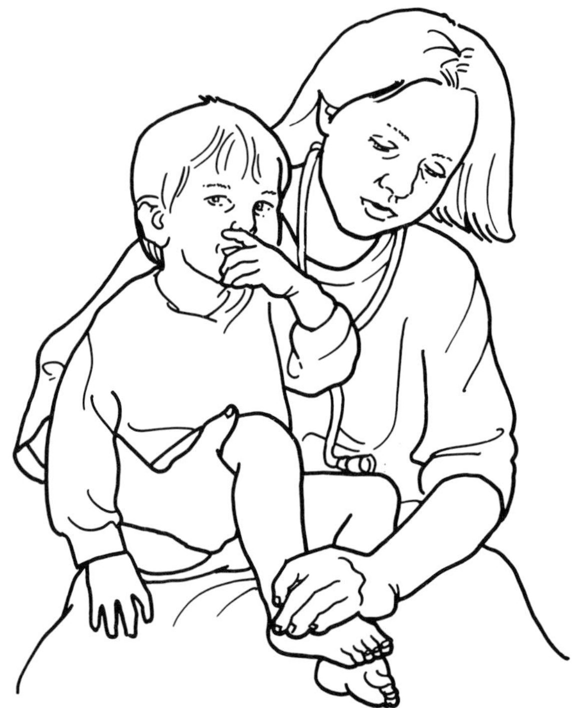

Fig. 1.4: *Gain the child's confidence and trust.*

the subsequent physical examination is made much easier. Young children may have a fear of the unknown, fear of separation from parents, and fear of having an injection or 'needle', often superimposed on feelings of anxiety and malaise if unwell. Children must be given an adequate opportunity to adjust themselves to their new surroundings. Any concerns that children express should be taken seriously and discussed openly, and the explanations which are given in response to these concerns should be understandable and reassuring. This will help them to relax and cooperate. Toys are distractors for toddlers and it is useful to be able to produce a toy with which the child might like to play. As long as the child's taste in toys is judged accurately, the manoeuvre will be a success and the child may even be impressed! This will gain his/her confidence rapidly. Pleasant talk and friendly gamesmanship will usually overcome the fear expressed by the terrified four-year-old clinging to mother!

When a child is undressed and lying on a couch awaiting examination, first physical contact with that child should be in a manner which will allay anxiety. It may be appropriate to touch the child gently while still talking to the child or the parents (Fig. 1.4). The child must be informed always of what the next stage in the examination involves. Uncomfortable procedures, such as throat or rectal examination, should be performed last.

History plus visual clues

The older child should be allowed to describe his/her own symptoms. To be able to take a good history from a child can be a challenge as well as being informative. In allowing children an opportunity to participate, an assessment of their level of intelligence and social maturity can be obtained while boosting their own self-confidence. If the child is capable of relating the history, the entire interview should be conducted with him/her, with reference to the parents for confirmation of particular facts, such as dates or times, as appropriate. It is surprising how often useful information is gained by patiently guiding the child through the history. Knowledge of the intellectual limitations of the child is important when interpreting the story, in order to judge the reliability and significance of each feature described. When the child is too frightened, too ill or too young, the history will need to be taken from the parents. The interaction between children and their parents is often relevant to understanding any psychogenic element in the symptoms, particularly if the complaint is one of abdominal pain. In order to lessen the level of anxiety, the child must always be informed of what is going to happen next, whether it be in terms of further treatment, investigation or hospital admission.

While listening to the presenting complaints, the clinician must begin to formulate the first tentative diagnosis or a short list of differential diagnoses. This is in preparation for clues which may be waiting later in the history or during the clinical examination. Visual clues should be sought during this early phase of the interview. Much can be gained from studying the appearance or behaviour of the child long before the physical examination begins.

Preliminary diagnosis

The goal during the interview is to reach a tentative or preliminary diagnosis. If correct, this eliminates innumerable irrelevant alternatives even before the physical examination is conducted. In addition, it acts as a mental 'signpost', directing the interview along a certain path by allowing predictions to be made for a particular diagnosis about other features which might be present in the history.

Predicted clues from the history

The predicted clues from the history are derived directly from the preliminary diagnosis and enable the child and parents to be cross-examined about specific features for which you are looking. Some general background information may be required as well, such as maternal, perinatal or family history, but it is important not to become too preoccupied with these areas unless they are directly relevant to the problem. It is easy to become distracted collecting unnecessary information.

Sometimes cross-examination will reveal clues which suggest an alternative diagnosis. Should this occur, reappraisal of the evidence already obtained may allow formulation of a revised diagnosis. Further direct questions may then be required to document the predicted features of the new diagnosis. This process is represented by circle A in the flow chart. It is reasonable to proceed around the circular path as often as is necessary to reach a firm preliminary diagnosis. Obviously, with greater experience, fewer circuits will be needed before a confident diagnosis is made.

Predicted physical signs

The preliminary diagnosis allows prediction of the physical signs which should be sought on examination. These signs may be positive or negative, because sometimes it is essential that certain important alternatives are eliminated.

Goal-oriented examination

The first step in any examination is to perform a screening check of the entire body, concentrating on areas not directly related to the likely diagnosis. This collects important background information and on occasions may reveal a surprise. If it is done first, it is less likely to be forgotten. After the relatively brief general examination, the organ or system in which the predicted physical signs are to be found, is examined. In this way, the preliminary diagnosis is either substantiated or refuted. There is a greater chance of elucidating subtle signs, and of detecting other more obvious signs which are rarely elicited, if the examiner is looking for particular features. A good example of a rare but important sign is perineal anaesthesia; it is obvious when sought but not when looked for routinely, yet it is an essential clue to the diagnosis of a neurogenic bladder.

The goal-oriented examination will usually confirm the preliminary diagnosis if the hypothesis is correct. With the diagnosis correctly ascertained, management can begin immediately. Occasionally, confirmation of the diagnosis depends on further corroboration by laboratory investigations, such as x-rays or blood tests.

Diagnosis in doubt

If the findings of goal-oriented examination do not support the preliminary diagnosis, or if unexpected signs are found, it is necessary to reconsider the diagnosis. This is shown in circle B. If an alternative diagnosis seems more probable after the initial findings, the parents and child must be questioned again for further clues in the history which might support a new diagnosis (circle A). Subsequent physical examination is then directed at new predicted physical signs derived from the new tentative diagnosis.

With greater experience, less time will be spent back-tracking (circles A and B) and progression to the diagnosis will be rapid. All that is needed to master this technique is (1) some knowledge, and (2) an idea of possible diagnoses. If either of these prerequisites is missing, the clinical evidence will not be recognized, i.e. relevant symptoms and signs will be missed, or their significance will not be appreciated.

Further Reading

Fulginiti V.A. (1981). *Pediatric Clinical Problem Solving*. Baltimore: Williams and Wilkins.

Green M. (1986). *Pediatric Diagnosis. Interpretation of Symptoms and Signs in Different Age Periods*, 4th edn. Philadelphia: Saunders.

Jones P.G., Woodward A.A., eds. (1986). *Clinical Paediatric Surgery. Diagnosis and Treatment*, 3rd edn. Melbourne: Blackwell Scientific.

MacMahon R.A., ed. (1984). *An Aid to Paediatric Surgery*. Edinburgh: Churchill Livingstone.

Spitz L., Steiner G.M., Zachary R.B. (1981). *A Colour Atlas of Paediatric Surgical Diagnosis*. London: Wolfe Medical.

2 Is the baby normal?

Some knowledge of the aetiology and patterns of congenital malformation is helpful to answer the question, 'Is the baby normal?'. This knowledge enables the clinician to perform a more specific 'screening' examination of the neonate, and anticipates the physical signs of those abnormalities which may be present.

EMBRYOLOGY

How common are congenital anomalies?

Nearly two thirds of all pregnancies are affected by serious abnormalities which lead to spontaneous abortion in the first three to four weeks, often before the pregnancy has been confirmed. Half of these have a chromosomal abnormality. Almost 10% of pregnancies abort in the embryonic stage, from inborn errors or gross malformations. The surviving fetuses now represent about 30% of the original number of fertilized ova, but a few still harbour a defect such that 3–4% of babies born have an abnormality (Fig. 2.1).

What types of abnormality are there, and when do they occur?

There are four main groups of congenital lesions: inborn errors affecting the fertilized ovum; abnormalities occurring at the time of the three germ layers; abnormalities of organogenesis; and defects in fetal movement or compression (Fig. 2.2). Genetic or chromosomal anomalies are present from the one-cell stage, and cellular or germ layer defects occur between one and three weeks after conception. These two groups account for the enormous drop in survival during the early weeks of pregnancy. Only a small percentage of conceptuses with these defects survive to birth.

Between three and 10 weeks' gestation, the basic shape and organs of the embryo form, and this is when most surgical malformations arise. Anomalies occurring during embryogenesis may be caused by innate genetic defects or by extrinsic teratogens (e.g. rubella or other congenital infections, x-rays, drugs, chemicals or maternal dietary

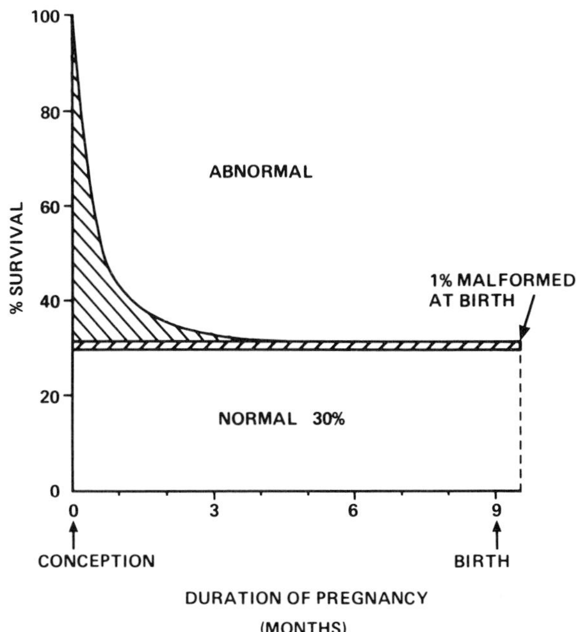

Fig. 2.1: *The survival of fertilized ova relative to the normal duration of pregnancy.*

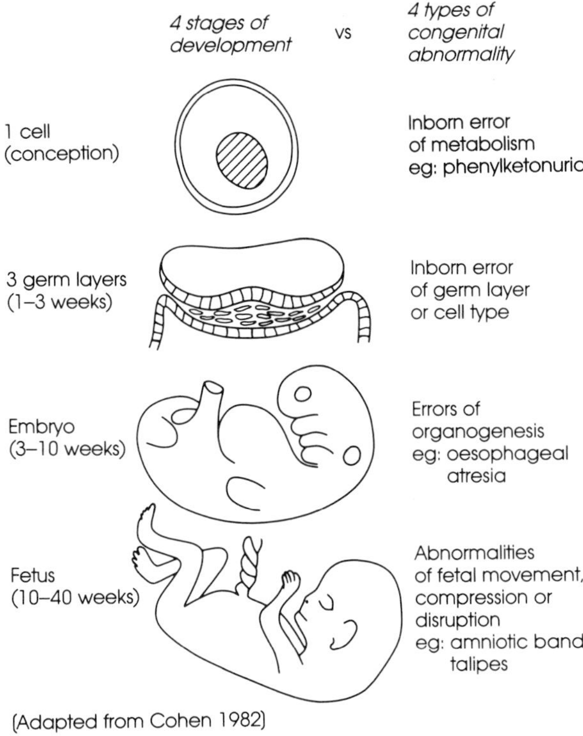

Fig. 2.2: *The four stages of development and the types of congenital anomaly which occur at each stage.*

abnormalities). Knowledge of the causation of many surgical malformations is poor because the embryonic stage is the most difficult phase of pregnancy to study. Despite this limitation, there are several important principles of surgical anomalies which are essential if the clinical situation at birth is to be understood.

(1) Anomalies are often multiple, because several organs may be sensitive to the same teratogenic influence. If one major anomaly is present, look for others.
(2) Multiple anomalies are related to each other in time or space. Different parts of the body may be sensitive to a particular extrinsic teratogen or mutation because they are all undergoing rapid cell division and morphogenesis at the same time. Conversely, several organs in the same part of the body may be affected by a 'field' anomaly of morphogenesis.

A good example of time-related defects is congenital rubella: the group of organs involved depends on the age of the embryo at infection. The heart, eyes and teeth will be affected at six weeks, while at nine weeks the ear will be involved, leading to deafness, but the eye is spared.

The 'VATER' association is a further example of time-related defects, where the following abnormalities are seen in combination:

V – vertebral anomaly, e.g. sacral agenesis, hemivertebrae
A – anorectal anomaly
T – tracheo-oesophageal fistula
E – (o)esophageal atresia
R – renal anomaly, deficiency of the radius.

Imperforate anus often provides an example of space-related anomalies since it is commonly associated with other pelvic abnormalities, such as sacral agenesis, deficiency of sacral nerves and pelvic floor muscles, and urogenital anomalies.

(3) The genetic control of morphogenesis is a multi-tiered hierarchy within which only certain abnormalities are possible and only a few are common. In other words, there is not an infinite array of possible defects, but only a small number of common lesions sufficiently compatible with survival to reach birth. One never finds a baby with antlers(!), but pre-auricular skin tags do occur. The commonest form of abnormal morphogenesis is incomplete development (Fig. 2.3). This is a normal process in which only the timing is disrupted. Less common is redundant morphogenesis, where the normal process has been partially or completely duplicated. Truly aberrant morphogenesis is rare, because the abnormality will usually lead to death well before birth.

Does it matter if the baby is dysmorphic?

Yes! Where one major anomaly is observed, the presence of others must be sought. Dysmorphism may indicate that the child has a number of malformations which may be well enough known to be called a 'syndrome'. A syndrome is a collection of features or defects which is recognized as belonging to the one entity. Individual syndromes are rare and may carry unwieldy eponymous names which make them an anathema

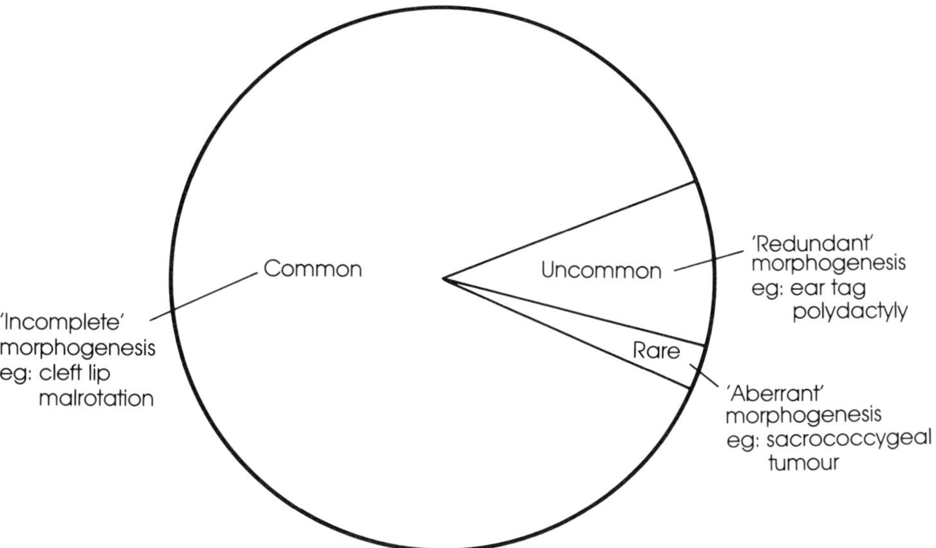

Fig. 2.3: *The different types of abnormal morphogenesis that are possible.*

to the average student or clinician, although obsessive/compulsive learners seem drawn to them. Their real importance is that definitive diagnosis of the syndrome will allow other features of the syndrome not yet identified to be actively sought, usually after consultation with a geneticist or reference book. Moreover, the prognosis will be predicted more readily than in complex cases without recognized syndromes, since outcome usually has been well defined by previously reported cases. This information is essential in the perinatal period so that the parents can be given a realistic outline of the future. The inevitable fatality of certain syndromes may enable proper discussion about the most appropriate treatment to be offered. In some cases, accurate syndrome identification also permits the cause and risk to future pregnancies to be determined.

How do I know if the baby has a syndrome?

The principles required by the average clinician are simple, although consultation with an expert colleague is advisable for confirmation. Where a baby has several obvious malformations, the clinician should be alerted to the possibility of a syndrome being present and seek further evidence of this. The areas of the body in which minor abnormalities occur frequently are easily accessible in the neonate and should be carefully scanned (Fig. 2.4). Facial features obviously need to be assessed in the context of the appearance of the parents. Minor anomalies are important because their presence has a strong correlation with the

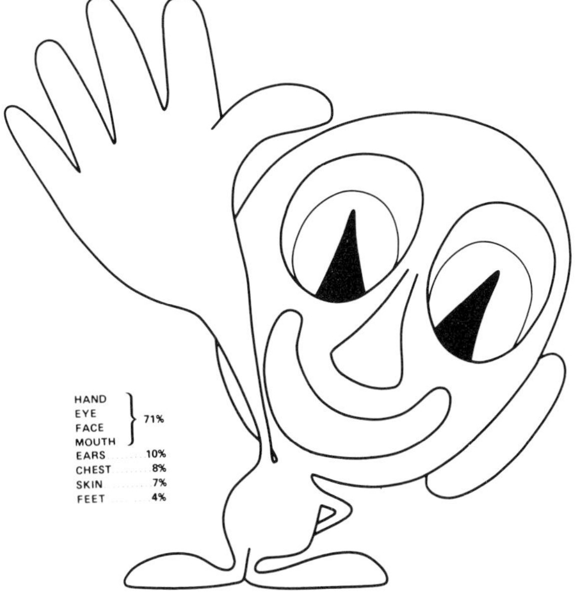

Fig. 2.4: *The relationship of recognizable minor anomalies to the parts of the body.*

existence of major malformations. The finding of a number of minor anomalies in addition to major defects adds weight to the possibility that a syndrome is present.

It is important that the clinician is not daunted by lack of detailed knowledge of individual syndromes. A search for time-related internal defects, space-related defects and minor anomalies of the face and hands will usually yield significant information, even when performed by inexperienced examiners.

SURGICAL ASSESSMENT OF THE NEONATE

This section describes those aspects of the general clinical assessment of the neonate which are commonly relevant to the infant with a surgical condition. It does not include a full description of the medical or neurological examination, but concentrates on features which a surgeon may be required to assess, or upon which he may be asked to provide an opinion.

The examination of a neonate should be performed under a heat lamp or in a warm quiet environment appropriate to the infant's needs, to avoid heat loss. Lighting must be adequate and the reflected light should not obscure subtle changes in skin colour. The entire surface of the baby must be observed, but care should be taken to avoid excessive handling of the sick infant. Much information can be obtained by careful observation with minimal disturbance to the infant.

General examination

Many abnormalities can be detected at birth by simple clinical examination provided that a systemic approach is adopted, such as the scheme outlined below.

First look for obvious major anomalies which require immediate measures to avoid unnecessary morbidity, e.g. a child with gastroschisis should be wrapped in plastic foodwrap to prevent excessive evaporative heat loss. If there are no external abnormalities which require immediate attention, commence examination by observing the overall posture and activity of the child. Does the appearance match the gestation? Next, observe the infant breathing. Is there tachypnoea, respiratory distress or cyanosis? Look for sternal retraction. Does the infant seem to be 'working hard' with breathing? Once respiratory distress is recognized, its cause should be established promptly. Details of how this is achieved are provided in Chapter 20. It should not be forgotten that distension of the abdomen exacerbates respiratory distress by elevating the diaphragm and interfering with the mechanics of ventilation.

The colour of the skin, sclera and mucous membranes should be noted, looking for jaundice, pallor or cyanosis. Turn now to inspection of the head. Feel the anterior and posterior fontanelles and the suture lines. Assess head size (Chapter 10), measure head circumference, inspect the eyes, test the patency of each nostril and look at the hard palate for evidence of a cleft (Chapter 11). Is the tongue normal in size or excessively large? Is there excessive salivation? Study the shape of the face: are the ears in the correct position and is the distance between the eyes normal? Are the pinnae fully developed and is there an external auditory meatus? Is the lower jaw normal or underdeveloped?

The neck of the neonate is relatively short but should be inspected for abnormal skin lesions or deeper swellings (Chapter 9), such as a cystic hygroma or sternomastoid tumour.

Is the chest wall normal and is chest expansion symmetrical? Is air entry equal on both sides? Listen to the lung fields for breath sounds. If these are abnormal, percuss the chest. The liver, which is relatively large in the neonate, is percussible in the right lower chest. Dullness of the chest (other than the liver) suggests fluid. Hyper-resonance may indicate a pneumothorax, in which case breath sounds will appear distant on auscultation. If chest movement and breath sounds are normal, next listen to the heart. The rapid heart rate of the neonate makes auscultation difficult for the inexperienced clinician, but an attempt should be made to detect murmurs and abnormalities in rhythm. Confirm the location of the heart to exclude situs inversus.

Move to the abdomen. Here, three questions should be answered: (1) Is the abdomen distended (or scaphoid)? (2) Are there any abnormal masses palpable? (3) Is there evidence of perforation or peritonitis? Observation of the contour of the ventral abdominal wall of many normal newborn infants provides the experience necessary to judge minor degrees of abdominal distension. Gross abdominal distension is obvious even to the untrained eye and usually indicates bowel obstruction (Chapter 21). Several organs are normally palpable in the abdomen: the liver, kidneys, bladder and less commonly the spleen can be identified in most babies (Chapter 15). The prominence of the vertebral column enables the pulsation of the overlying aorta to be felt easily. Clues to the presence of peritonitis include redness and oedema of the skin of the ventral abdominal wall, tenderness to palpation and increasing distension. A localized perforation may become apparent as a fixed tender mass.

The distal part of the umbilical cord rapidly dessicates and shrivels up to become the black rigid umbilical stump, but remains attached for about one week before separating from the umbilicus itself. Swelling at the umbilicus is common in the first weeks after separation, but usually disappears as the umbilical cicatrix contracts. In most babies, there are three vessels in the umbilical cord: the presence of only two vessels may be related to other congenital anomalies. Failure of the umbilicus to contract after involution of the fetal vessels will produce an umbilical hernia (Chapter 6).

Next examine the inguinoscrotal and perineal regions (Chapters 4 and 5). What sex is the child (Chapter 22)? Look for groin swellings indicating inguinal herniae. In boys, identify the position of the testes to determine whether they are fully descended. Remember, transinguinal descent occurs at about seven months gestation. Inspect the foreskin and location of the urethral meatus. A dorsal hood of foreskin and chordee is suspicious of hypospadias.

In both sexes, look for the anus. Two questions must be answered: (1) Is it in the correct position? (2) Is it patent? If the anus is absent in the male, carefully inspect the median raphe of the perineum, scrotum and central surface of the penis for a fistulous opening which may be stained black with meconium. In the female, part the labia to inspect the vestibule for an opening. Where the anus is anteriorly displaced, its patency must be established (Chapter 21).

Examine the limbs for congenital dislocation of the hip, club foot and other orthopaedic anomalies (Chapter 13). Count the fingers and toes. Inspect the skin for lesions: certain hamartomata are not present at birth but become apparent in the first weeks of life as slightly elevated red or purple lesions (e.g. strawberry naevi) whereas others (e.g. port wine stains) are present at birth and do not change.

Finally, turn the infant over to examine the back. Run your fingers down the spinous processes and confirm the presence of the sacral segments and coccyx. Look for midline swellings and sinus openings. While the infant is held prone in your hand, test for muscle tone and posture.

Assessment of gestational age

The gestational age is an important factor in determining the infant's ability to adapt to the extra-uterine environment. The best estimate of age comes from the mother's dates (when known) or from the antenatal ultrasound. Clinical assessment of the stage of development provides an adequate but less accurate estimate of gestation, but is important in confirming the mother's dates. Knowledge of the birth weight alone is inadequate as it is unable to distinguish the infants with intra-uterine growth retardation from those with prematurity. It is important to distinguish these two groups as they have different neonatal problems and requirements. Furthermore, it should be recognized that any assessment of gestational age is only approximate, but if the guidelines described below are followed it should be possible to determine the gestation to within about three weeks (Table 2.1), an error which is entirely acceptable from the therapeutic point of view.

Ears

Two features of the ear make it useful in the assessment of gestational age: (1) the amount of cartilage present; and (2) the form of the pinna.

Before 34 weeks, there is no cartilage in the pinna and it feels thin and soft and will stay folded if deflected forwards. After 34 weeks, increasing

Table 2.1 ASSESSMENT OF GESTATION

Ears	Cartilage
	Form (in-curving)
Breast	Breast tissue
	Nipple and areola
Sole creases	
Skin	Thickness
	Fat deposition
	Desquamation
Genitalia	Testes
	Scrotum
	Labia majora and clitoris
Vernix	
Hair	
Skull	
Posture	Resting posture
	Recoil of extremities
	Muscle tone (horizontal suspension)

cartilage is laid down, making the ear more elastic so that by term it stands away from the head and, if folded forward and released, springs back to its original position promptly (Fig. 2.5).

In-curving of the edge of the superior part of the pinna commences at about 34 weeks and proceeds downwards towards the lobe. If no in-curving is evident, the gestation is likely to be less than 34 weeks. Where in-curving is well defined and has reached the lobe, the baby is near term (Fig. 2.6).

Breast

The fetal development of the breast is similar in both sexes. Before 34 weeks, the areola and nipple are barely visible and there is no palpable breast tissue. At about 34 weeks gestation, the areola becomes raised and the nipple well defined. Two weeks later, the breast tissue begins to increase in size to form a nodule 1–2 mm in diameter, and by term this breast nodule has reached 6–10 mm in diameter (Fig. 2.7).

Sole creases

Until 32 weeks, the soles are smooth and without skin creases. Creases first appear on the anterior part of the sole, and by 36 weeks cover the anterior half of the sole. At term, the creases extend posteriorly to include the heel (Fig. 2.8).

Genitalia

In the male, the testes are not palpable outside the inguinal canal until after 28 weeks of gestation, when they commence their descent into the scrotum. They are usually in the scrotum by 37 weeks (Fig. 2.9).

There are no rugae in the scrotum until 28 weeks and only a few appear in subsequent weeks until 36 weeks, at which stage they become prominent, particularly in the anterior half of the scrotum. At term, the scrotum is pendulous (Fig. 2.10).

The clitoris is prominent and the labia majora small, poorly developed and widely separated until 36 weeks. In the last month before term, the labia majora enlarge to nearly cover the clitoris. At

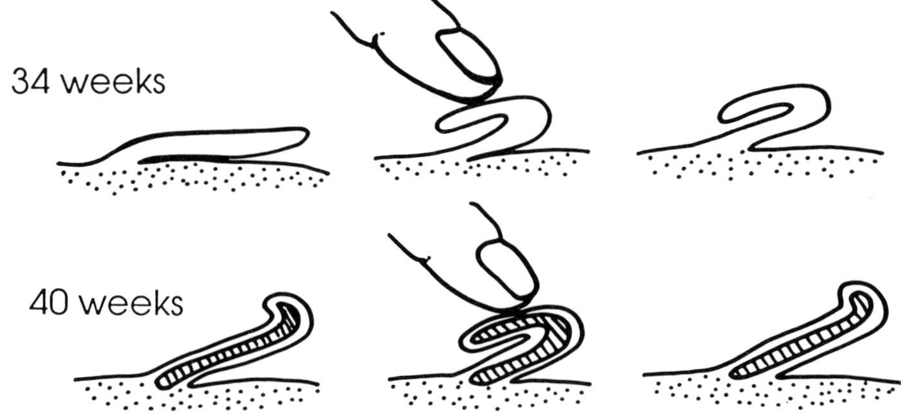

Fig. 2.5: *Assessment of ear cartilage development. At 34 weeks, the pinna will remain folded while at 40 weeks, the cartilage provides elastic recoil.*

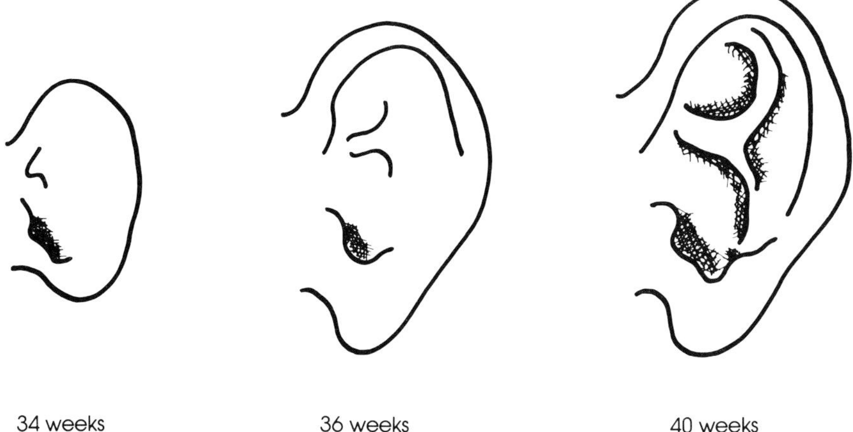

Fig. 2.6: *The development of the folds of the pinna relative to gestational age.*

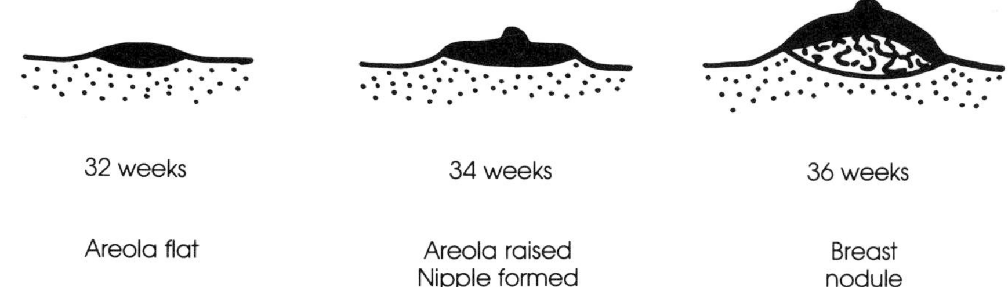

Fig. 2.7: *Breast bud development compared with gestational age.*

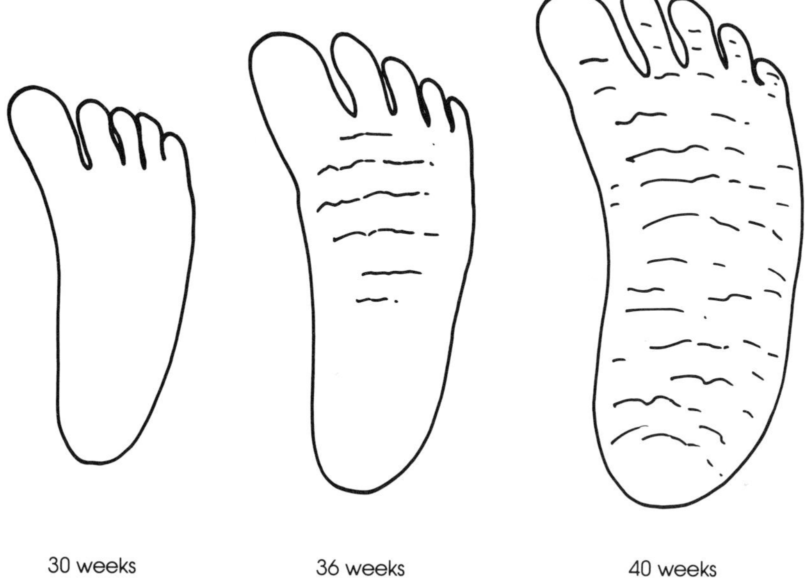

Fig. 2.8: *The appearance of sole creases with gestation.*

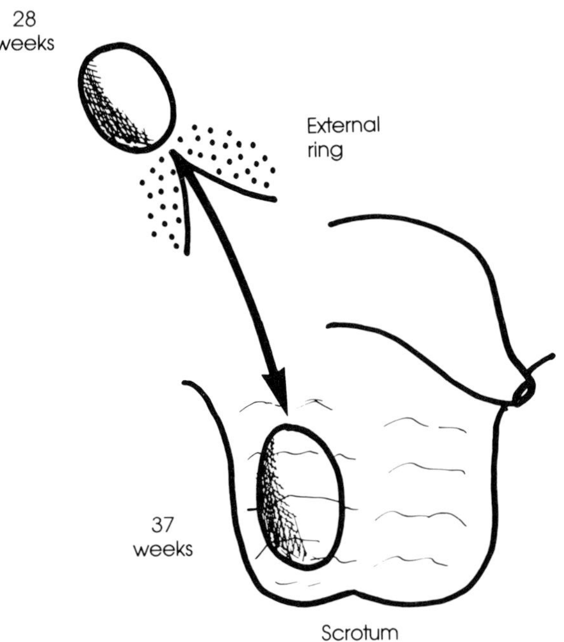

Fig. 2.9: *The timing of testicular descent through the external ring of the inguinal canal and down into the scrotum.*

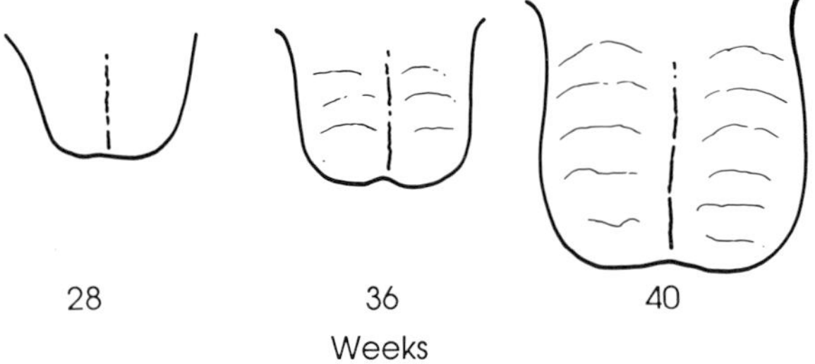

Fig. 2.10: *Scrotal development related to gestational age.*

birth, both the labia minora and clitoris are concealed (Fig. 2.11).

Neurological development

A full neurological examination of a neonate in the first hour of life is not usually appropriate or in the best interests of the infant, but three characteristics can be readily assessed: (1) resting posture, (2) recoil of the limbs, and (3) muscle tone during horizontal suspension. The assessment of nervous development may be affected significantly by perinatal mishaps, such as asphyxia.

(1) Muscle tone first appears in the lower extremities. Until 28 weeks, the infant will lie in an extended position (Fig. 2.12). Hip flexion develops first, and by 34 weeks the infant assumes a 'frog' position. The arms are flexed by 36 weeks.

(2) Recoil to the resting posture after extending the limb can be seen to follow the acquisition of the flexed posture of that limb. Recoil of the legs begins at 34 weeks and that of the arms by about 36–38 weeks.

(3) Horizontal suspension can be performed during weighing of the infant. The manoeuvre tests tone in the trunk and extremities. The infant is allowed to hang in the prone position (face down) over the hand of the examiner with the arms and legs dangling (Fig. 2.13). Until 34 weeks, the infant appears hypotonic and the limbs hang straight. After this time, there is some flexion of the limbs and straight-

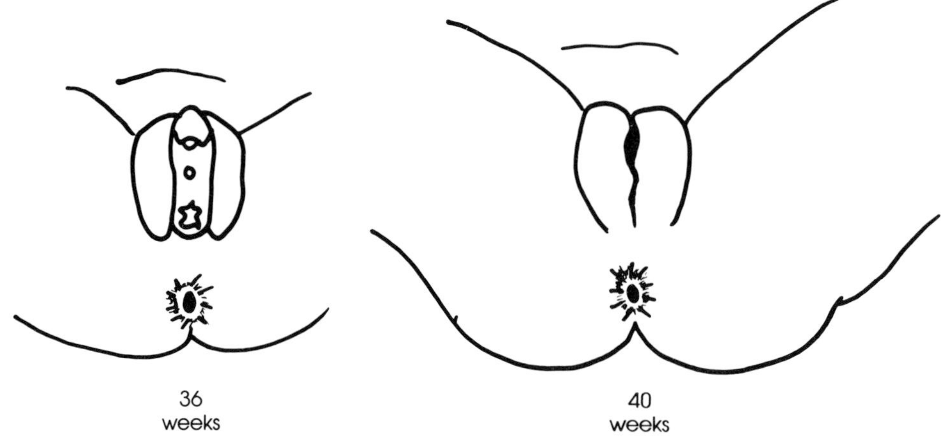

Fig. 2.11: *Development of the female labia to cover the clitoris as the fetus matures.*

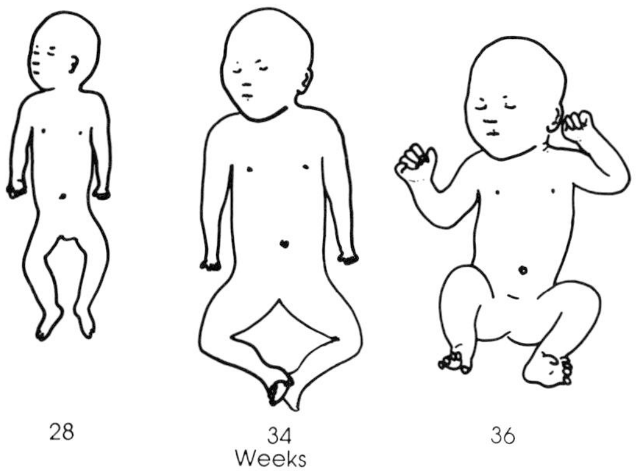

Fig. 2.12: *Limb posture according to gestational age.*

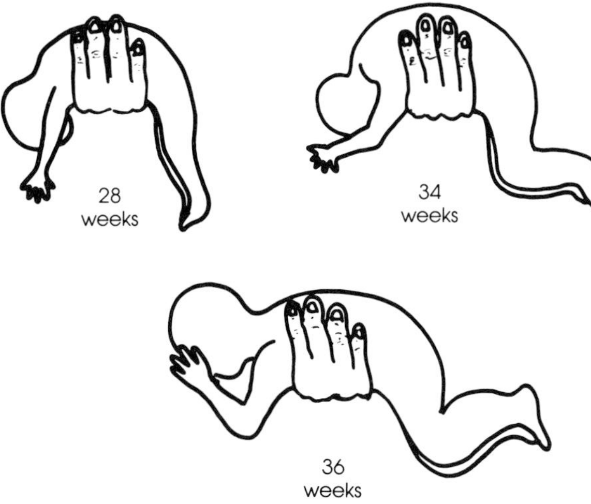

Fig. 2.13: *Horizontal suspension to test limb and truncal muscle tone.*

ening of the body. The head cannot be raised effectively until term at which stage the limbs are tightly flexed.

GOLDEN RULES

(1) If one major anomaly is present, look for others.
(2) If multiple major and minor anomalies are found in the same infant, there may be an identifiable 'syndrome'.
(3) The identification of a particular syndrome enables the prediction of further anomalies not yet discovered, as well as providing prognostic information.
(4) Congenital anomalies are related to each other in time (different organs sensitive to teratogenic influence at the one time) or space (several adjacent organs deformed in a 'field' abnormality).
(5) Morphological development is commonly incomplete, uncommonly redundant, and only rarely aberrant.
(6) The most accurate indication of gestation is the mother's dates.

Further Reading

Avery G.B. (1981). *Neonatology. Pathophysiology and Management of the Newborn*, 2nd edn. Philadelphia: J.B. Lippincott & Co.
Brock D.J.H. (1982). *Early Diagnosis of Fetal Defects.* Edinburgh: Churchill Livingstone.
Cohen M.M. (1982). *The Child With Multiple Birth Defects.* New York: Raven Press.
Filston H.C., Izant R. (1978). *The Surgical Neonate, Evaluation and Care.* New York: Appleton-Century-Crofts.

3 Abdominal pain: Is it appendicitis?

Abdominal pain is extremely common in children and may reflect a variety of conditions (Table 3.1). Often, the cause cannot be determined, or is caused by pathology unrelated to the abdomen. Pain which lasts for more than four to six hours, which is becoming worse or is associated with persistent vomiting or prolonged diarrhoea, should be taken seriously and a surgical cause excluded. If appendicitis is the cause, it is best treated before peritonitis develops. Therefore, examination of the abdomen is directed at localizing the likely origin of the pain and detecting the presence of peritonitis. Peritonitis is a surgical emergency and should almost always be treated by operation within hours of diagnosis. When a child presents with persistent or worsening abdominal pain, every effort must be made to obtain a clinical diagnosis.

Table 3.1 DIFFERENTIAL DIAGNOSIS FOR ACUTE ABDOMINAL PAIN

Very common	Acute appendicitis
	Non-specific viral infection (mesenteric adenitis)
	Gastro-enteritis
	Constipation
	Urinary tract infection
Less common	Intussusception
	Lower lobe pneumonia
	Intestinal obstruction – congenital (1%)
	– adhesions (2%)
	Urinary tract obstruction
	Strangulated inguinal hernia
Rare	Henoch-Schönlein purpura
	Primary peritonitis
	Pancreatitis
	Hepatitis
	Diabetic ketoacidosis
	Lead poisoning
	Acute porphyria
	Herpes zoster
	Sickle-cell anaemia
	Haemophilia (retroperitoneal haematoma)

Frequently, the child with significant abdominal pain is anxious and scared. His fear that palpation of his abdomen will cause him further suffering may make him appear uncooperative. Patience and skill are needed to assess the abdomen accurately in order to avoid the disaster of not recognizing significant intra-abdominal pathology. Where the child is old enough to understand, each stage of the examination must be explained before it is commenced so that the child knows what to expect. The clinician must appear understanding, sympathetic and gentle, and it is helpful to develop a rapport with the child before commencing palpation of the abdomen. Interesting toys, a torch or stethoscope may act as a distractor during examination in the smaller child. Most children are cooperative if they are comfortable with the situation and if they see that they are not going to be hurt unnecessarily.

In the vast majority of children with abdominal pain of unknown cause, the symptoms resolve spontaneously over several hours. At the other end of the spectrum, abdominal pain may reflect significant pathology and necessitate precise clinical assessment before the appropriate therapeutic measures can be undertaken. In young children, infection outside the abdomen (e.g. lung, hip) may be interpreted as abdominal pain. This pain must be distinguished from pain arising within the abdomen. As a general rule, conditions which cause peritonitis need surgery, and therefore one of the more important aspects of the examination of the abdomen is the ability to detect the presence of peritonitis.

The age of the patient is helpful in diagnosing acute abdominal disease because some disorders are confined largely to specific age ranges (Fig. 3.1). Intussusception occurs rarely in children over three years of age and when it does, may signify the existence of a pathological lesion as the lead point. Appendicitis is uncommon below the age of three, but in the older age groups becomes the predominant condition requiring surgery.

Knowledge of the age of the patient, supplemented by a detailed history of the onset, duration, location and characteristics of the pain and related symptoms, provide substantial diagnostic evidence even before physical examination is commenced. This allows a physical examination directed at confirming or refuting the provisional diagnosis and obviates the need for many unnecessary laboratory and radiological investigations. For example, a history of lower abdominal pain lasting several days, with general malaise, recent diarrhoea and the passage of mucus rectally, suggests a diagnosis of untreated appendicitis causing a pelvic abscess, and so the clinician should perform a digital rectal examination to feel a tender swelling bulging from the anterior rectal

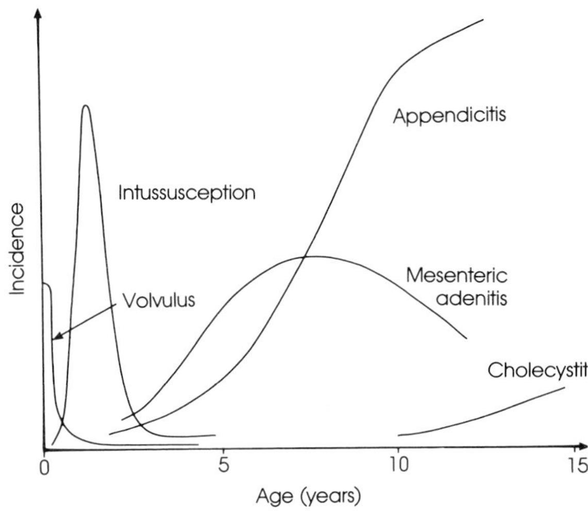

Fig. 3.1: *Influence of age on the incidence of acute abdominal disease.*

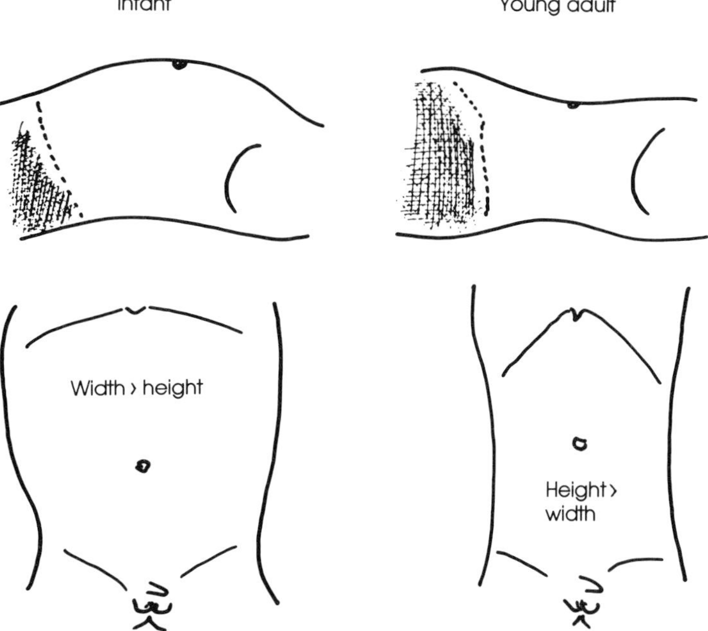

Fig. 3.2: *The different shape of the infant's abdomen compared with that of a young adult; not only is it more protuberant but it is also much wider than it is long.*

wall. A seven-month-old child with episodes of screaming and pallor accompanied by vomiting should be subjected to a careful examination of the abdomen in search of an intussusception mass. Failure to make the appropriate provisional diagnosis after taking a history will usually result in failure to detect the key physical sign which will tend to confirm the diagnosis. The importance of a careful history cannot be over emphasized.

GENERAL CONSIDERATIONS

Physical characteristics of the abdomen in children

The shape of the abdomen in an infant differs from that of an older child in three respects:

(1) It is more protuberant (Fig. 3.2).
(2) It is wider (Fig. 3.2). In the infant, the abdomen tends to bulge between the costal margin and the iliac crest. Consequently, most surgical incisions in children are horizontal rather than vertical.
(3) The pelvis is shallow. This means that, in infants, the bladder is an abdominal organ which extends to the umbilicus when full. The shallow pelvis also allows extensive information to be gained by rectal digital examination. The fingertip is able to reach the pelvic inlet, to palpate the internal ring in the case of a strangulated hernia, and to palpate the reproductive organs in the female.

The posterior abdominal wall is not flat but has a prominent midline ridge due to the vertebral bodies (Fig. 3.3). This makes the aorta and the transverse colon easy to feel compared with other organs, such as the adrenal glands, which lie to the side of the vertebral column.

In infancy, the relatively horizontal direction of the ribs contributes to the normal liver edge being palpable below the costal margin.

The attachment of the membranous layer of the subcutaneous tissue (Scarpa's fascia) to the fascia lata of the thigh produces the inguinal skin crease. This crease is located below the inguinal ligament, which may be a trap in the localization of herniae in infants, especially between 6 and 18 months. The inguinal ligament is palpable through the subcutaneous tissue about 1 cm above this skin crease.

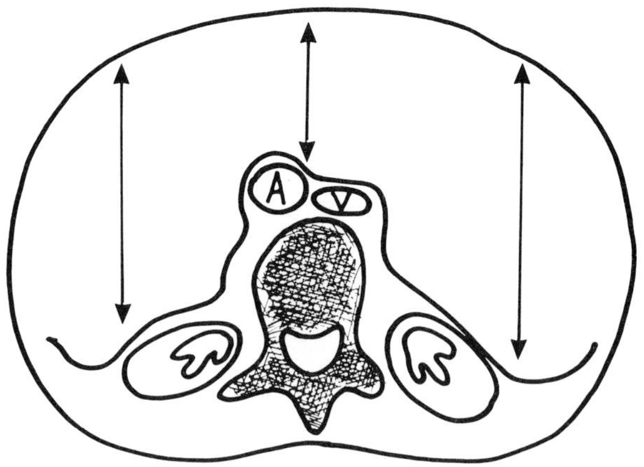

Fig. 3.3: *A cross-section of the abdominal cavity to show the anterior prevertebral organs compared with those situated laterally.*

In the infant, the processus vaginalis is often patent and any fluid that collects in the peritoneal cavity (e.g. blood, pus or meconium) may track down through the processus and produce a discoloured scrotum (Fig. 3.4).

The muscles of the ventral abdominal wall contract during crying and make examination of the abdomen difficult. Therefore, the abdomen is best palpated with the child relaxed or between episodes of crying, and can be done most easily lateral to the rectus muscle where the abdominal

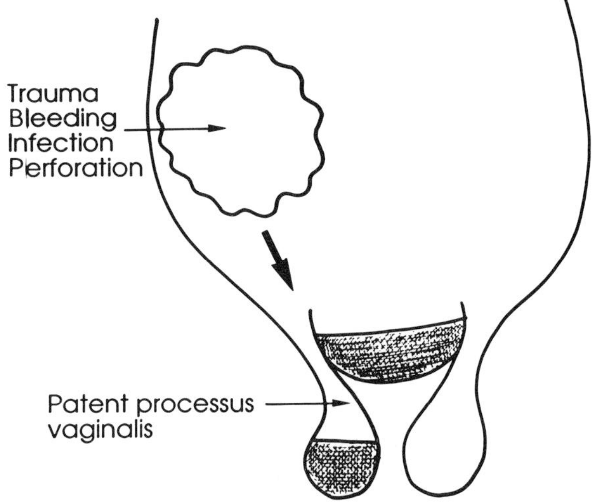

Fig. 3.4: *The downward tracking of fluid (blood, pus or intestinal contents) to the most dependent parts of the peritoneal cavity.*

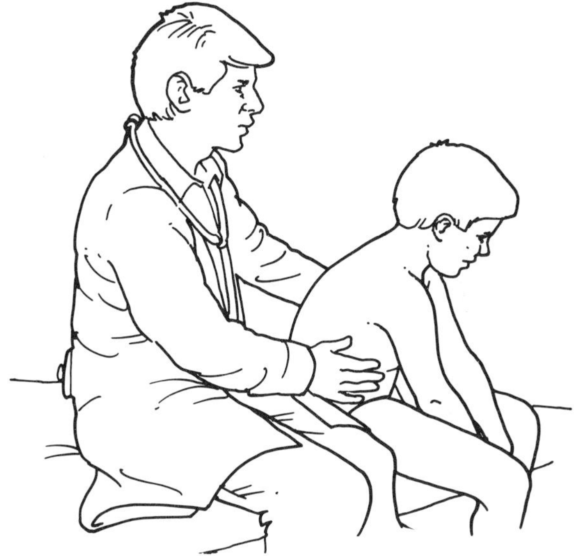

Fig. 3.5: *Overcoming the tight abdominal muscles by examination with the child sitting up and leaning forward.*

musculature is thinnest. In pneumonia, some degree of splinting of the abdominal muscles may occur but is overcome by examining the child as he leans forward in the sitting position (Fig. 3.5). This manoeuvre is useful also when there is difficulty evaluating the amount of tenderness in a child with suspected peritonitis.

The location of pain

Inflammation or distension of the bowel or its coverings causes pain which is transmitted through two separate pathways. Distension of the bowel and inflammation of the visceral peritoneum stimulate sympathetic pathways, and the perceived location is dependent on the level of bowel involved (Fig. 3.6). As a general rule, pain arising in the fore-gut projects to the epigastrium, in the mid-gut to the umbilicus, and in the hind-gut to the infra-umbilical or hypogastric region. As with most autonomic pathways, localization of pain is not precise and the distribution described serves as a rough guide only. Localized distension with peristalsis against obstruction causes colic, whereas inflammatory lesions produce constant pain, usually in association with anorexia and nausea. It is visceral pain which so commonly causes the vomiting seen early in the development of appendicitis and other inflammatory lesions of the abdomen.

In contrast, irritation of the parietal peritoneum supplied by segmental somatic nerves is localized, sharp, continuous and made worse by movement. Not all parts of the parietal peritoneum are subserved by the segmental nerves, which supply in addition the muscles of the ventral abdominal wall. Irritation of the pelvic peritoneum produces no abdominal wall guarding. Rectal examination may be the only way to diagnose pelvic peritonitis.

Referred pain is not recognized commonly in children, but when appreciated may provide valuable clues as to the underlying pathology. Irritation of the underside of the diaphragm by blood or pus may produce pain referred to the shoulder tip. The explanation for this is that the phrenic nerve which supplies the diaphragm is largely made up of fibres from the fourth cervical nerve root, of which other fibres are cutaneous to the shoulder region. Biliary colic is rare in children but may produce pain in the back, below the inferior angle of the right scapula. Uterine and rectal pain may be referred to the lumbosacral region of the back, while loin pain emanating from the kidney may radiate to the ipsilateral testis. The close proximity of the ovary to the obturator nerve as it courses on the lateral pelvic wall, accounts for the pain radiating to the inner aspect of the thigh in ovarian disease.

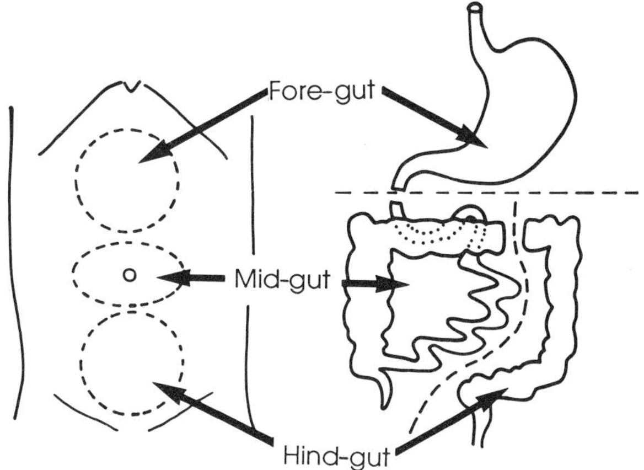

Fig. 3.6: *Surface projection of referred pain from the gastro-intestinal tract.*

Masses palpable in the normal abdomen

Faeces may be palpable in the colon and can be distinguished from pathological masses in that they are indentable (see Chapter 15, Fig. 15.2). Their distribution follows the line of the colon and it must be remembered that the sigmoid colon may lie in the right iliac fossa. The lower pole of the right kidney is often palpable with deep inspiration as the diaphragm pushes the kidney downwards. The liver causes the right kidney to assume a slightly lower position than the left. The liver in infancy is often palpable two to three finger breadths below the right costal margin. Further details are found in Chapter 15.

THE HISTORY

The characteristics of the pain must be established (Table 3.2). Even in the small child who is unable to provide a history, useful information regarding the nature of the pain can be obtained from the parents. They are aware of the duration of the illness and, where the pain has been severe and colicky, will have observed the child cry out and perhaps draw up his legs. Refusal to feed, objection to movement or handling, and the presence of associated symptoms (e.g. vomiting and diarrhoea), are useful observations. The large, watery stools of gastro-enteritis must be distinguished from the small, mucous stools of pelvic appendicitis or intussusception.

Table 3.2 CHARACTERISTICS OF THE PAIN

1. Time of onset	– duration
2. Location	– at onset
	– at examination
	– 'referred' pain
3. Severity	– mild to severe
	– progression
	– alleviating factors
	– exacerbating factors
4. Type	– colicky
	– constant
5. Associated symptoms	

Duration of pain

Knowledge of the duration of pain and the normal rate of progression of pathological processes is the key to assessment of physical signs. In malrotation with volvulus, infarction of the entire mid-gut can occur within several hours. In appendicitis, the inflammatory process may proceed to gangrene and localized perforation, but this is uncommon within 18 hours. By contrast, pain which has been present for a week without evidence of peritoneal irritation is not likely to be appendicitis.

Shifting of pain

Movement of pain away from a vague central location to one or other side is often indicative of the development of parietal peritoneal signs (see the section on appendicitis). The extension of pain from a lateral position to involve the whole abdomen is suspicious of extension of the pathology to other parts of the peritoneal cavity. For example, after a blow to the left upper abdomen which causes splenic injury, pain may be first located in the left hypochondrium but progresses to generalized abdominal tenderness with continued bleeding. Pain commencing in the right iliac fossa which extends across the midline may indicate extension of peritonitis due to a ruptured appendix.

Type of pain

The difference between splanchnic and somatic pain has already been described. Obstruction of a hollow viscus causes sharp spasms of 'colic' between which the patient suffers a dull ache. The interval between episodes of colic becomes less pronounced as the obstruction progresses. Not all abdominal pains are caused by intra-abdominal disease: when the features do not seem typical of appendicitis, extra-abdominal causes should be considered (Fig. 3.7).

Exacerbating and relieving factors

The child with colic is restless and may writhe around unable to obtain a position of comfort. On the other hand, the child with peritonitis will remain still and dislike being disturbed or handled. If he walks he will do so slowly, bent forward with his hands holding his abdomen in an attempt to prevent movement of the peritoneal surfaces

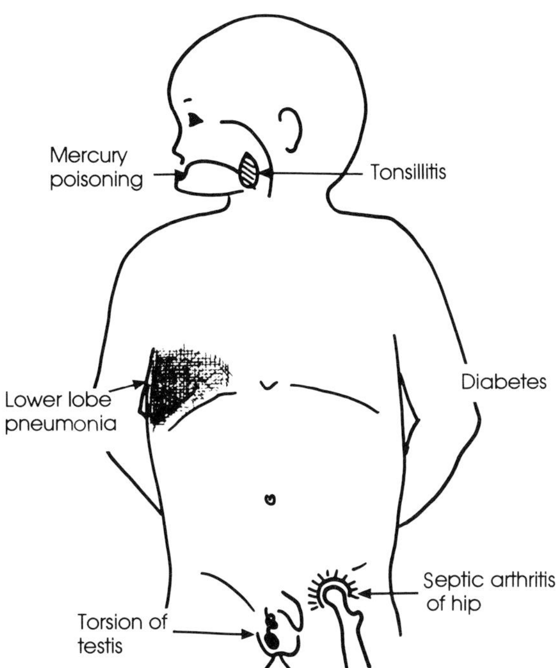

Fig. 3.7: *Extra-abdominal illnesses causing abdominal pain.*

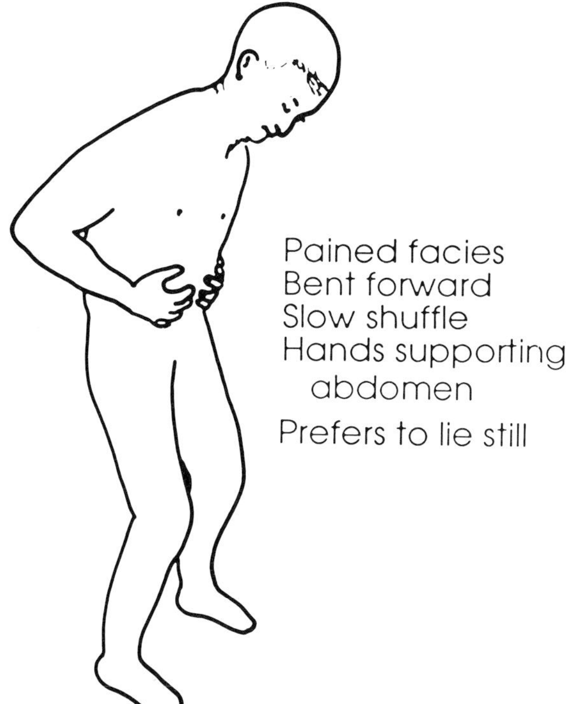

Fig. 3.8: *The 'appendix shuffle'. Movement of adjacent peritoneal surfaces causes pain and is minimized by adopting this posture whilst walking.*

(Fig. 3.8). It will hurt to cough, sneeze, vomit or to take a deep breath. Where the inflammation involves the pelvis, micturition and defaecation will exacerbate the pain. In toddlers, pneumonia may masquerade as abdominal pain which is made worse by deep inspiration and relieved by breathing quietly. It is caused by abdominal muscle contraction to splint the diaphragm.

Associated features

Vomiting commonly accompanies abdominal pain in children because autonomic reflexes stimulate vomiting in response to any inflammation or severe pain. The significance of the symptom is determined by:

(1) the relationship of its onset to the development of pain;
(2) its frequency;
(3) the nature of the vomitus.

In appendicitis, vomiting generally commences several hours after the onset of pain. It is unusual for it to appear before the pain except in the very small child where the time of onset of the pain may be difficult to ascertain. In acute colic of the ureter, the onset of vomiting coincides with that of pain, both being sudden and dramatic. In obstruction of the intestinal tract, the onset of vomiting is dependent on the level of obstruction. Where the obstruction is high (e.g. duodenum or upper small bowel), vomiting commences early but where the obstruction is low (e.g. distal small bowel or colon), it may be a day or longer before vomiting appears.

The frequency of vomiting correlates with the severity of the pathology. For example, in acute appendicitis, severe vomiting is often associated with rapid progression of abdominal signs and may indicate an obstructed appendix which is likely to perforate early. On the other hand, in distal intestinal lesions (e.g. intussusception) the degree of vomiting may not be impressive and may belie the seriousness of the underlying pathology. Proximal obstruction of the bowel is associated with frequent and forceful vomiting.

It is essential to determine whether the vomiting contains bile (Table 3.3). The first clue to the life-threatening condition of malrotation with volvulus may be bile-stained vomitus. In this con-

Table 3.3 RELATIONSHIP BETWEEN TYPE OF VOMITUS AND ITS UNDERLYING CAUSE

Vomitus	Cause	Reason
Bile-stained	Malrotation with volvulus	Duodenum obstructed just beyond the ampulla
Gastric contents, then bile	Gastro-enteritis	Inflamed stomach or secondary to pain/ileus
Gastric contents, then bile, then faecal fluid	Intestinal obstruction	Fluid collection above distal block
Not bile-stained	Pyloric stenosis	Pylorus blocked (*above* ampulla)
Blood (including 'coffee grounds')	Oesophageal varices Gastritis Gastro-oesophageal reflux	Portal hypertension Infection/corrosion/aspirin ingestion Oesophagitis

dition, there is obstruction at the second part of the duodenum from twisting of the mid-gut. Where volvulus is suspected, early confirmation of the diagnosis by barium study and treatment by operation is required. Severe gastro-enteritis with profuse vomiting can also produce bile-stained vomiting. In intestinal obstruction, the vomitus is initially of gastric contents, followed by bile-stained material and, ultimately, yellow/brown faeculent fluid.

In congenital hypertrophic pyloric stenosis, pyloric outlet obstruction means the vomitus contains no bile. In patients with a long history, development of gastritis may cause the vomitus to be blood-tinged, a feature also seen with other causes of gastritis. Copious quantities of fresh blood in vomitus is suggestive of oesophageal varices or acute gastritis caused such as that by aspirin ingestion (Table 3.3).

The pattern and character of bowel actions may indicate the diagnosis (Table 3.4). In acute gastro-enteritis, there is dramatic onset of loose stools which, in young children, may result in loss of continence. The volume of stool passed is usually considerable and may be associated with vomiting and colicky abdominal pain ('cramps'). It is unusual for the symptoms to persist for more than 24–48 hours. The passage of a small volume of loose motions, shortly following the onset of pain, is a feature of appendicitis in many children, especially when the appendix is retro-ileal. Persistence of 'diarrhoea' with or without the passage of mucus in the presence of low abdominal pain, is suggestive of a pelvic abscess, of which the most common cause is an unrecognized pelvic appendicitis. In intussusception, small amounts of loose motions, which may subsequently be tinged with blood and mucus, are passed (Table 3.4). The significance of blood in the bowel actions is discussed in more detail in Chapter 16.

PREPARATION FOR EXAMINATION

The child should be positioned so that he is comfortable and in a way which facilitates full

Table 3.4 RELATIONSHIP BETWEEN ABNORMAL STOOLS AND THEIR UNDERLYING CAUSE

Stools	Cause	Reason
High volume and watery	Gastro-enteritis	Primary effect on absorption
Small volume and mucousy	Appendix abscess	Secondary irritation of the rectum
Initial evacuation then blood ± mucus	Intussusception	Mass induces reflex emptying and vascular compression leading to venous congestion

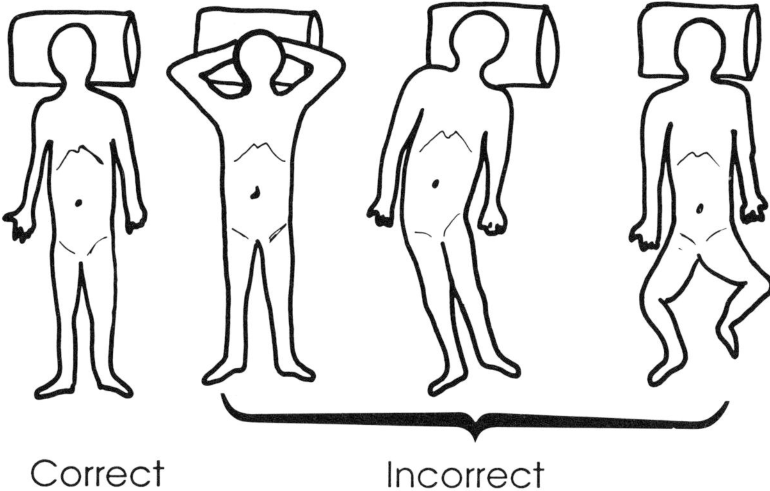

Fig. 3.9: *The position of a patient for examination of the abdomen.*

examination of the abdomen. An explanation of each manoeuvre gains the confidence of the child and provides reassurance which helps the child to relax. The examination must be performed in a warm room, particularly in the case of an infant or small child where heat loss can occur quickly. If the examination is to take place in the ward, the curtains should be pulled to avoid distractions and provide privacy. Most pubertal and many younger children are hesitant to remove their clothing unless privacy is assured. The clothing should be removed to expose the abdomen, chest and external genitalia. Testicular torsion and strangulated hernia will be overlooked unless this is done, since in these conditions the pain may be referred to the iliac fossa and flank. The child has to be lying comfortably in a supine position with a pillow behind the head. He must be symmetrical with his legs together and arms at his side (Fig. 3.9). Failure to ensure that the child is correctly positioned may result in an erroneous assessment of the site and severity of tenderness, muscle tone and guarding.

IS THERE PERITONITIS?

In the child with acute abdominal pain, one of the most important questions is whether the child has peritonitis. The infant is less able than the adult to contain the spread of intraperitoneal sepsis because the greater omentum is small and immature. Peritonitis in this group progresses rapidly and, if untreated, may result in septicaemia and death. The presence of peritonitis is an indication for surgery in virtually every situation. It is imperative, therefore, that the clinician is familiar with the signs of peritonitis, which in the infant or young child may be difficult to elucidate.

Clinical assessment of peritonitis or inflammation of the peritoneum, involves the demonstration of pain produced by movement between adjacent inflamed peritoneal surfaces. Certain clues may be obtained from the history. The child may be reluctant to move about because movement makes the pain worse. He may refuse to run, and will walk stooped forward clasping his abdomen with his hands (Fig. 3.8). An older child may go to bed where he will prefer to lie motionless (Fig. 3.10). An infant may protest at being handled and refuse feeds. During the drive to hospital, the child may complain that every time the car goes over a bump the pain is made worse.

Contraction of the diaphragm causes the abdominal wall to move with respiration. Such movement is painful in peritonitis, and the child will use the chest wall muscles in breathing to a greater degree in an effort to keep the abdomen still. This is assisted by tonic contraction of the abdominal wall muscles which, in a thin child, is

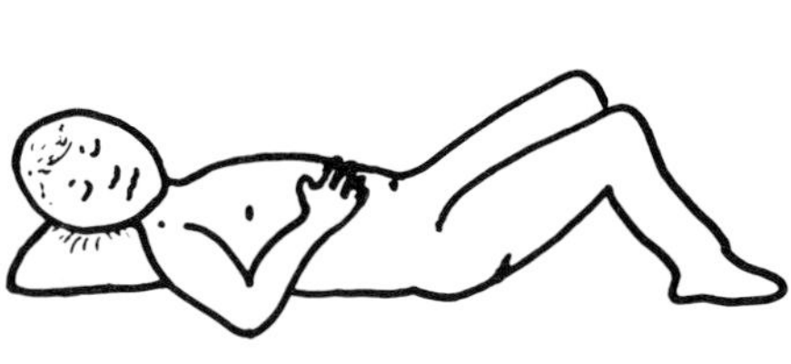

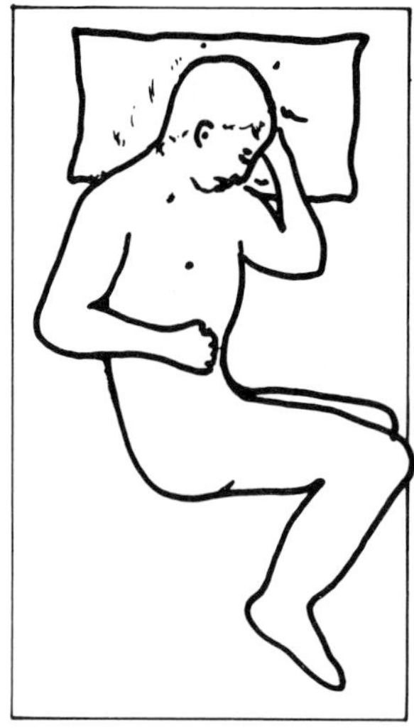

Fig. 3.10: *The posture of a child with peritonitis.*

seen as prominence of the rectus abdominis muscles at rest in an abdomen which moves little with respiration.

The child should be asked to puff out his abdomen as far as he can. In the absence of peritonitis, this is a painless manoeuvre but the child with peritonitis is either unable or unwilling to protrude his abdomen. Likewise, in peritonitis, attempts to draw in the abdomen and 'be as thin as possible' will result in severe pain (Fig. 3.11). The voluntary excursion of the abdomen is reduced. Coughing and sitting up cause similar discomfort, which adds support to the findings above.

The tests so far described are dependent on the cooperation of the patient to move the peritoneal surfaces. The following tests detect peritoneal irritation more directly, and of these, the detection of guarding is the most specific and sensitive.

A child with a sore abdomen fears palpation as he anticipates that it will increase the pain he is suffering. For this reason, it is imperative to gain as much information as possible before palpating the abdomen. A useful test is to hold the child firmly on each side of the chest wall with the fingers and palms of the hands, and to shake the chest from side to side. The pressure on the chest wall causes no discomfort, but if there is peritonitis, the shaking will cause pain in the abdomen. A similar manoeuvre can be conducted by holding the pelvis below the iliac crest firmly between the hands (Fig. 3.12) and assessing the degree of discomfort caused by shaking the pelvis

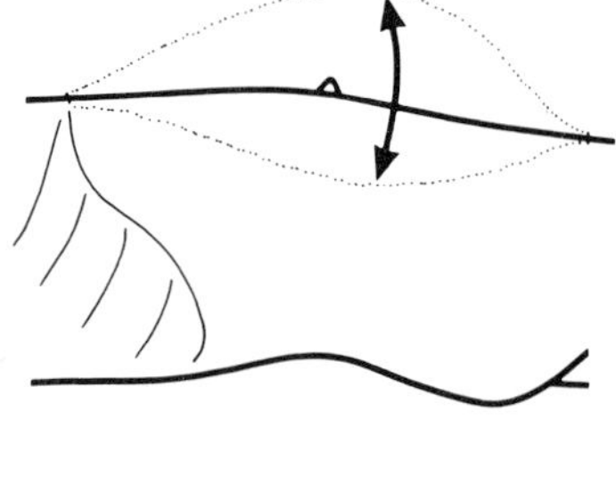

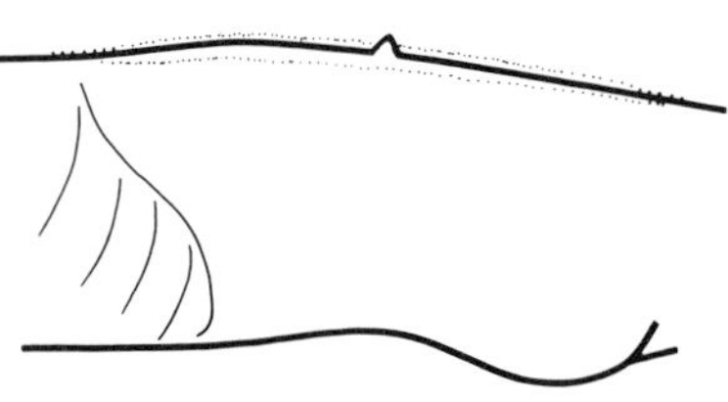

Fig. 3.11: *The effect of peritonitis on abdominal excursion.*

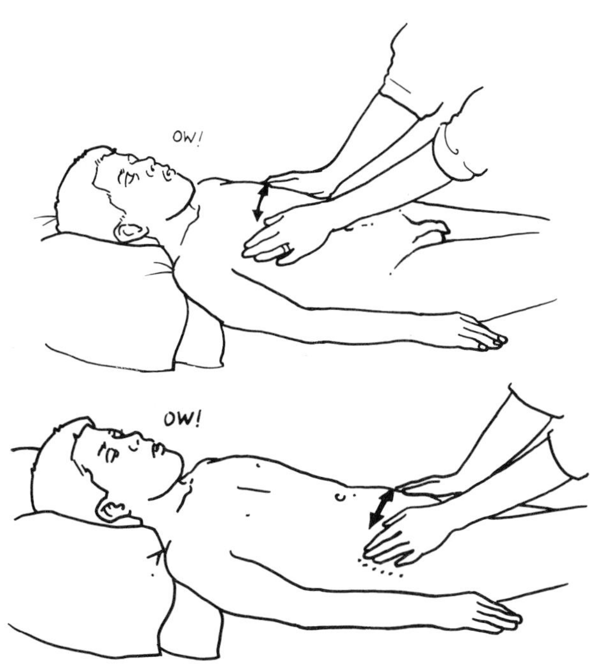

Fig. 3.12: *Is peritonitis present? Shaking the chest or pelvis from side to side will cause the child to grimace with abdominal pain.*

quickly in a lateral direction. Initially, the pelvis is rocked gently to avoid excessive discomfort in the child who has peritonitis.

The existence of involuntary contraction ('guarding') of the muscles of the abdominal wall is determined by gentle palpation starting with the region of the abdomen in which the least tenderness is anticipated. For example, where a child complains of maximal pain in the right iliac fossa, examination should start below the left costal margin. It is essential that initial palpation is extremely gentle in order to : (1) maintain the confidence of the patient and enable him to remain relaxed until the degree of tenderness has been established; and (2) detect subtle differences in muscle tone. Guarding is sometimes described as being either 'voluntary' or 'involuntary'. Voluntary guarding is conscious tightening of the abdominal wall musculature as a protective device in anticipation of tenderness. It suggests apprehension, but may or may not signify underlying peritoneal irritation. Involuntary guarding is a reflex spasm of the muscles, even in the absence of

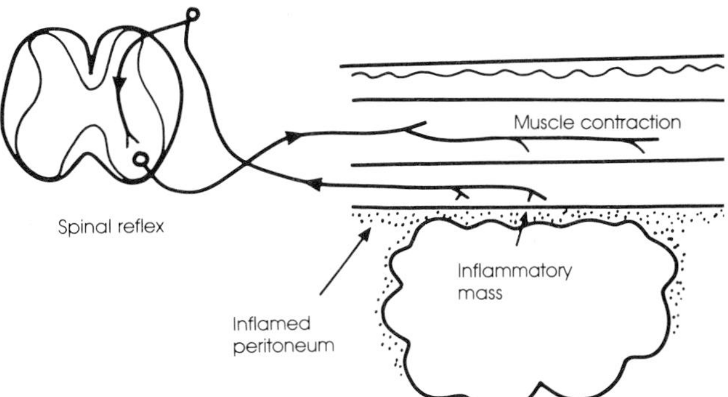

Fig. 3.13: *Guarding: the involuntary reflex contraction or spasm of anterior abdominal wall muscles when the anterior parietal peritoneum is inflamed. Spasm persists even when the child is asleep or distracted.*

palpation, in an attempt to immobilize the adjacent parietal peritoneal surface (Fig. 3.13). The tips of the fingers should gently test the tension in the muscles as they progress around the abdomen. If abdominal wall spasm and tenderness are present, the patient has peritonitis and no further palpation is needed. The most sensitive areas for demonstrating guarding are lateral to the rectus abdominis muscle (Fig. 3.14), and it is often useful to assess muscle tone on both sides simultaneously (Fig. 3.14). Each side is palpated alternately to allow detection of minor differences in tone. If the first journey around the abdomen elicits little tenderness, the process should be repeated with firmer palpation but is unlikely to reveal much more information. The exception to this is seen when deep palpation in one area causes pain in an

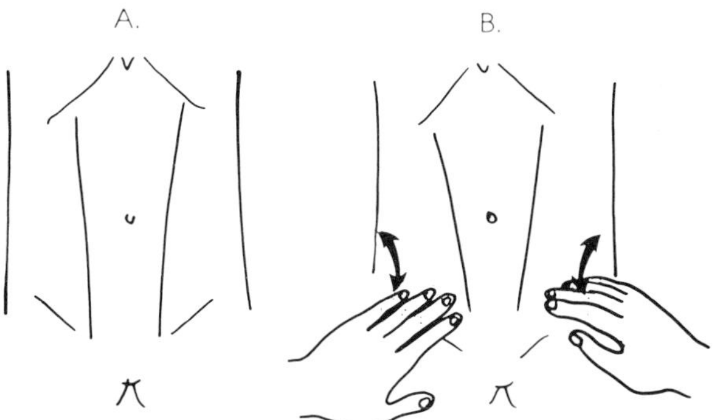

Fig. 3.14: *Muscular guarding is best assessed lateral to the rectus abdominis muscle (A). Subtle differences in muscular tone can be detected by simultaneous palpation of both sides (B).*

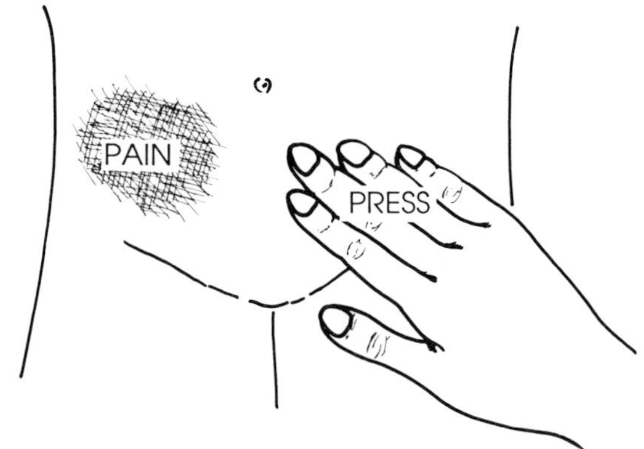

Fig. 3.15: *Rovsing's sign: deep palpation of the left iliac fossa causes pain in the right iliac fossa.*

adjacent area, the most well-known example of which occurs in appendicitis where deep palpation of the left iliac fossa may cause sharp pain in the right iliac fossa (Rovsing's sign) (Fig. 3.15). This occurs because deep indentation of the peritoneal cavity in the left iliac fossa causes displacement of loops of bowel in the region of inflammation in the right iliac fossa (Fig. 3.16).

Where the child refuses to relax, or it is suspected that guarding is voluntary, percussion of the abdomen identifies those with rebound tenderness and genuine guarding. In children, percussion produces a vibration of the underlying tissues which is not dampened by the obesity often present in adults.

The child under three years of age may be uncooperative and extremely difficult to examine. Severe abdominal pain from peritonitis may be the reason he refuses to allow his abdomen to be palpated, yet it is this child who needs an accurate diagnosis. Assessment can be facilitated by:

(1) diverting the child's attention by allowing him to play with a torch, a stethoscope or a colourful toy, and waiting until he is fully distracted before surreptitiously palpating his abdomen;
(2) re-examining him when he is asleep, since guarding does not disappear with sleep and if he has peritonitis gentle palpation will waken him;
(3) allowing the mother to cuddle the child facing her chest, and when he has settled in that position gently palpating the abdomen while standing behind the child.

Auscultation of the abdomen is of limited usefulness in children as the presence of bowel sounds does not rule out peritonitis.

If the focus of inflammation is in the pelvis and has not spread to involve the rest of the peritoneal cavity, there may be little evidence of peritonitis on palpation of the ventral abdominal wall. On rectal examination, however, movement of the peritoneal reflection of the rectum will cause severe pain. In many children, rectal examination is a painful procedure in itself, so it must be clear that the pain is from peritoneal movement and not from the anal canal. This can be determined by keeping the finger in the rectum stationary until the child adjusts to the discomfort of the anal canal before palpating the rectal wall. Generous application of lubricant and slow introduction of the finger lessen the initial pain caused by stretching the anal canal.

The second major sign of peritonitis is tenderness. Tenderness is most marked in the region of the primary pathology (Fig. 3.17), but as the process extends to involve other parts of the peritoneal cavity, the tenderness becomes more widespread. Progression and extension of tenderness are suggestive of peritonitis. Tenderness is most marked if the inflammation is close to the area palpated (Fig. 3.18).

The demonstration of rebound tenderness as performed in an adult is not justified in the child because it provides unreliable information and, if peritonitis is present, is cruel. Rebound tenderness elicited by gentle percussion is a more valuable sign (Fig. 3.19).

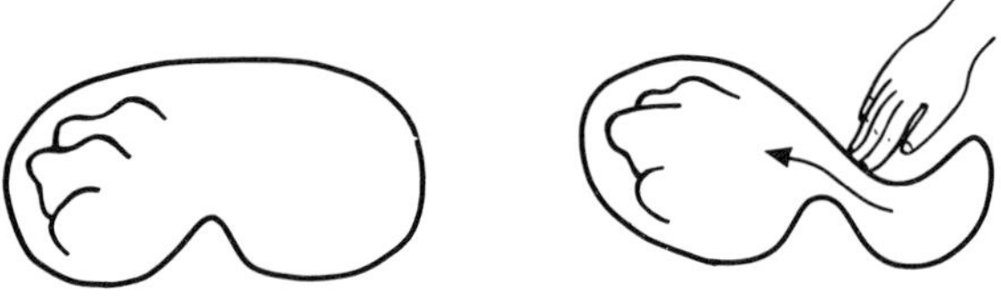

Fig. 3.16: *The explanation of Rovsing's sign: movement of uninvolved bowel on the left disturbs inflamed structures on the right near the appendix, causing pain.*

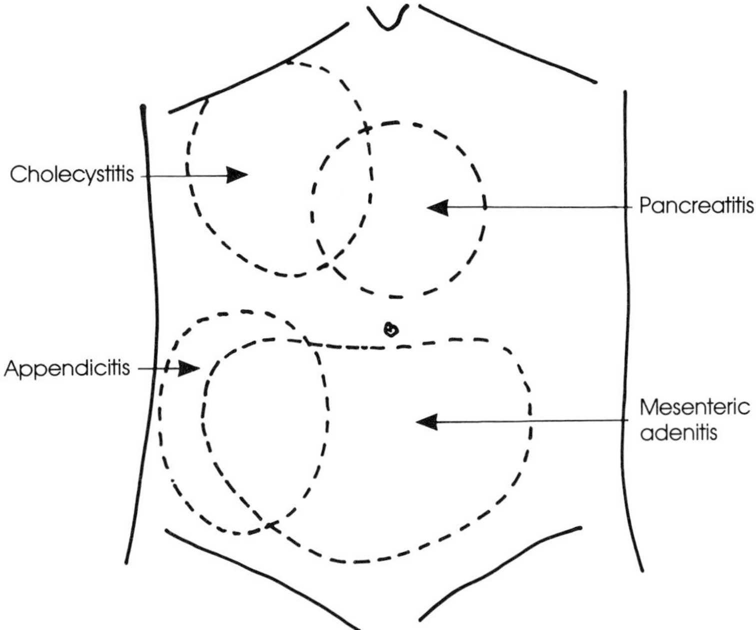

Fig. 3.17: *Sites of maximal tenderness of abdominal diseases.*

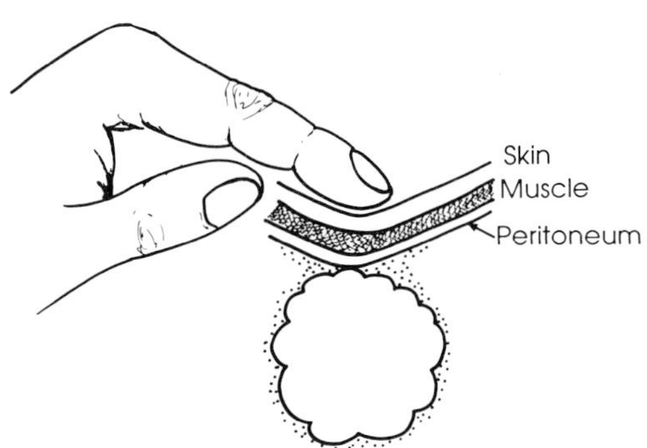

Fig. 3.18: *Local tenderness: pain on touching/moving inflamed tissues (which are usually close to the anterior abdominal wall).*

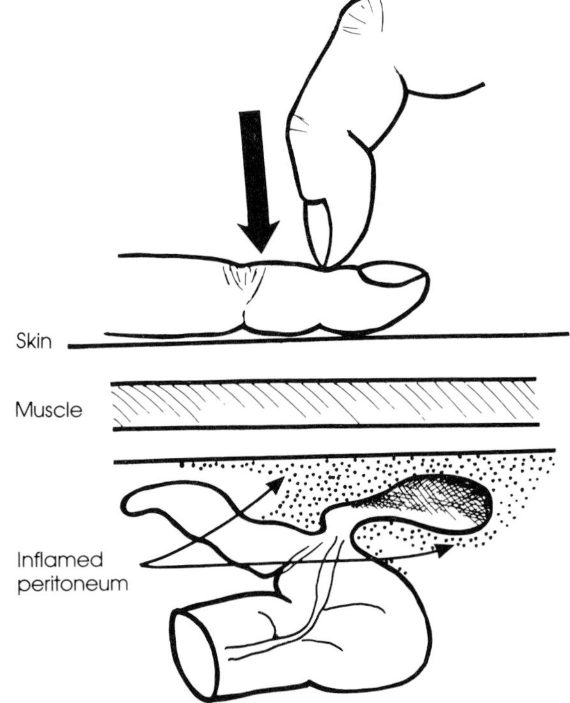

Fig. 3.19: *Rebound tenderness: caused by the sudden movement of inflamed peritoneal surfaces. Best elicited by gentle percussion because this produces minimal pain. Sudden release after deep palpation is too coarse to localize the site of disease and is unnecessarily painful.*

NON-SPECIFIC SIGNS OF PERITONITIS

Facial expression will show the child to be in pain. The complexion may be pale or flushed. Sometimes the cheeks are red in association with perioral pallor. In early peritonitis, and in the young child, the face may provide few clues. There is usually vomiting at some stage of the history, although it may have stopped by the time of presentation. Pyrexia, fetor, and furred tongue may be present but are not specific to peritonitis. A tachycardia is usually present, but a normal pulse rate appropriate to the age of the child does not rule out peritonitis.

In long-standing peritonitis, the signs of septicaemic shock develop. Loops of intestine become distended and paretic, causing abdominal distension. The abdomen is silent on auscultation. Vomiting of small bowel contents develops and the respiratory rate becomes rapid. It is unfortunate if signs have progressed to this stage before a diagnosis of peritonitis is made.

APPENDICITIS

Appendicitis commences with a dull continuous central abdominal pain which moves after 6–24 hours to the right iliac fossa where it is perceived as being more severe and sharper in nature. The pain is accompanied by anorexia and nausea, and in most children vomiting occurs. There may be some alteration in bowel habit.

There is an anatomical and physiological basis for these symptoms. The appendix is an appendage of the mid-gut so that inflammation of the organ involves the splanchnic fibres of the mid-gut and produces periumbilical discomfort (Fig. 3.6). Also, visceral pain causes anorexia and nausea to which the child is particularly sensitive and, in combination with developing ileus, vomiting is frequent. When inflammation progresses to the adjacent parietal peritoneum, pain is perceived as being more sharply localized and severe. This accounts for the apparent shift in the localization of the pain from the periumbilical region to the right iliac fossa (Fig. 3.20).

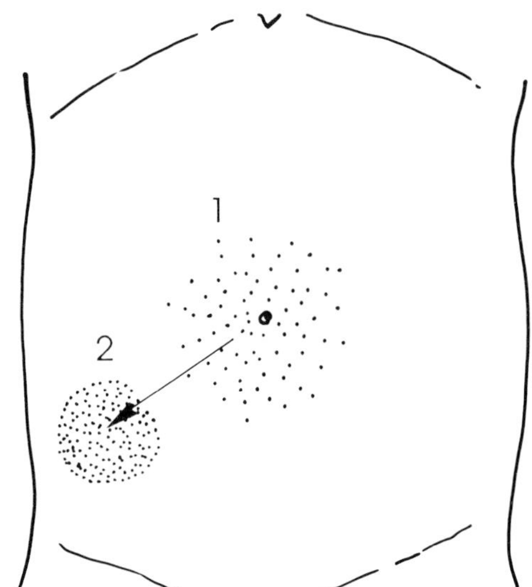

Fig. 3.20: *The shifting of pain in appendicitis. Initial distension of the appendix causes referred visceral pain felt around the umbilicus (1). Extension of the inflammation to the peritoneum adjacent to the appendix allows better localization of the pain to the right iliac fossa (2), producing an apparent shift.*

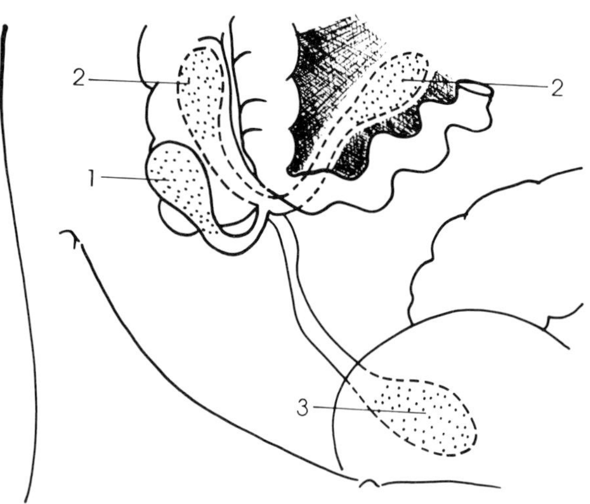

Fig. 3.21: *The three presentations of appendicitis depending on its location: (1) anterior right iliac fossa – obvious signs; (2) posterior right iliac fossa (behind the caecum or ileum) – vague signs; (3) pelvis – 'invisible signs'.*

The appendix arises from the caecum immediately adjacent to the ileocaecal valve. It is a thin, tubular structure 7–10 cm in length, and the tip can occupy a number of positions in relation to the caecum (Fig. 3.21). The clinical presentation of appendicitis depends on the position of the appendix (Table 3.5). Where it lies anterior to the caecum, it produces obvious signs of local tenderness and guarding because of adjacent peritoneal irritation; diagnosis is easy and can be made at an early stage. The posterior appendix may lie behind the caecum, the ascending colon or the terminal ileum (Fig. 3.21). The pain remains localized to the right iliac fossa, but there may be no evidence of guarding or parietal peritoneal irritation. Tenderness to deep palpation is not as marked as might be anticipated from the history or general

Table 3.5 THE THREE PRESENTATIONS OF APPENDICITIS

Right iliac fossa anterior to bowel	**Right iliac fossa posterior to bowel**	**Pelvis**
Obvious right iliac fossa tenderness	Vague deep tenderness	Vague suprapubic tenderness
Guarding	± guarding	*No* guarding
Rebound tenderness	May develop mass or perforation before diagnosis ± Limp	Per rectum – tenderness/mass ± Urinary symptoms ±'Diarrhoea' Commonly perforated before diagnosis
→ Easy and early diagnosis	→ Hard, delayed diagnosis	→ Hardest, late diagnosis
Anterior peritoneum inflamed early	Posterior peritoneum or psoas inflamed (→ limp), but few anterior abdominal wall signs	Pelvic peritoneum inflamed (→ bladder and rectal irritation), but few anterior abdominal wall signs

signs of toxicity. The inexperienced clinician may be misled by the apparent paucity of signs. Where the appendix occupies a position in the pelvis, the area of maximal tenderness is vague and lower than McBurney's point. There is *no* guarding of the peritoneum of the lower abdomen. Clues to the presence of pelvic appendicitis include:

(1) complaints of pain in the abdomen during micturition (this is not urethral dysuria but is pain caused by movement of the peritoneum over the bladder);
(2) passage of loose bowel actions owing to irritation of the rectum by the adjacent inflammatory mass;
(3) marked tenderness anteriorly on rectal examination.

When should a rectal examination be performed in suspected appendicitis?

Where the diagnosis of appendicitis is obvious from the history and clinical findings, and the decision to perform an appendicectomy has been made, there is no advantage in performing a rectal examination. In all cases where there is doubt about the diagnosis, where other diagnoses are entertained or where pelvic appendicitis is likely, a rectal examination is indicated. The examination is unpleasant to the child and, if useful information is to be obtained, it must be performed gently and with care. In children under three years of age, the lubricated little finger is used, whereas in older children, the index finger is preferred. The finger must be introduced slowly and carefully, with the child in the left lateral position with the knees bent up towards the chest (see Fig. 3.22). An alternative method in the infant is to have the child supine with the legs flexed at the hip (see Fig. 3.22); while the left hand is lifting the legs upwards, the little finger of the right hand performs the examination.

The examination itself causes pain in the anal canal, and this has to be distinguished from deep

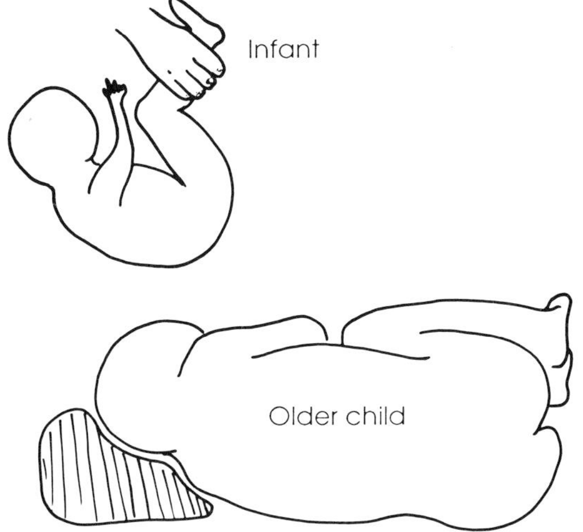

Fig. 3.22: *The positions for digital examination of the rectum.*

pelvic pain. After introducing the finger, it is kept still for several seconds until the child becomes comfortable before palpating in each direction for abnormal masses or localized tenderness.

Appendicitis in children under five years

Appendicitis is rare in the child under five years of age and, when it occurs, is often difficult to diagnose and more likely to present once peritonitis has developed. The young child cannot communicate his symptoms or localize the site of tenderness well. He appears uncooperative and refuses to allow examination of his abdomen. For this reason, an irritable and unwell child with abdominal pain who is difficult to examine must be taken seriously, and every effort made to determine whether there is peritonitis.

How can the site of maximal pain and tenderness be identified in children?

The child can be asked to point with one finger to the place which hurts the most (Fig. 3.23). In most cases, the child points to McBurney's point, which lies one third of the way between the anterior superior iliac spine and the umbilicus and is recognized as the surface landmark of the base of the appendix. In the child who is difficult to assess by palpation, the area of maximal tenderness can be located by gentle percussion.

Do there have to be signs of a localized peritonitis before a diagnosis of appendicitis is made?

It is in the patient's interest that a diagnosis is made on clinical grounds before peritonitis develops. Peritonitis is a sign of advanced disease and, in most cases, a history consistent with appendicitis, combined with marked localized tenderness in the right iliac fossa, provides sufficient grounds for a diagnosis of appendicitis to be made.

Has the child who presents with a generalized peritonitis got appendicitis?

Once generalized peritonitis has developed, there are few clinical clues specifically to implicate the appendix, although in all children except babies, appendicitis is the commonest cause of peritonitis. The guarding may be most pronounced in the right iliac fossa, and the history may be of pain which, in its early stages, was predominantly confined to the right iliac fossa. It is appropriate to treat the patient with peritonitis as having appendicitis, unless specific features point to an alternative diagnosis.

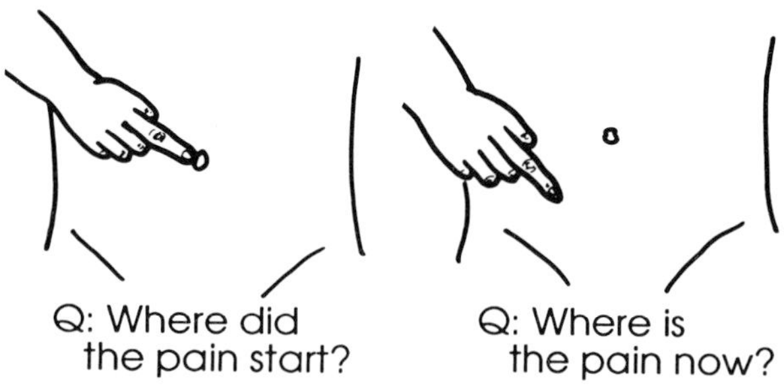

Q: Where did the pain start?

Q: Where is the pain now?

Fig. 3.23: *The pointing test in locating the site of abdominal pain in children.*

When does diarrhoea occur with appendicitis?

If the inflamed appendix lies against the rectum, the irritation it causes produces a mild diarrhoea. Retro-ileal and retrocaecal appendicitis may also produce loose bowel actions. If the appendix perforates, the infected material released collects in the most dependent parts of the peritoneal cavity – the retrovesical pouch in the male, and the retro-uterine recess in the female – and a pelvic abscess develops. As the abscess increases in size, it causes irritation of the rectum and can be palpated as a bulge of the anterior rectal wall. The abscess causes small and frequent loose stools containing mucus, which is a direct result of irritation of the rectal mucosa. The pelvic abscess takes several days or weeks to develop, and there may be no clear history of antecedent abdominal pain. Persistent small volume diarrhoea and the passage of mucus in a vaguely unwell child should signal the possibility of a pelvic collection.

Does appendicitis produce a fever?

In most children with appendicitis, the temperature is slightly elevated (37.5–38°C). A normal or slightly subnormal temperature does not preclude the diagnosis of appendicitis – nor does a grossly elevated temperature (39–40°C), although this is unlikely unless peritonitis is present. Unfortunately, most of the other conditions from which appendicitis must be distinguished are inflammatory or infective in nature and produce elevation of the temperature.

A MASS IN THE RIGHT ILIAC FOSSA

Appendicitis may produce a mass in the right iliac fossa (Fig. 3.24). If there is overlying guarding, it may be extremely difficult to palpate until the patient is anaesthetized; where there is no guarding, it can be felt as a tender, immobile mass deep to the muscles of the ventral abdominal wall. It is an inflammatory phlegmon of an infected appendix, stuck by inflammatory exudate to adjacent oedematous loops of small bowel and greater omentum. Depending on the patient's ability to localize infection, and on whether the appendix perforates, the mass will resolve, develop into an appendix abscess or cause generalized peritonitis.

In girls, a large ovarian cyst may be palpable as a smooth surfaced mass in the right iliac fossa. The mass is non-tender and mobile, unless there is torsion of its pedicle. It may disappear over the pelvic inlet into the pelvis, and be ballotable by bimanual examination between the rectum and the anterior abdominal wall. If torsion has occurred, the mass is tender and there are signs of peritoneal irritation in a girl with severe pain and no fever.

In the child under two years of age, the mass may be an intussusception. The sudden onset of a colicky pain with drawing up of the legs, pallor, lethargy and short duration of symptoms with or without rectal bleeding, would be suggestive of intussusception; a longer history of four or five days, with generalized anorexia, malaise and marked abdominal tenderness would make one more suspicious of appendicitis.

In the older child, a relatively painless, fixed mass in either iliac fossa would raise the possibility of lymphoma, in which case there may be evidence of weight loss, fever, lymphadenopathy or hepatosplenomegaly. Rare causes of a right iliac fossa mass include Meckel's diverticulitis, Yersinia lymphadenitis, tuberculosis, actinomycosis, duplication cyst and lymphangioma. Children with cystic fibrosis may develop a mass from ileal obstruction with viscous contents.

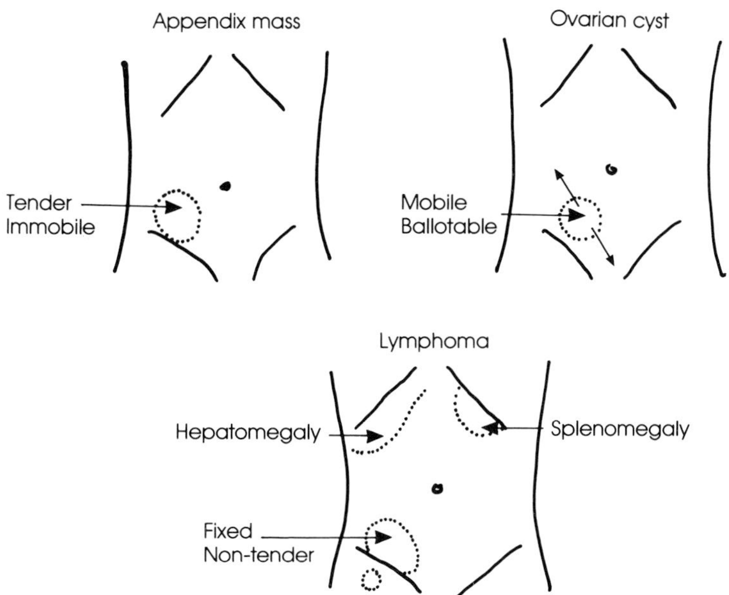

Fig. 3.24: *The right iliac fossa mass.*

OTHER PATHOLOGIES IN SUSPECTED APPENDICITIS

Viral enteritis ('mesenteric adenitis')

In addition to the localized collection of lymphoid tissue seen in the terminal ileum (Peyer's patches), there are numerous lymph nodes at the mesenteric edge of the bowel and within the mesentery of both small and large intestine. These nodes are particularly prominent in the mesentery of the terminal ileum and right colon. Infection by a number of enteric organisms, for example, *Yersinia* or *Campylobacter*, cause enlargement and even suppuration of these nodes. It is likely that many viral organisms, yet to be isolated or identified, also cause mesenteric adenitis. Infection with these organisms causes diffuse tenderness of the abdomen and signs which may be compatible with early acute appendicitis (Fig. 3.25). Tenderness is often maximal in the right iliac fossa, and is simply a reflection of the location of the enlarged nodes. The inflamed ileum becomes distended with fluid and gas such that deep palpation may produce a succussion splash. In mesenteric adenitis, there may be other signs of viral infection with puffiness around the eyes and a slight conjunctivitis, headache, generalized aches and pains, and rhinorrhoea. There may be some moderate enlargement of cervical, axillary and inguinal lymph nodes, but it should be acknowledged that in most normal children these nodes are palpable. The temperature may reach 40°C, but usually returns to normal within 48 hours. Despite abdominal pain and fever, the child is often hungry – unlike the situation in appendicitis. The disorder is self-limiting with all symptoms resolving within three or four days. With serial examination of the abdomen, the area of maximal tenderness may vary and, in most cases, there is no evidence of peritonitis. If the clinical signs are suggestive of peritonitis, operation is indicated. When in doubt, the child can be admitted to hospital and the examination repeated in a few hours.

Gastro-enteritis

This common condition is characterized by vomiting and diarrhoea. The diarrhoea usually commences as the first symptom or shortly after the onset of vomiting. There may be associated abdominal pain which tends to be cramping and diffuse. In the majority of children, symptoms are improving within 24–72 hours. Persistence of either vomiting or diarrhoea should make one suspicious of alternative diagnoses, of which ap-

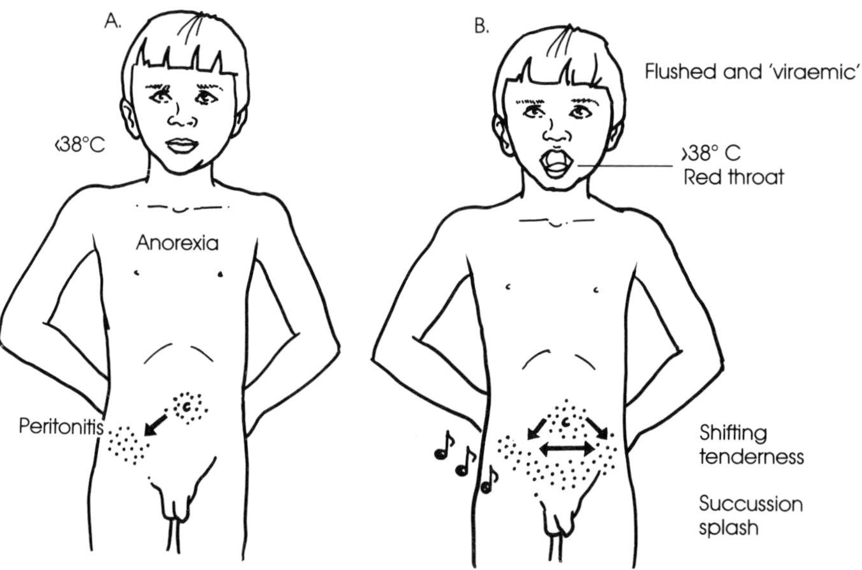

Fig. 3.25: *The differences between appendicitis* (A), *and mesenteric adenitis* (B). (*Adapted from* Hull *and* Johnston 1981).

Table 3.6 RARE CAUSES OF ABDOMINAL PAIN

Condition	Features
1. Primary peritonitis	Nephrotic syndrome – *Pneumococcus* – *Streptococcus* Seen in three- to six-year-olds
2. Pancreatitis	Secondary to steroid treatment for – nephrotic syndrome – collagen disease Mumps Trauma
3. Diabetic ketoacidosis hyperglycaemia	
4. Henoch-Schönlein purpura	Diffuse anaphylactoid vasculitis – gastro-intestinal tract bleeding – colicky pain Buttock and leg purpura Dorsal foot oedema Joint pains Haematuria Intussusception occurs in 2–3%
5. Haemophilia	Retroperitoneal, Mesenteric } haematoma
6. Sickle-cell anaemia	Common in negroes
7. Herpes zoster	Adolescents Cutaneous manifestations
8. Lead poisoning	Common after exposure to sun, therefore in summer Colicky pain, constipation, vomiting Anaemia with basophilic stippling
9. Abdominal epilepsy/migraine	
10. Porphyria	Urine turns red-brown on standing
11. Rectus abdominis haematoma	Trauma ± bleeding disorder

pendicitis is one. Rectal examination should exclude pelvic appendicitis masquerading as enteritis.

Constipation

Poor diet, a constitutional predisposition and poor bowel training, may all contribute to constipation. There is usually a long history of infrequent passage of hard bowel actions. The pain is often colicky and may be relieved by a bowel action. Examination of the abdomen reveals faecal material on both sides of the colon. There is no peritonitis. Digital examination of the rectum will reveal a capacious rectum full of faecal material.

Urinary tract infection or obstruction

These conditions may produce abdominal pain and be difficult to separate from appendicitis. A high index of suspicion and urinary examination will exclude this important cause. The child has a higher fever and fewer localizing signs than is caused by appendicitis (see Chapter 14 for details).

Rare conditions

Occasionally, abdominal pain may be the first manifestation of one of the conditions listed in Table 3.6.

GOLDEN RULES

(1) Symptoms suggestive of significant intra-abdominal pathology are: (i) pain persisting for more than four hours; (ii) pain increasing in intensity; and (iii) persistent vomiting, even in the absence of pain.
(2) Beware peritonitis: the most important aspect of the examination of the abdomen is exclusion of peritonitis.
(3) Beware of the uncooperative child: the child may have peritonitis and fear palpation of the abdomen.

(4) The clinical aim in appendicitis is to recognize early, localized peritonitis.
(5) The commonest lump in the acute abdomen is faeces (which are indentable on palpation).
(6) The sigmoid colon (which contains faeces) is often palpable in the right iliac fossa.
(7) Visceral pain is referred to the epigastrium, umbilical region or hypogastrium according to involvement of the fore-gut, mid-gut or hind-gut, respectively.
(8) Irritation of the anterior parietal peritoneum produces pain via segmental somatic nerves and causes guarding of the ventral abdominal wall musculature subserved by the same segment.
(9) Inflammation of the posterior parietal peritoneum does not cause guarding of the ventral abdominal wall musculature.
(10) The infant's abdomen is more protuberant, wider and has a shallower pelvis than that of the older child or adult.
(11) Narcotic analgesia should be given to a child with abdominal pain only once a definite clinical diagnosis or decision to operate has been made.
(12) Abdominal pain may be the presentation of pathology originating outside the abdomen.
(13) The abdominal signs of peritonitis are pain on movement of the abdomen, reluctance to protrude or indraw the abdomen, involuntary guarding and rigidity of the abdominal wall musculature, and rebound tenderness to percussion.
(14) Late signs of peritonitis include abdominal distension, and signs of septicaemia.
(15) Beware diarrhoea persisting for more than 24 hours; it may reflect a pelvic abscess which can be palpated by rectal examination.

Further Reading

Apley J. (1975). *The Child with Abdominal Pains*, 2nd edn. Oxford: Blackwell Scientific Publications.
Cope Z. (1972). *The Early Diagnosis of the Acute Abdomen*, 14th edn. Oxford: Oxford University Press.
Hull D., Johnston D.I. (1981). *Essential Paediatrics*. Edinburgh: Churchill Livingstone.
O'Donnell B. (1985). *Abdominal Pain in Childhood*. Oxford: Blackwell Scientific Publications.

4 Inguinoscrotal lesions

Abnormalities of the male genitalia are extremely common and comprise a large part of general paediatric surgical practice. Accurate diagnosis of these disorders depends on a sound understanding of normal development, which provides the clinician with anatomical information as well as an appropriate list of differential diagnoses.

EMBRYOLOGY

In the human fetus, sexual differentiation begins at about eight weeks gestation, at which time the urogenital ridge contains the developing gonad, mesonephros and the genital ducts. The Wolffian (mesonephric) duct develops into the vas deferens, epididymis and seminal vesicle under the stimulation of testosterone, while the Müllerian (paramesonephric) duct regresses under the action of a newly described glycoprotein hormone, Müllerian inhibiting substance. The testis has descended to the internal inguinal ring by 14–17 weeks of gestation, where it remains quiescent until about 28 weeks (Fig. 4.1). Then there is rapid descent through the inguinal canal into the scrotum and by 35–40 weeks descent is complete.

During descent through the inguinal canal into the scrotum, the testis is preceded by an outgrowth of peritoneum, the processus vaginalis, which invades the gubernacular mesenchyme (Fig. 4.2A). When descent is complete, the processus proximal to the testis obliterates (Fig. 4.2B). Failure of this obliteration is the cause of infantile herniae and hydroceles. Partial involution of the proximal processus without complete obliteration of the lumen, results in an encysted hydrocele (Fig. 4.2C) or scrotal hydrocele (Fig. 4.2D). Total failure of involution at the level of the internal inguinal ring leads to a hernia (Fig. 4.2E and F). In the more common situation, only the proximal processus remains patent and the hernia presents as a lump at the external ring. Occasionally, the entire processus vaginalis remains widely patent and the hernia presents clini-

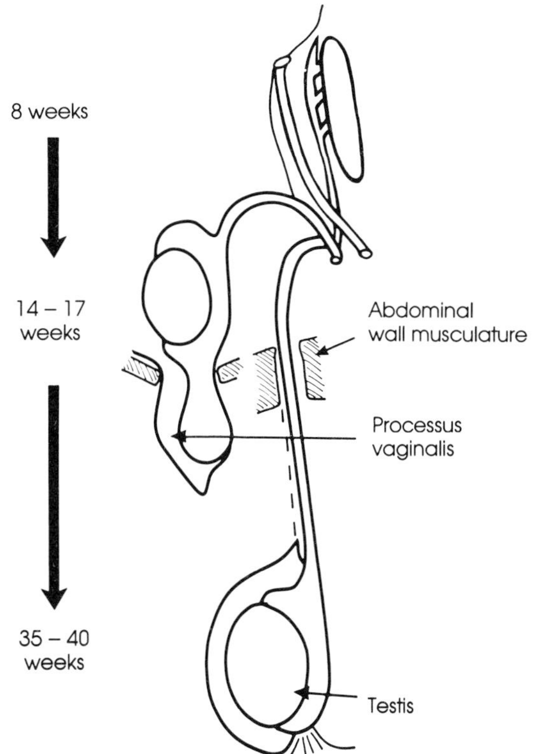

Fig. 4.1: *The timing of testicular descent.*

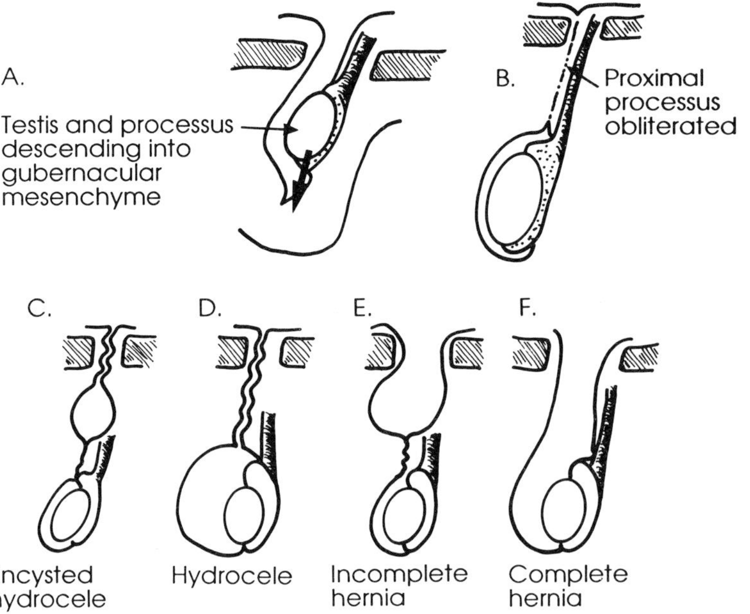

Fig 4.2: *The mechanism of testicular descent through the inguinal canal (A), and obliteration of the processus vaginalis (B). Incomplete obliteration leads to an encysted hydrocele (C), a scrotal hydrocele (D), an incomplete hernia (E) or a complete hernia (inguinoscrotal hernia) (F).*

cally as a swelling extending from the external ring into the scrotum ('inguinoscrotal' or 'complete' hernia) (Fig. 4.2F). Involution of the processus begins as soon as the testis has descended; delay in this process of obliteration may result in a hernia because, after birth, increases in abdominal pressure (with crying etc.) push the small bowel into the still patent processus and keep it open. A premature infant, therefore, is more likely to have incompletely descended testes and patent hernial sacs.

THE UNDESCENDED TESTIS

Testicular descent is a complex process initiated by hormones and executed by mechanical events; abnormalities of either of these may cause undescended testes. The hormonal signals are not known completely, but testosterone appears to be responsible for the second phase of descent through the inguinal canal into the scrotum. Therefore, in children with undescended testes, one needs to consider androgen deficiency, even though it is much more common for maldescent to be caused by mechanical abnormalities.

Anatomical landmarks for the undescended testis

The key to the clinical assessment of undescended testes is determination of their location. Undescended testes are arrested in the line of descent, or deviated to an 'ectopic' or abnormal position. Rarely, the testis may remain inside the inguinal canal or abdomen, in which case it will be impalpable. A testis which has descended beyond the external ring but has not reached the scrotum will be deviated from the normal line of descent by the bony prominence of the pubic tubercle to lie lateral to the external ring (the commonest site for an ectopic testis). Here, it overlies the external oblique aponeurosis midway between the pubic tubercle and anterior superior iliac spine (Fig. 4.3). In this location, the testis remains invested by the external spermatic fascia, and the 'pouch' this layer so forms is sometimes referred to as the superficial inguinal pouch. If the testis cannot be palpated lateral to the external ring, there are three rare sites in which an ectopic testes may be located. They are:

(1) lateral to the scrotum in the thigh (femoral testis);

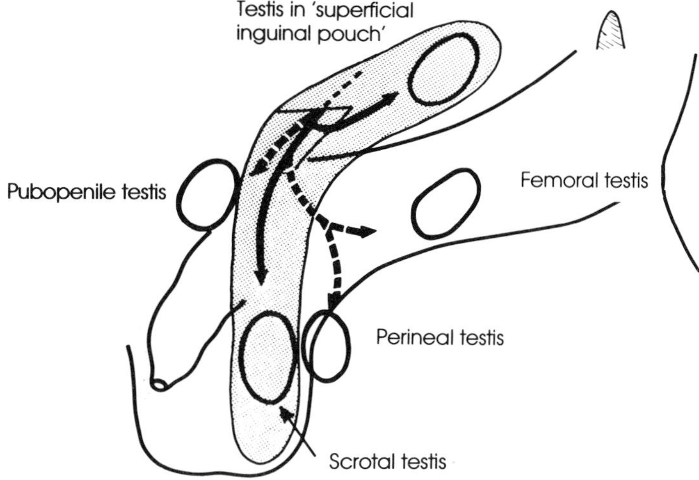

Fig. 4.3: *The surface anatomy of the inguinal region and the arc along which the testis normally is located.*

(2) medial to the external ring (pubopenile testis);
(3) behind the scrotum (perineal testis).

It is important to identify the position of the external ring and inguinal ligament to establish the anatomical location of the undescended testis (Fig. 4.4). The pubic tubercle marks the inferior margin of the external ring, and the inguinal ligament extends laterally from there to the anterior superior iliac spine. The skin crease most visible in the groin of small children *does not* correspond with the inguinal ligament, but rather the attachment of the superficial abdominal fascia (Scarpa's fascia) to the fascia lata.

In small children, there is a tendency to underestimate how far above the scrotum is the superficial inguinal pouch, either leading to failure to locate a testis in the superficial inguinal pouch, or to the misdiagnosis of an inguinal lymph node for a testis.

In the neonate, descended testes are easy to see, since the scrotum is flaccid and the skin very thin. Even at birth, the midpoint of the normal testis is at least 4 cm to 6 cm below the superior border of the pubis. In some premature children, the testes may not have completed descent by birth and may still be in the inguinal canal or pubic region. By

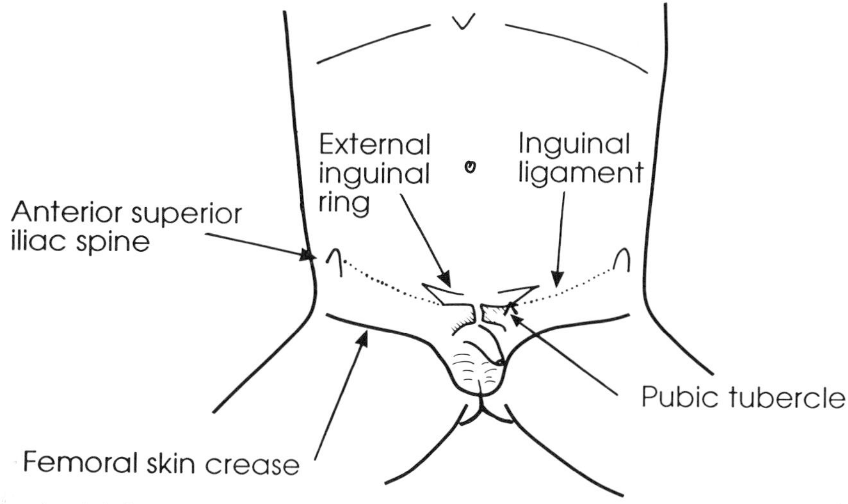

Fig. 4.4: *The relationship of the bony landmarks and external rings to the skin creases.*

three to six months, however, these 'stragglers' will be resident in the scrotum, allowing truly undescended testes to be distinguished from normally descended testes.

The cremasteric reflex

The spermatic cord contains the cremaster muscle, which modulates testicular temperature by retracting the testis from the scrotum. An active cremaster muscle causes a retractile testis, which may mimic an undescended testis when the testis is not found in the scrotum. The muscle is sensitive to circulating testosterone, with greater contractility of the muscle being observed when testosterone concentrations are low. When the testosterone concentration in the serum is high, contractility of the cremaster muscle is suppressed. During childhood, serum testosterone concentrations are high for the first few months after birth and at the onset of puberty (Fig. 4.5). Between the ages of about two and eight years, serum testosterone concentrations are low, equivalent to those found in girls. During this time,

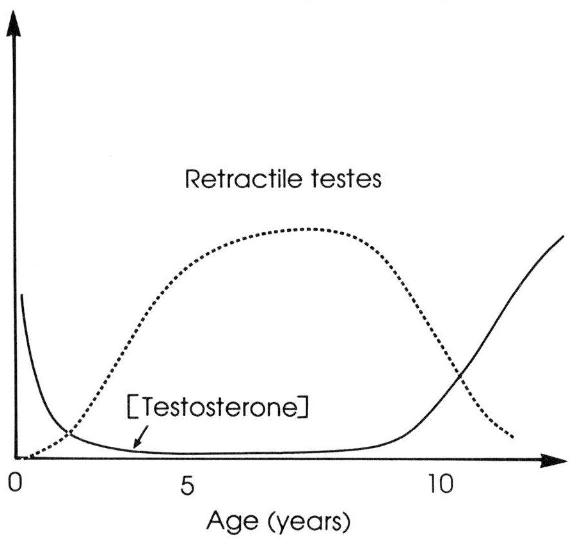

Fig. 4.5: *The reciprocal relationship between the serum testosterone concentration and retractility of the testis.*

the contractility of the cremaster is enhanced markedly and leads to a high incidence of retractile testes in childhood. Since many children have a screening examination for undescended testes in the early primary school period when retractile testes are common, the distinction between true maldescent and retractile testes may be difficult.

There are certain criteria which should be met before a testis can be described as being retractile (Table 4.1). The testis should have been in the scrotum earlier in childhood, and there may be a history of it being visible low in the scrotum at birth. The testis must reside there at some time during the day; usually, it is best seen at bath time when the warmth of the water suppresses cremasteric contraction and allows it to be fully descended. It should be possible to manipulate the testis to the bottom of the scrotum without undue tension on the cord. A testis that will only reach the top of the scrotum is maldescended. After manipulation of the testis to the bottom of the scrotum, the spermatic cord should not be so tight that the testis immediately springs back out. In other words, the retractile testis should remain in the scrotum for a few minutes after manipulation. Where the testis is fully descended only when the spermatic cord is stretched tightly, maldescent must be assumed to be present. Finally, the testis should be normal in size, which implies that its development is not impaired by its position. This is a useful clinical point, since an undescended testis tends to become hypoplastic and smaller than a normal contralateral one.

Table 4.1 CRITERIA FOR THE DIAGNOSIS OF A RETRACTILE TESTIS

1. Testis can be manipulated to the bottom of the scrotum
2. Testis remains in the scrotum after manipulation
3. Testis resides spontaneously in the scrotum some of the time
4. Testis is normal in size

History

Most boys with undescended testes present when someone notices that one or both sides of the scrotum appears to be empty. Knowledge of the location of the testes at birth is helpful. Where there were fully descended testes at birth, the empty scrotum of later childhood is likely to be caused by retractile testes. This can be confirmed by asking about the position of the testes at times of relaxation of the cremaster, such as at bath time or after sleeping in a warm bed.

Physical examination

Examination of the scrotum is aided when there is no stress or tension, and the room is warm: anxiety and cold stimulate the cremasteric reflex. The best way to avoid stress in a boy is to explain what is being done and to examine the genitalia gently. Inspection of the scrotum with the child standing will reveal whether it is large and contains testes, or whether it is small and flat, suggesting the testes are not normally resident within it.

An alternative method is to get the small child to squat on the examining couch (Fig. 4.6A). This position causes automatic relaxation of the cremaster muscle and allows the testes to be seen in the scrotum. Older boys can be asked to sit on the couch, with the knees pulled up against the chest (Fig. 4.6B).

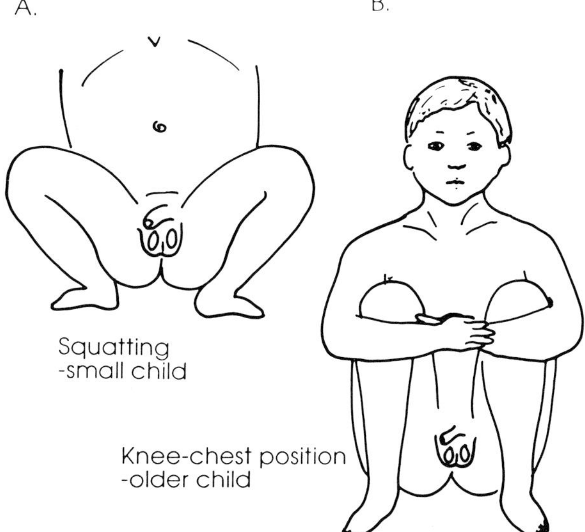

Fig. 4.6: *Techniques to eliminate the effects of cremasteric contraction. Retractile testes appear in the scrotum when the small child squats (A) and the older boy sits in the knee-chest position (B).*

Often, when a normal child lies supine, the testes can be seen within the scrotum. In others, the scrotum may be difficult to see completely and, if there is cremasteric retraction, the testes may be lying near the upper part of the scrotum or higher, where they are concealed by the skin because of the increased subcutaneous fat (Fig. 4.7A). Without touching the scrotum itself, the pubic skin can be retracted cranially, a manoeuvre which often reveals the testes (Fig. 4.7B). It

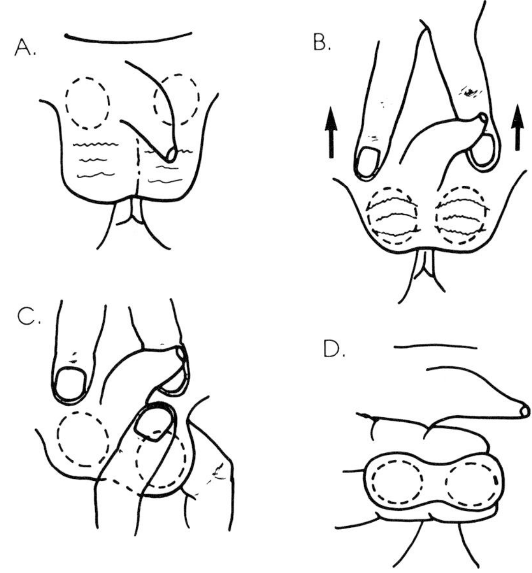

Fig. 4.7: *The technique of examining retractile testes.*

should be remembered that a testis is easy to see and feel only because of the extreme thinness of the skin of the scrotum. When the testis is in any other position, it is not only difficult to feel but also difficult to see (Fig. 4.8). If the scrotum is pulled up over the pubis to reveal the testis, it can then be palpated by the other hand and gently pulled caudally (Fig. 4.7C). Parental anxiety can be dramatically relieved by the demonstration of both testes in the scrotum (Fig. 4.7D).

Where the testis is truly undescended, the first step is to locate its position. The flat of the hand is placed gently over the inguinal region in the area of the superficial inguinal pouch (Fig. 4.9A). By gently rolling the finger-tips round and round, the testis usually can be felt as a mobile, spherical structure between the subcutaneous fat and the abdominal wall muscles. The mobility of the testis in the superficial inguinal pouch is such that it is easily overlooked unless the flat of the hand is used. This prevents the testis slipping out unnoticed from under the examiner's fingers.

Once the testis is located, attempt to deliver it

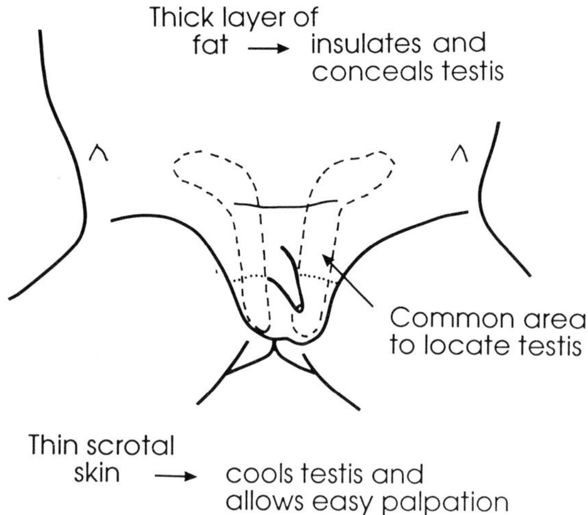

Fig. 4.8: *The relationship between the position of the testis and the overlying skin.*

into the scrotum. Begin lateral to the known position of the testis, using the fingers of one hand to press firmly against the abdominal wall, and attempt to 'milk' the testis towards the scrotum like a plough (Fig. 4.9B). If the testis can be manipulated to the pubis, it can then be snared through the thin scrotal skin by the opposite examining hand. The testis is held by compression of the spermatic cord, immediately proximal to the testis, rather than by holding the testis itself which

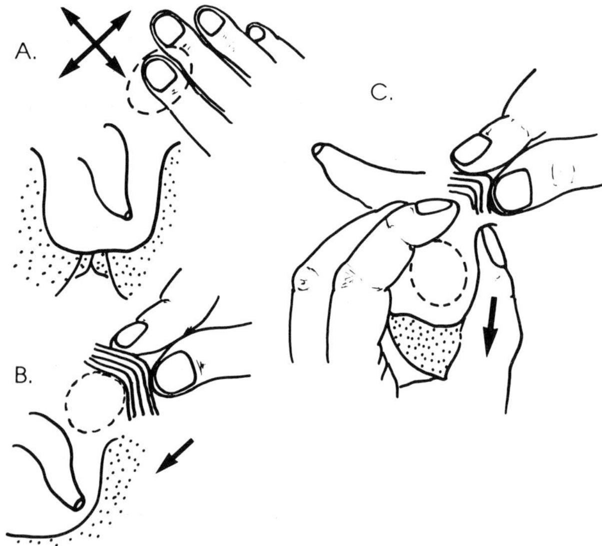

Fig. 4.9: *The technique of locating and delivering to the top of the scrotum an undescended or retractile testis.*

would be painful to the child (Fig. 4.9C). By grasping the spermatic cord through the scrotal skin, the testis can be pulled down into the normal scrotal position and an estimate made of the degree of descent. This should be determined by the relationship of the testis to the scrotum (i.e. high, medium or low), and compared with the contralateral testis. An alternative procedure is to measure in centimetres the distance between the midpoint of the testis and the superior pubic crest. If the testis is descended normally, this should be at least 4 cm to 6 cm. A palpable testis is defined as being undescended if it is impossible to manipulate it into the scrotum to a distance of more than 4 cm below the pubic crest, or into the lower scrotum.

The impalpable testis

The testis may be completely impalpable, which suggests that it is either inside the inguinal canal or abdomen, or less commonly, absent. Although deep palpation over the inguinal canal may cause some discomfort, the intracanalicular testis is not palpable unless it can be 'milked' out of the external ring. Nevertheless, testes within the abdomen or the inguinal canal are rare, and in the majority of boys with undescended testes, a testis is palpable. The commonest reason for failure to feel a testis is failure to locate it in the superficial inguinal pouch, probably because the clinician is misled by (1) the position of the skin creases, (2) the mobility of the testis, or (3) a thick layer of subcutaneous fat which conceals the testis.

Two important clues should be sought if the testis cannot be found. First, the pubis adjacent to the external ring should be palpated carefully to feel for the emergent spermatic cord. An ectopic testis in a rare position may be traced by following the cord from the external ring (Fig. 4.10) to the testis. Secondly, the size of the contralateral testis is helpful in assessing whether the testis is absent or impalpable because of its location within the inguinal canal or abdomen (Fig. 4.11). If one testis is absent (it may have undergone atrophy secondary to torsion during prenatal or perinatal descent), the contralateral organ undergoes compensatory hypertrophy, which may be apparent on clinical examination. It is important to remember

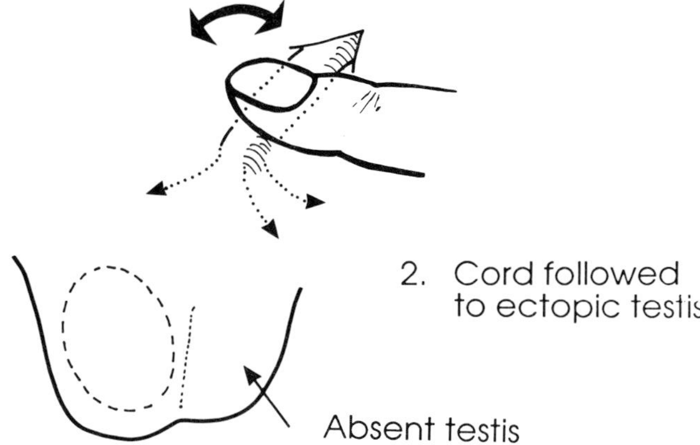

Fig. 4.10: *Locate the missing testis by first locating the spermatic cord.*

that the size of the normal testis changes little between six months and 10 years until the onset of puberty, when it grows rapidly. The hypertrophied testis is conspicuous once this fact is appreciated.

THE ACUTE SCROTUM

The term 'acute scrotum' describes the scrotum with acute pain and swelling, or other signs of inflammation. There are four main causes, which include torsion of the testis or one of its appendages, epididymitis (or 'epididymo-orchitis'), and idiopathic scrotal oedema (Table 4.2).

Table 4.2 CAUSES OF THE ACUTE SCROTUM

Condition	Frequency (%)
Torsion of a testicular appendage	60
Torsion of the testis	30
Idiopathic scrotal oedema	<10
Epididymitis	<10

Torsion of the testis is the most important cause of the acute scrotum, but is less common than its minor counterpart, torsion of a testicular appendage. Testicular torsion occurs most frequently at two ages: first in the perinatal period, when the whole tunica and contents twist ('extravaginal torsion'), and secondly at puberty, when an excessively mobile testis twists inside the tunica vaginalis ('intravaginal torsion') (Fig. 4.12). Extravaginal torsion occurs at, or shortly after, testicular descent into the scrotum, when the processus vaginalis is not fixed tightly to the scrotal fascia. After the first few months, torsion becomes relatively less common again, until the approach of puberty, when rapid enlargement of the testis predisposes to twisting in those testes which are not anchored by a normal mesorchium. The peak incidence at 13 years corresponds to the high circulating testosterone levels and rapid growth of the testis at that time. Testicular torsion needs to be recognized quickly, as immediate operation is required to avert infarction of the organ. Infarction is the presumed cause of the absent testis after perinatal torsion.

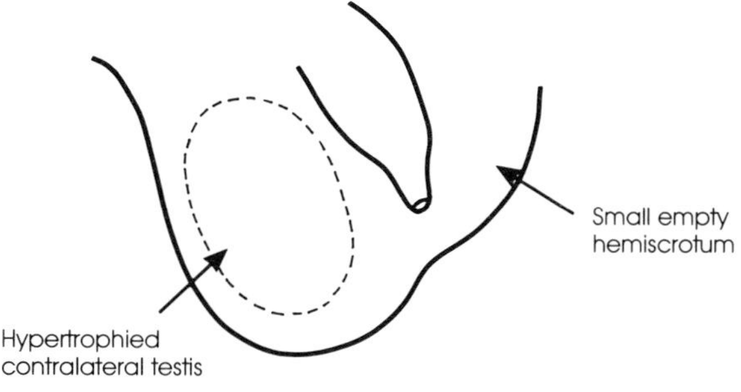

Fig. 4.11: *Hypertrophy of the contralateral testis is a sign of atrophy of the testis.*

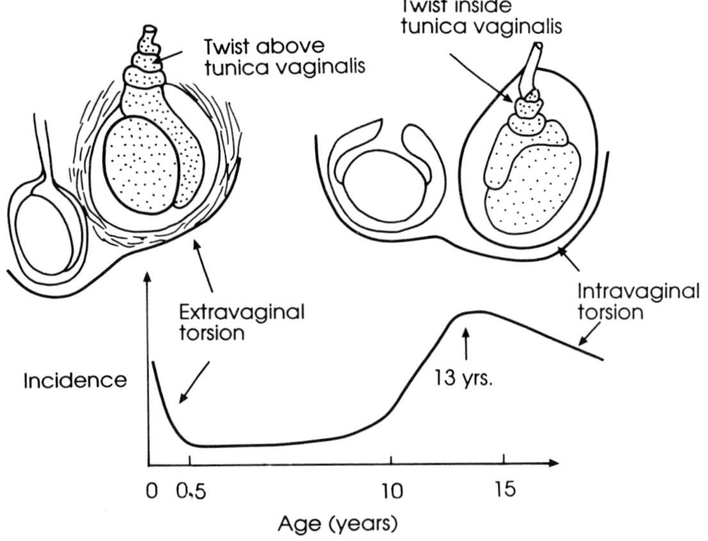

Fig. 4.12: *The relationship of the incidence of extravaginal and intravaginal torsion of the testis to age.*

Torsion of a testicular appendage is the commonest cause of an acute scrotum in childhood. The hydatid of Morgagni, or 'appendix testis', situated near the upper pole of the testis, is a normal remnant of the cranial end of the Müllerian duct (Fig. 4.13) which readily undergoes torsion because of its long stalk. Torsion can occur at any time during childhood, but peaks at 11 years when low oestrogen levels signal the onset of puberty (Fig. 4.14). Because of its origin from the Müllerian duct, the hydatid may enlarge with oestrogen stimulation (as does the uterus) and predispose to torsion.

Epididymitis (epididymo-orchitis) is an uncommon cause of the acute scrotum in modern paediatrics. It usually results from reflux of infected urine via the vas deferens, and may be associated with significant urinary tract malformation. The infection reflects its origin from the urine with *Escherichia coli* being the commonest organism isolated. Epididymitis with urinary tract malformation and infection occurs commonly in

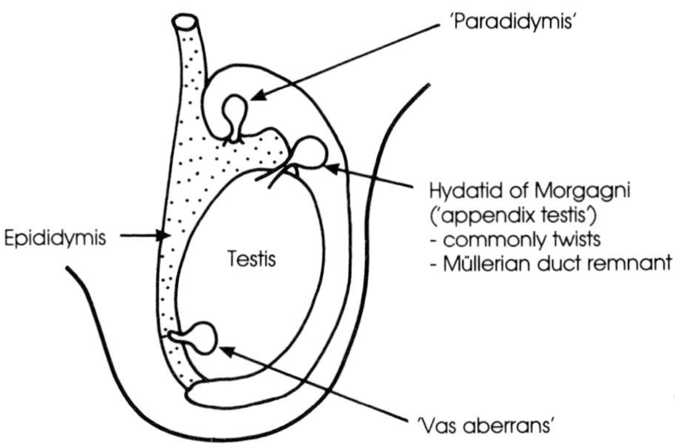

Fig. 4.13: *The testicular appendages.*

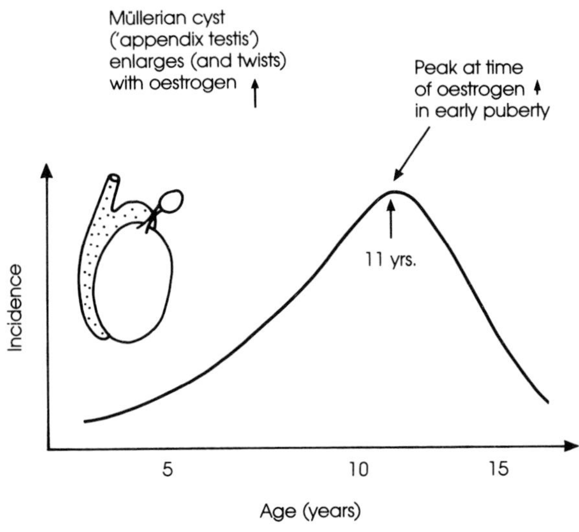

Fig. 4.14: *The relationship of the incidence of torsion of the hydatid of Morgagni to age and oestrogen secretion.*

small infants, but is rare thereafter (Fig. 4.15). The narrow vas deferens, lack of semen or secretions, and successful treatment of urinary infections with antibiotics all may contribute to the rarity after infancy. Beyond puberty, the disease becomes

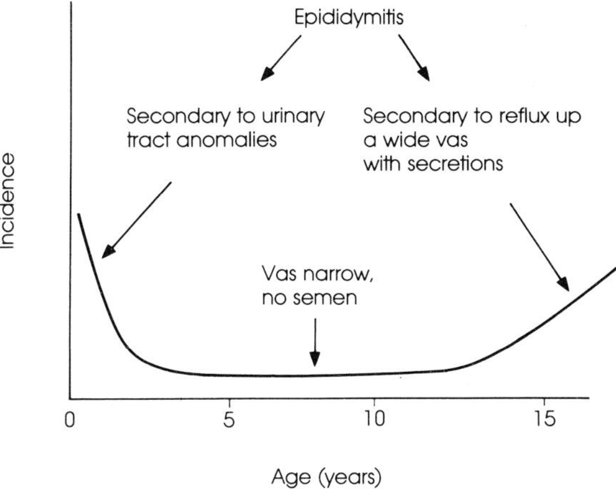

Fig. 4.15: *The relationship of the incidence of epididymitis to age.*

more common, as the size of the vas deferens and the volume of secretions increase. The testis may be seeded by blood-borne organisms, but this is exceptionally rare. The mumps virus has little affinity for the testis until after sexual maturation.

Acute idiopathic scrotal oedema is probably an allergic-type inflammation of the perineum, caused perhaps by a local reaction to an insect bite or sting. It is self-limiting and requires no intervention once recognized.

The history

The symptoms of an acute scrotum are similar regardless of the aetiology. In infancy, there may be crying, distress, fever and vomiting. The child is brought for consultation because his mother finds the swollen, red scrotum when changing his nappies. In older boys, particularly adolescents, there may be vague iliac fossa pain, or pain in the loin or flank. This is a vital point because boys of this age are reluctant to remove their underpants because of embarrassment. Furthermore, where there is referred pain, the patient himself may not be aware of the scrotal abnormality, and the torsion may be concealed from the unwary examiner (Fig. 4.16). Usually, however, there is marked local pain and tenderness in the scrotum, with or without vomiting. These symptoms suggest severe disturbance of testicular blood supply. In some children, there is a history of trauma to the scrotum, but characteristically this is minor and vague; it represents an attempt by the boy or his parents to relate the onset of symptoms to a specific event, when in reality the minor trauma merely draws attention to the already abnormal scrotum.

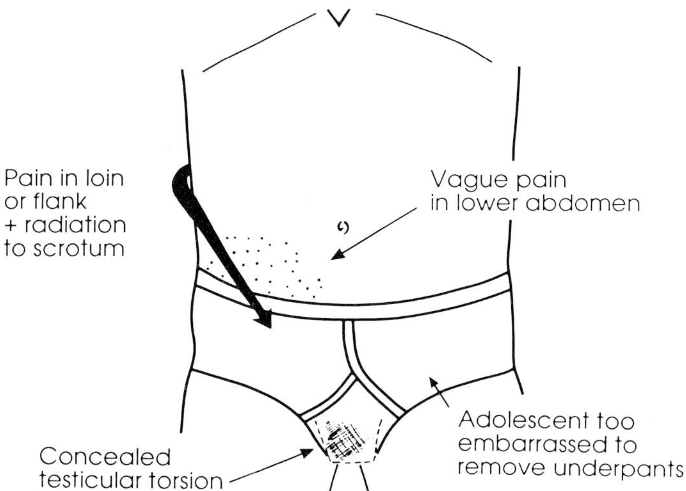

Fig. 4.16: *Referred pain in torsion of the testis may conceal the true cause.*

Physical examination of the scrotum

Signs are well localized to the scrotum, except in extravaginal torsion or where torsion occurs in an undescended testis. These two latter conditions produce an acutely tender lump and inflammation higher in the scrotum, or even in the groin, which has to be distinguished from a strangulated inguinal hernia (see below). The first step in the examination, therefore, is to determine whether the swelling involves the testis. A normal testis palpable below the swelling indicates that the abnormality is not torsion, but is more likely to be a hernia or one of its variants.

The next point in the examination is to determine whether the testis or its adjacent structures are involved, since these cases should have immediate surgical exploration unless a clear alternative diagnosis is made. With this caveat in mind, an accurate diagnosis should always be attempted, as this may negate the need for surgical exploration in a few cases.

The hemiscrotum is often red, swollen and oedematous in both testicular torsion and torsion of an appendage (Fig. 4.17). There is a variable amount of pain and tenderness of the testis, depending on the degree of oedema and ischaemia. Where infarction of the testis has occurred already, pain may be surprisingly minimal.

The testis that has undergone torsion assumes a location high in the scrotum, secondary to the shortening effect of torsion of the cord on its intravaginal length (Fig. 4.18). An additional sign which may indicate testicular torsion is the orientation of the contralateral testis, which may hang

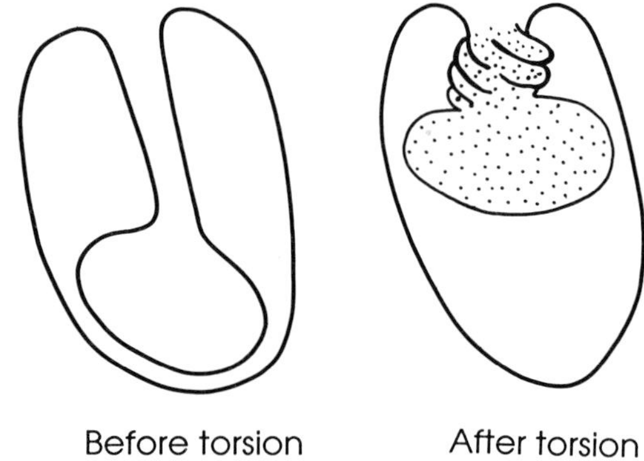

Fig. 4.18: *Torsion of the intravaginal spermatic cord causes the testis to ride up within the scrotum.*

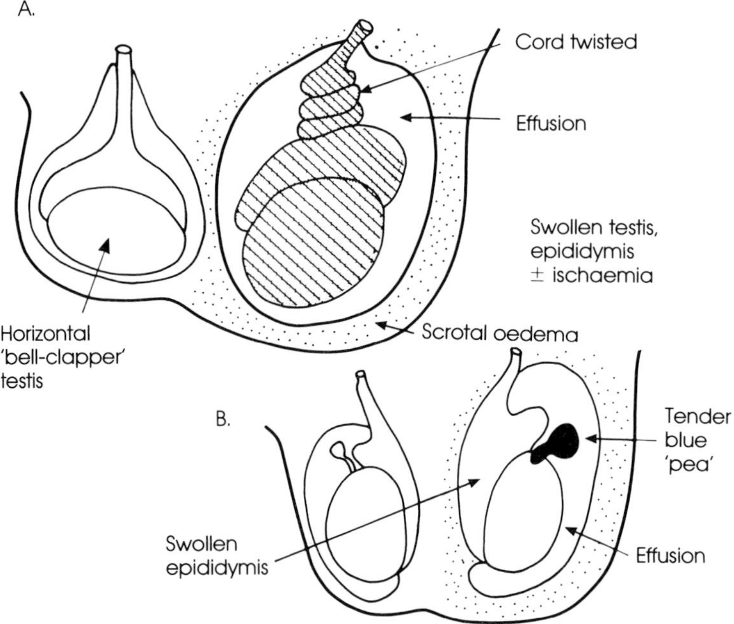

Fig. 4.17: *Comparison of the signs of torsion of the testis* (A) *with those of its appendages* (B).

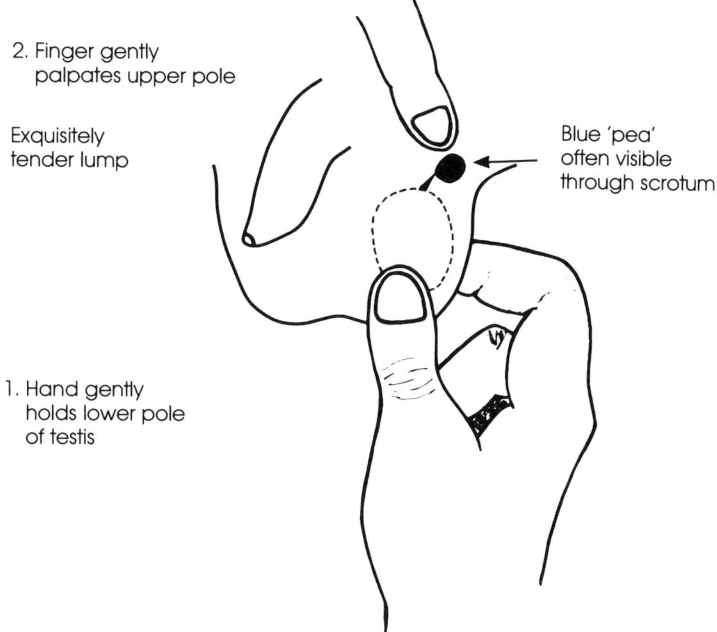

Fig. 4.19: *The technique for identifying torsion of the hydatid of Morgagni.*

loosely within the processus vaginalis like a 'bell clapper'.

The pathognomonic sign of a twisted hydatid of Morgagni is a visible blue-black spot seen through the scrotal skin near the upper pole of the testis. This is present when (1) the secondary scrotal oedema and inflammation is minimal or absent, and (2) the torsion has produced haemorrhage in the pedunculated cyst. Should the cyst undergo infarction without haemorrhage, the diagnosis may be missed. Even at surgical exploration, a pale, infarcted cyst looks trivial, and many cases of apparent 'epididymo-orchitis' are probably examples of bloodless infarction of the hydatid.

A swollen, tender hydatid can be palpated at the upper pole of the testis when scrotal oedema is minimal (Fig. 4.19). One hand gently supports the testis while the other hand touches the upper pole. The presence of a localized, exquisitely painful lump the size of a pea, near the upper pole of the testis, confirms torsion of the hydatid; the rest of the testis is non-tender.

The physical signs of epididymitis are non-specific, although the cord may be conspicuously swollen and tender (Fig. 4.20). The presence of a known urinary tract anomaly (e.g. recto-urethral fistula in a baby with imperforate anus), a proven urinary tract infection, recent urethral instrumentation and involvement of both testes, are all suggestive features. The non-specific signs and rarity of epididymitis outside these special circumstances means that the diagnosis should be made at operation, rather than by clinical assessment.

Idiopathic scrotal oedema can be distinguished from torsion in most patients (Fig. 4.21). The oedema and inflammation are superficial, have the appearance of an allergic wheal, and are not confined to one hemiscrotum. The perineum, thigh or penis (including the foreskin) is involved in continuity. Occasionally, the first sign is oedema of the foreskin and penis; this rapidly extends to the scrotum which in turn becomes swollen and turgid. The diagnosis is confirmed when the testis can be displaced gently out of the scrotum into the superficial inguinal pouch, where its normal size and consistency can be determined. This manoeuvre is relatively painless, unlike the situation in testicular torsion where even gentle manipulation of the testis causes exquisite pain. A subtle sign which may be seen in idiopathic scrotal

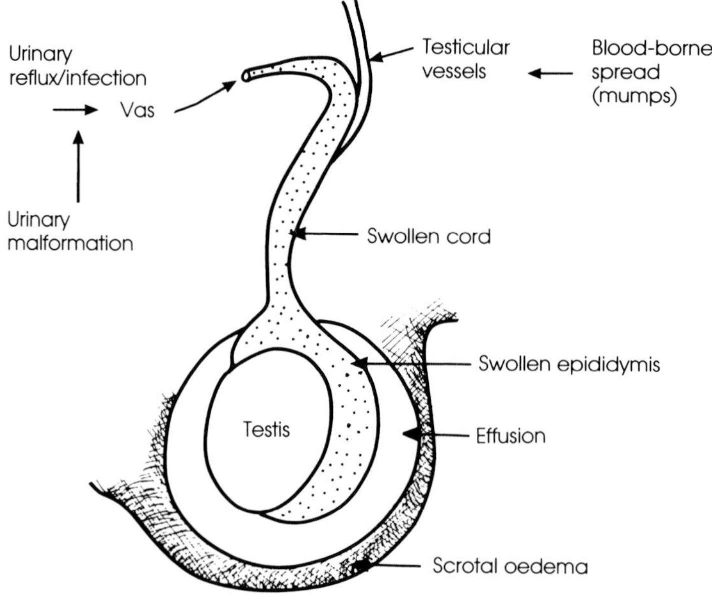

Fig. 4.20: *Epididymitis.*

oedema is slight erythema which extends over the entire groin and perineum.

THE PAINLESS, SWOLLEN SCROTUM

The common causes of painless swelling of the scrotum are a complete inguinal hernia (inguino-scrotal hernia) and a hydrocele (Table 4.3). The common hydrocele is caused by intraperitoneal fluid trickling down through the narrow processus vaginalis and collecting around the testis (Fig. 4.22). The fluid gravitates down the processus during the waking hours, when intra-abdominal pressure is elevated by crying and general activity. When the child sleeps, the fluid is absorbed into the adjacent tissues, reducing the size of the collection by morning. Since the condition occurs when the processus has not quite closed, it is most frequent in infancy. Further involution of the processus leads to spontaneous resolution in most children. It needs to be distinguished from an inguinal hernia which reaches the scrotum, because the treatment of the two conditions is so different.

There are three main criteria which are needed to diagnose a hydrocele (Table 4.4). The upper limit of the swelling must be defined by palpation of the neck of the scrotum between finger and

Table 4.3 CAUSES OF A SWOLLEN SCROTUM

Common:	Hydrocele Complete inguinal hernia
Uncommon:	Haematocele Varicocele
Rare:	Testicular tumour

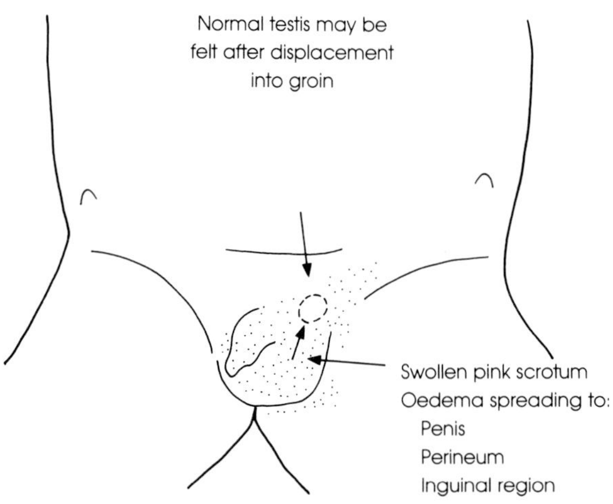

Fig. 4.21: *Features of idiopathic scrotal oedema.*

Table 4.4 CRITERIA FOR DIAGNOSIS OF A HYDROCELE

1. 'Can get above it' – normal narrow cord above the swelling
2. Brilliant transillumination – but a hernia also may transilluminate
3. Cannot be emptied on pressure – quick emptying implies a wide neck

thumb. The narrow processus contains no bowel and is not palpable as a separate structure. The collection of clear fluid is brilliantly transilluminable, although care needs to be taken because even the bowel in a hernial sac will transilluminate dimly. In a hydrocele, transillumination of the scrotum will cast the shadow of the testis and cord within the hydrocele against the wall of the scrotum (Fig. 4.23). The other useful sign is inability to empty the fluid on firm but gentle compression of the scrotum. Where the swelling is reduced by compression, the neck must be wide and the diagnosis of a hernia can be made. This sign is also useful in identifying the uncommon hernia which contains greater omentum in the neck of its sac; large amounts of fluid are produced within the sac giving it the appearance of a hydrocele, but the fluid is emptied readily on compression (Fig. 4.24) as the omentum is pushed out of the neck of the sac.

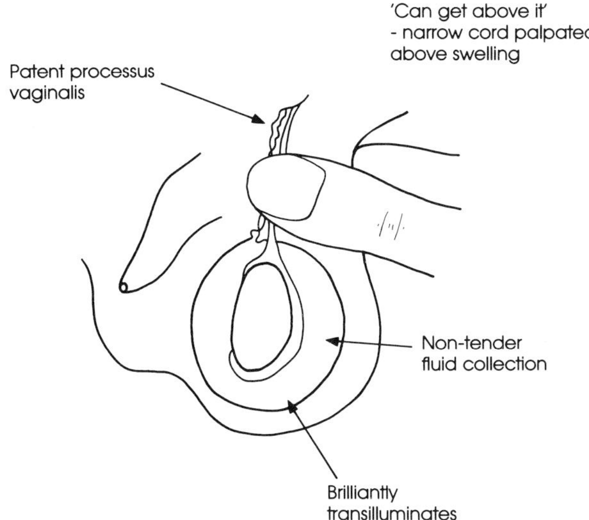

Fig. 4.22: *Signs of a hydrocele of the scrotum.*

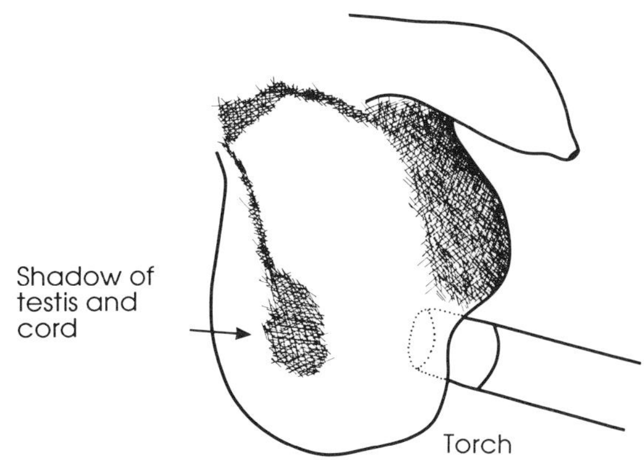

Fig. 4.23: *In the large hydrocele, transillumination of the scrotum will cause the shadow of the testis and cord to be cast against the wall of the scrotum.*

Uncommon causes of a scrotal swelling include a varicocele and a haematocele. The varicocele is nearly always on the left side, and occurs in tall, young adolescents when the valves in the testicular veins become incompetent. The lump surrounds the testis and feels like a 'bag of worms'.

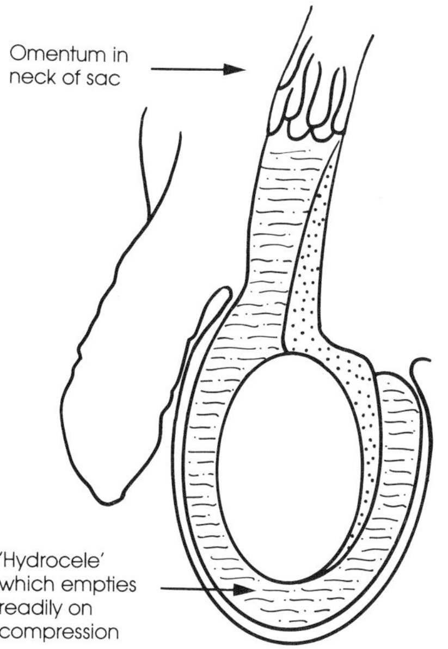

Fig. 4.24: *Signs of a 'fluid hernia', where omentum occupies the neck of the sac.*

The boy may complain of mild discomfort or a dragging sensation. Examination needs to be performed with the boy standing and then lying down; the varicose pampiniform plexus fills with blood on standing, or on cough impulse, but may be completely impalpable when lying down. In small boys, the appearance of a varicocele should alert the examiner to the possibility of a renal tumour with secondary compression and occlusion of the testicular veins.

A haematocele is a collection of blood in the processus vaginalis and may result from direct trauma to the scrotum. It is uncommon in childhood, but can be recognized by bruising of the scrotal tissues – in contrast to testicular torsion where the overlying skin is inflamed.

Rarely, a testicular tumour presents as a painless scrotal swelling. The testis is enlarged, irregular and less tender than normal, and may be surrounded by a secondary hydrocele. Where a tumour is suspected, the central abdomen needs to be palpated to identify secondary spread to the para-aortic lymph nodes.

THE GROIN LUMP

An indirect hernia is the commonest cause of a groin lump (Table 4.5). In most children with inguinal herniae, the distal part of the processus vaginalis has closed off, so that the so-called 'incomplete' sac does not extend far beyond the exteral ring. The diagnosis can be made from the history and the exact anatomical location of the lump.

The history

There are four points which indicate an inguinal hernia: (1) the sudden appearance of a swelling in the groin of a baby, often during crying; in an older child, it may appear with coughing or walking (related to peaks of high intra-abdominal pressure); (2) the variability in the size of the swelling (bowel is able to enter or leave the sac); (3) the periodic disappearance of the lump (the contents may return completely to the abdomen); and (4) the apparent lack of pain, except when the bowel becomes stuck in the sac (incarceration) causing venous congestion and/or ischaemia (strangulation). Many others can point to the exact location of the swelling.

Physical examination

Lump present

When the lump is present at the time of consultation, the key point in the examination is to determine the exact position of the swelling in relation to the external ring (Fig. 4.25). The bony landmarks (anterior superior iliac spine and pubic tubercle) define the position of the inguinal ligament and the external ring, both of which are cranial to the most obvious skin crease in the groin (Fig. 4.4). Inguinal or femoral lymph nodes are more lateral in position, and may be associated with a primary septic focus in the lower leg or

Table 4.5 CAUSES OF A GROIN LUMP

	Condition	Distinguishing features
Common:	Indirect inguinal hernia	At the external ring/extending into the scrotum Reduces with taxis
	Hydrocele (encysted)	Transilluminates Moves down with testis traction
	Retractile/undescended testis	Scrotum is empty Can be pulled down
	Lymph node	Lump is lateral/below the external ring Primary infection in perineum/leg
Rare:	Direct inguinal hernia	Above/lateral to the external ring Very obvious cough impulse
	Femoral hernia	Below/lateral to the external ring

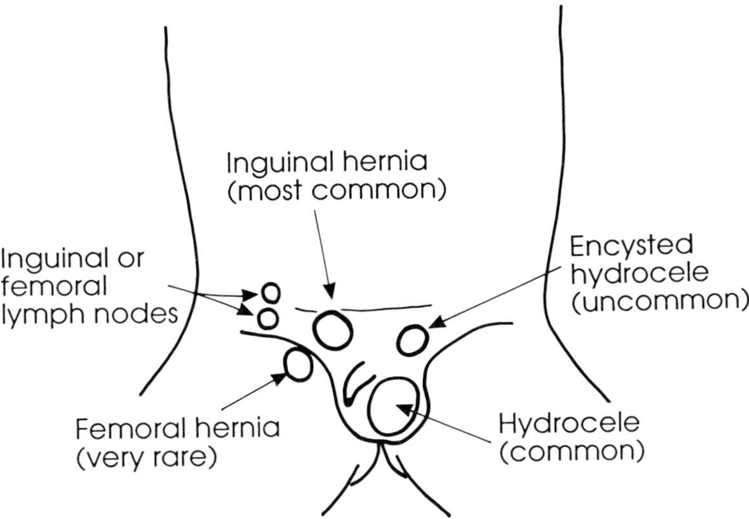

Fig. 4.25: *The differential diagnosis of a groin lump.*

perineum. The very rare femoral hernia is below and lateral to the pubic tubercle, closer to the femoral skin crease. The common hydrocele is within the scrotum, but the less common encysted hydrocele in the processus of the cord may be found at the external ring.

A rectractile or undescended testis located at the external ring can be confused with a hernia, an error that is avoided by palpation of a normally sited testis within the scrotum. Remember that an undescended testis may have an adjacent patent processus, and can present because of its associated hernia.

Palpation of the neck of the scrotum between the finger and thumb reveals whether the lump reaches the scrotum (Fig. 4.26). When the hernia extends into the scrotum, the fingers 'cannot get above it', an observation which distinguishes it from a hydrocele that does not extend up to and through the external ring.

The diagnostic feature of an inguinal hernia is the ability to reduce it by manual compression, a

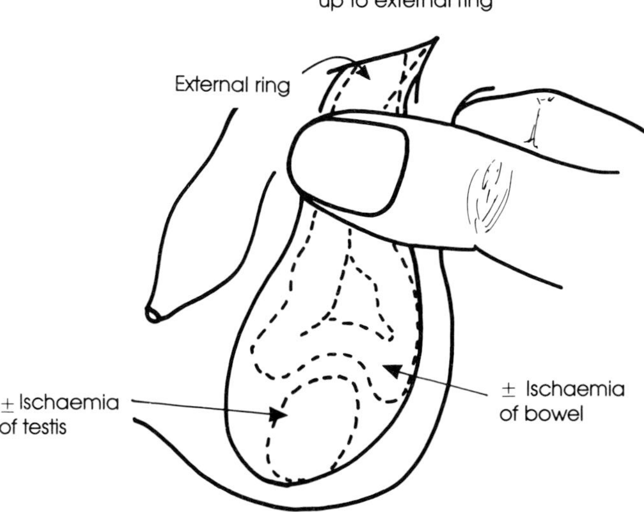

Fig. 4.26: *The clinical signs of a complete inguinal hernia.*

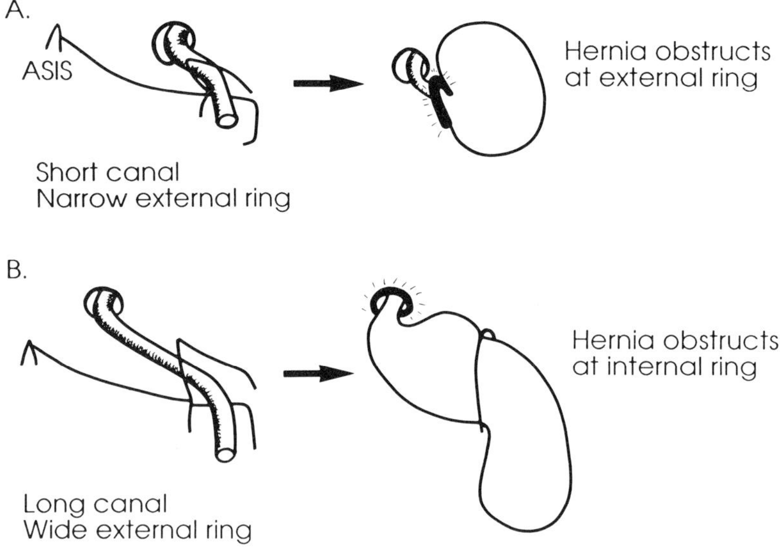

Fig. 4.27: *Comparison of infantile* (A) *and adult* (B) *inguinal herniae.*

manoeuvre known as 'taxis'. Most herniae reduce readily, and often spontaneously, without the need to resort to taxis. Sometimes, however, particularly in infants, an inguinal hernia becomes irreducible ('obstructed'), a term employed to indicate a hernia which fails to reduce spontaneously once the infant ceases straining or crying. In children, a hernia obstructs at the external ring, unlike the situation in adults where it obstructs at the internal ring (Fig. 4.27). Because the internal ring does not prevent reduction, compression of the hernia through the external ring leads to complete return of the hernial contents to the abdomen.

The external inguinal 'ring' is in reality a narrow V-shaped slit in the fibres of the external oblique aponeurosis, and may provide a barrier to the manual reduction of a hernia by taxis (Fig. 4.28), although in practice, most so-called irreducible herniae are reducible, given the right circumstances and technique. The child needs to be relaxed to allow the slit of the external ring to be pushed open; crying or straining causes contraction of the external oblique aponeurosis and narrowing of the external ring. The secret of the manoeuvre is to use the upper hand to disimpact the neck of the hernia from the narrow V-shaped apex of the external ring. This can be done by pushing the neck of the hernia caudally towards the scrotum. Meanwhile, the other hand compresses the fundus of the hernia gently but firmly. Gentle, sustained pressure, as opposed to forcible reduction, is more successful. Gentle rocking of the neck of the hernia from side to side, or up and down towards the scrotum, helps to free the bowel and its contents, allowing them to return to the abdomen – an event which often occurs suddenly and is accompanied by a gurgle.

Bowel which is stuck tightly within a hernial sac soon swells as its venous return is compromised. In time, this swelling impedes the arterial supply as well, and the bowel becomes ischaemic. An inflammatory reaction develops around the sac, manifested clinically by discoloration and signs of inflammation of the overlying skin. The lump is extremely painful even to gentle palpation, and the child may vomit. In a few instances, obstruction of the bowel produces generalized distension of the abdomen and further vomiting. If untreated, gangrene and perforation of the bowel ensues, causing peritonitis and septicaemia. Pressure of the hernial contents on the testicular artery at the neck of the sac may cause ischaemia of the ipsilateral testis. This sequence of events highlights the importance of recognizing and relieving an obstructed inguinal hernia promptly. All irreducible inguinal herniae in childhood should be considered as being potentially strangu-

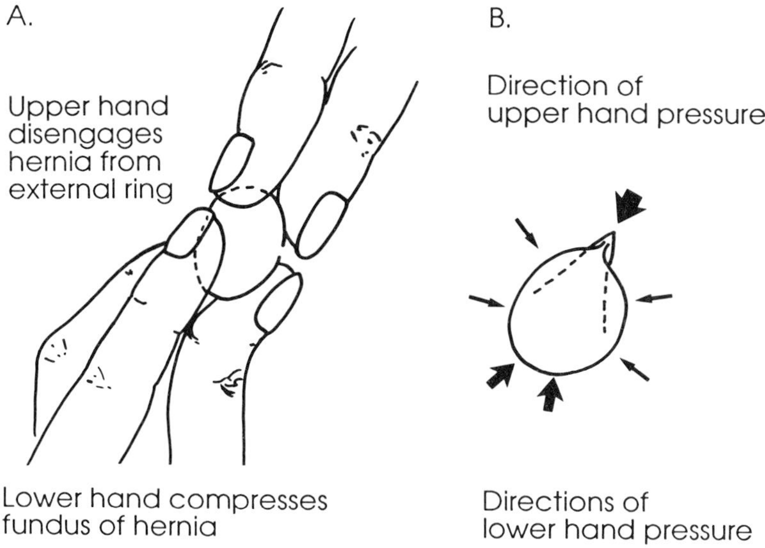

Fig. 4.28: *The technique of taxis for a strangulated left inguinal hernia.*

lated, and managed with appropriate urgency.

An encysted hydrocele in the cord may mimic an inguinal hernia where both are at the external ring (Fig. 4.29). The hydrocele is a slightly mobile, spherical cyst which transilluminates, but the feature which confirms its nature is its downward movement when traction is applied to the testis (Fig. 4.30). In contrast, the incarcerated hernia, which may also feel spherical and transilluminate (although to a lesser degree), is fixed at the external ring. If doubt persists, the clinician should attempt to reduce the lump by taxis, a manouevre which will confirm the diagnosis of a hernia.

Occasionally, after reduction of the bowel, a lump is still present at the external ring. Although small bowel is the usual content of a hernia, other viscera may be involved (Table 4.6), and in girls, the ovary is frequently present (Fig. 4.31). Since the processus is not required for gonadal descent in girls, an inguinal hernia is much less likely (one tenth as common as in boys) because obliteration of the processus occurs at an earlier stage. When an ovary is within the sac, the hernia may be of the 'sliding' type: the peritoneum adjacent to the ovary is pulled into the sac and drags the gonad with it. The attachment of the ovary and fallopian tube to the sac wall prevents it from being reduced by taxis.

On rare occasions in a girl, the sac may contain a testis. This occurs when there is a defect in androgen receptors leading to complete androgen

Table 4.6 CONTENTS OF AN INGUINAL HERNIA

Organ	Frequency	Comment
Small bowel	Very common	Incarceration leads to bowel obstruction
Large bowel	Uncommon	Occasionally appendix
Omentum	Uncommon	Sac contains fluid mimicking hydrocele
Ovary/tube	Common in girls	Sliding hernia – difficult to reduce
Testis	1/50 in girls	Presentation of complete androgen insensitivity syndrome

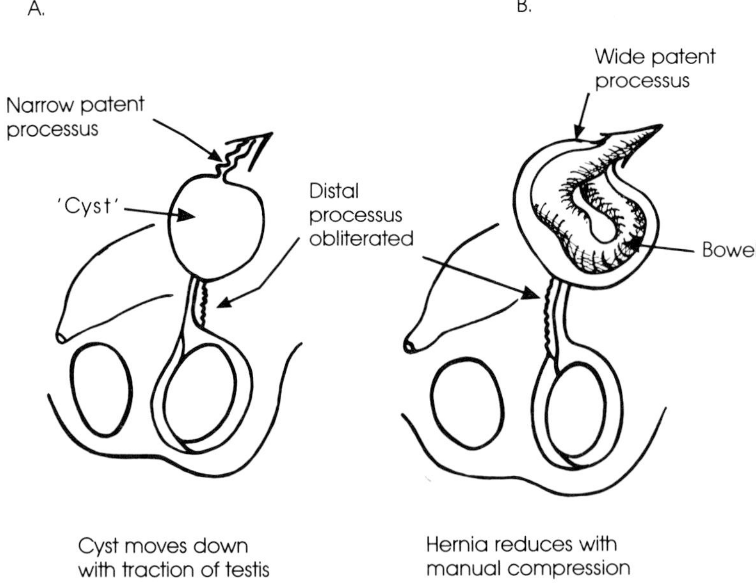

Fig. 4.29: *Comparison of the features of an encysted hydrocele of the cord* (A) *with an incarcerated inguinal hernia* (B).

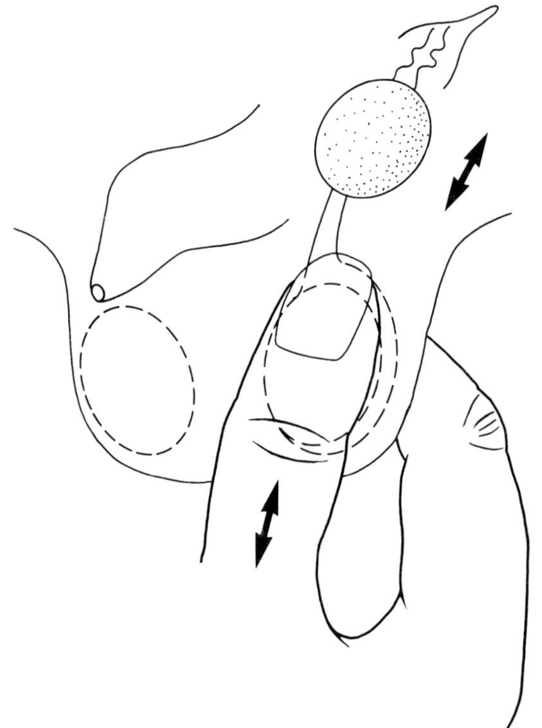

Fig. 4.30: *The method of demonstrating that an encysted hydrocele is part of the spermatic cord. Downward traction on the testis pulls the cyst down.*

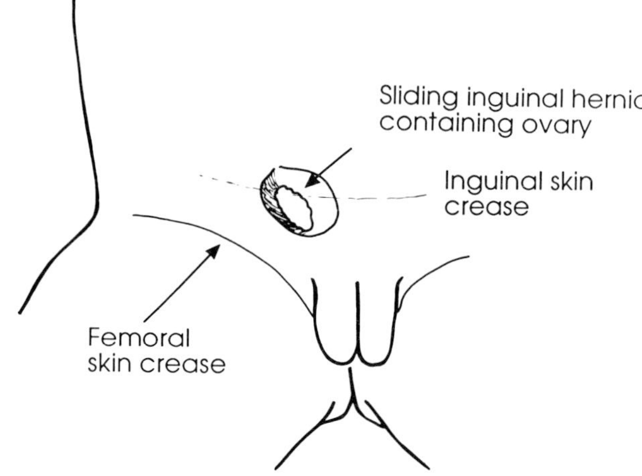

Fig. 4.31: *The features of an inguinal hernia in a girl when it contains an ovary.*

resistance. Despite normal or high androgen levels, the genitalia remain unaffected and develop a normal female appearance. This condition should be suspected when a girl presents with bilateral herniae which contain gonads.

Lump absent

In infancy, it is common that the hernia is not present at the time of consultation, and different techniques are required to demonstrate it. Even though the child may appear completely well, the correct diagnosis must be established because of the potential hazards of strangulation (Table 4.7); the hernia may re-emerge and strangulate at any time.

Table 4.7 THE THREE DANGERS OF A STRANGULATED INGUINAL HERNIA

1. Bowel ischaemia → gangrene → perforation + sepsis
2. Bowel obstruction → abdominal pain, vomiting, constipation
3. Spermatic cord compression → ischaemia → necrosis + secondary atrophy of the testis.

The first step is to ask the mother to point precisely to the site of the lump; this should confirm its proximity to the external ring. Sometimes, after being unable to demonstrate any hernia, the parents can be asked to mark the site of the lump on the skin with a marker pen when it next appears.

If the child is old enough, he should be examined standing and the external ring palpated during a cough. A cough impulse may be both felt and seen, provided the examiner's eyes are level with the groin (Fig. 4.32).

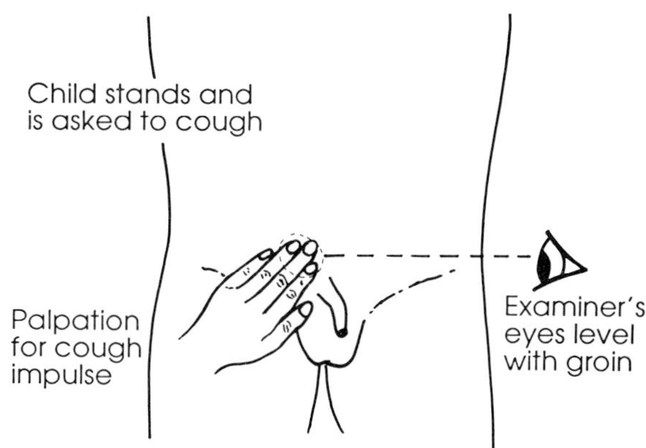

Fig. 4.32: *Examining for a cough impulse with the child standing.*

Small children or infants are not able to cough on demand. An alternative way to increase the abdominal pressure is by pressing gently but firmly on the abdomen (Fig. 4.33) using the flat of the hands or a closed fist. The hernia will commonly 'pop out' when the abdominal pressure rises, after which its characteristics can be determined by palpation.

Lastly, when the hernia cannot be demonstrated, the spermatic cord should be palpated carefully for the presence of an empty sac (Fig.

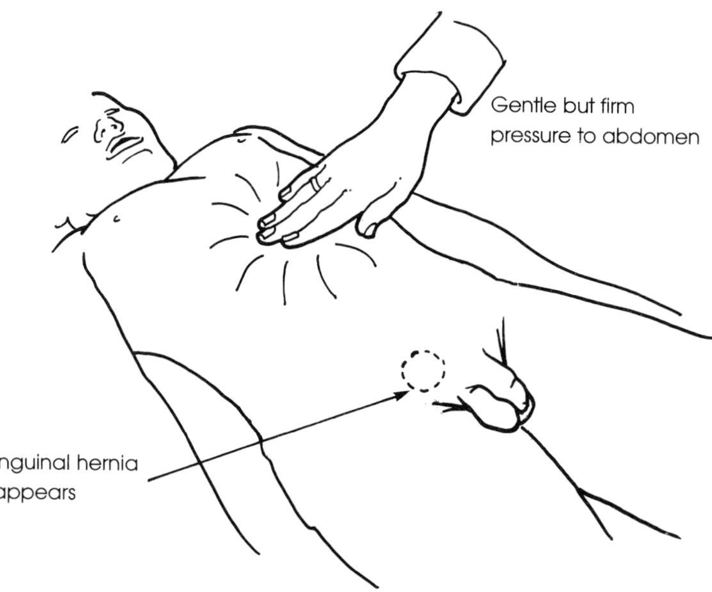

Fig. 4.33: A *method of increasing intra-abdominal pressure by direct compression.*

4.34). By rolling the cord against the pubis with the finger tips, the empty sac can be felt like multiple folds of silk sliding together ('the silk sign'). The thickened, rustling cord is compared with the contralateral side.

A clear history from the mother in the absence of a demonstrable hernia may be accepted as sufficient evidence of a hernia being present, justifying immediate referral to a paediatric surgeon.

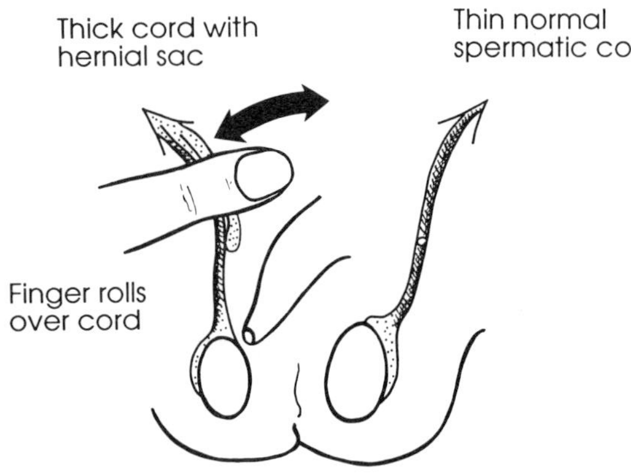

Fig. 4.34: *The 'silk sign'.*

GOLDEN RULES

(1) Beware epididymo-orchitis: it should never be diagnosed except by a paediatric surgeon.
(2) Torsion of a hydatid of Morgagni (testicular appendage) should not be diagnosed instead of torsion of the testis unless an exquisitely tender, blue 'pea' can definitely be seen and felt at the superior pole of an otherwise non-tender testis.
(3) Referral of a child with an acute scrotum for immediate exploration is the safest way to exclude torsion of the testis.
(4) Beware the encysted hydrocele of the cord: it may mimic an incarcerated inguinal hernia.
(5) Beware dull transillumination of a 'hydrocele': herniae often transilluminate dimly.
(6) Beware the retractile testis: it may mimic an undescended testis.
(7) Always identify the bony landmarks in the groin to determine the exact site of the external ring.
(8) Beware the impalpable testis: it is more likely to be concealed by subcutaneous fat than to be absent or intra-abdominal.
(9) Beware the groin skin crease: it marks the fascial attachment over the hip joint rather than the inguinal ligament.
(10) Beware the 'hydrocele' which empties on compression: it is a hernia containing omentum.

Further Reading

Koop C.E. (1976). *Visible and Palpable Lesions in Children*. New York: Grune & Stratton.

5 Abnormalities of the penis

Abnormalities of the penis are an important part of paediatric surgery because of their frequency. In addition, the emotional response of parents to perceived anomalies of their boys' genitalia can be extreme; the pressure this puts on the clinician may lead to hasty, inappropriate or even incorrect diagnosis and treatment. The range of anomalies is shown in Table 5.1.

THE NORMAL UNCIRCUMCISED PENIS

The loose foreskin protrudes well beyond the glans of the penis (Fig. 5.1). Postnatally, the foreskin is adherent to the glans for a variable period: in many primary school-age boys, the foreskin still is partially adherent. Nevertheless, retraction of the foreskin by parents or doctor is not necessary, since separation will occur spontaneously (often secondary to erections and masturbation by the boy himself).

SMEGMA DEPOSITS

If the foreskin separates from the glans around the coronal groove before the more distal foreskin is free, secretions and desquamation of keratin can accumulate as lumpy deposits of smegma (Fig. 5.1). The characteristics of smegma are:

(1) a bright yellow collection, because of its high cholesterol content (similar to xanthelasma);
(2) a lump covered by foreskin which is thin enough to allow the yellow colour to show through;
(3) absence of inflammation or infection when the

Table 5.1 PENILE ABNORMALITIES

Condition	Frequency	Cause
Smegma deposits	Very common	Adherent foreskin
Phimosis	Common	Chronic trauma to the foreskin → scar
Balanitis	Common	Acute infection under the foreskin
Paraphimosis	Common	Retraction of a tight foreskin
Meatal ulcer	Common	Acute trauma to the glans → ulcer
Meatal stenosis	Uncommon	Chronic trauma to the glans → scar
Hypospadias	Uncommon	Incomplete development of the urethra
Ambiguous phallus	Rare	Incomplete/inappropriate genital development

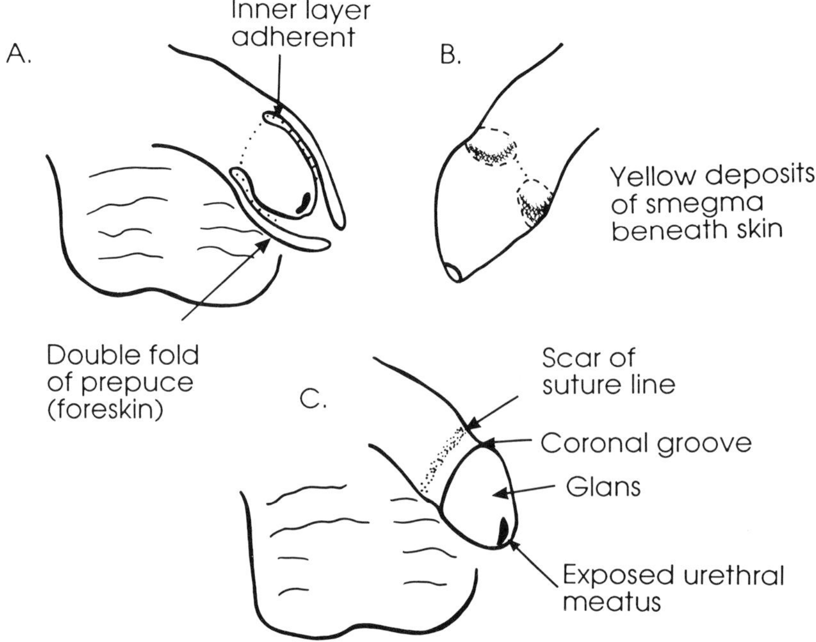

Fig. 5.1: *The normal anatomy of the uncircumcised (A) and circumcised (C) penis. Deposits of yellow smegma are common after partial separation of the foreskin (B).*

smegma is entirely contained within the congenital adhesions of the foreskin to the glans.

The diagnosis is important, because this trivial lesion requires no treatment but is misdiagnosed often as serious pathology, such as a 'cyst' or 'tumour' of the penis, resulting in unnecessary psychological trauma for the child and parents.

THE NORMAL CIRCUMCISED PENIS

The scar at the line of resection of the foreskin lies proximal to the coronal groove. The meatus on the tip of the glans is visible as a small vertical slit (Fig. 5.1).

EXAMINATION OF THE NON-ADHERENT FORESKIN

This is a simple manoeuvre where the finger-tips of one or both hands gently squeeze the foreskin over the glans and simultaneously pull the skin down the shaft of the penis (Fig. 5.2). If the skin is not adherent and there is no phimosis, the entire glans can be exposed. It is important to replace the foreskin in the normal position as soon as the examination is complete to prevent the development of paraphimosis.

Even minor phimosis or adherence will make

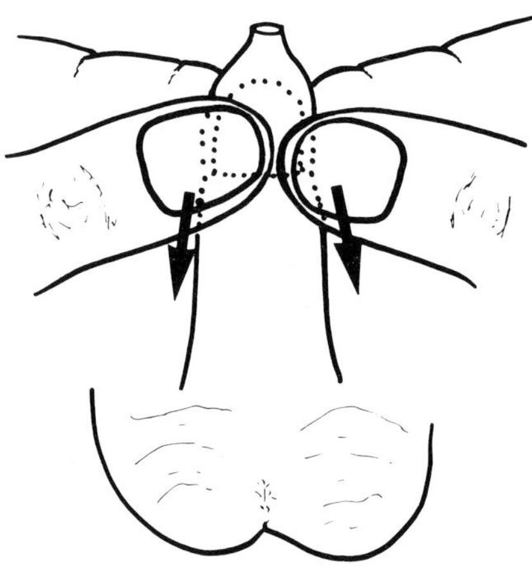

Fig. 5.2: *Retracting the non-adherent foreskin for phimosis or to expose the glans.*

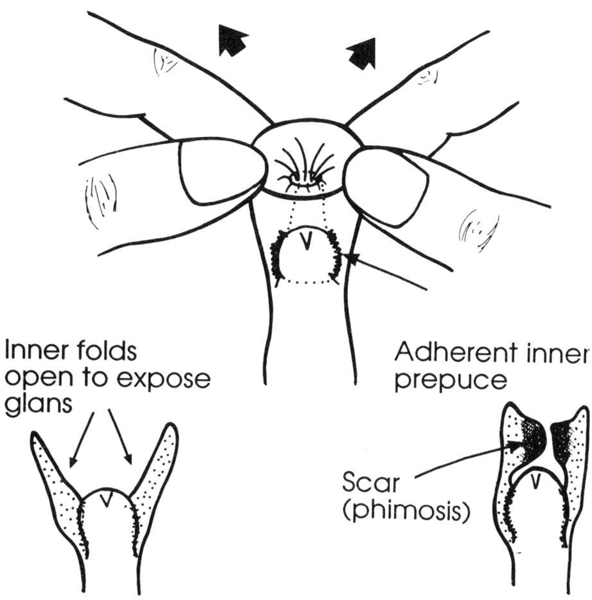

Fig. 5.3: *Examining the adherent foreskin for evidence of phimosis.*

retraction of the foreskin difficult and, unless force is used, will prevent exposure of the entire glans. Hence, this method of demonstrating retractibility of the foreskin tends to overdiagnose phimosis. Where there is difficulty distinguishing an adherent foreskin from phimosis, the method shown in Figure 5.3 should be used.

EXAMINATION OF THE ADHERENT FORESKIN

When the foreskin remains adherent to the glans, it may be difficult to retract in order to visualize the urethral meatus or to determine whether phimosis is present. By pulling the edges of the foreskin up with the tips of the fingers, the inner layer of the foreskin is stretched open and the glans can be seen (Fig. 5.3). If phimosis is present, the scarring of the foreskin prevents it being stretched open, and the examiner cannot see the glans. This method does not hurt the child and will separate readily the minor examples of phimosis which need no treatment from the more severe lesions requiring surgery.

PHIMOSIS

Phimosis is caused by scarring of the foreskin distal to the glans and occurs as a result of:

(1) tearing of the foreskin, from over-zealous retraction;
(2) chemical or physical irritation from ammoniacal dermatitis producing recurrent or chronic ulceration;
(3) infection under the foreskin (balanitis), sometimes from retained smegma.

Mild phimosis causes no symptoms apart from a narrow urinary stream. There may be evidence of scarring around the tip of the foreskin (Fig. 5.4) which can be assessed as shown in Figs 5.2 and 5.3.

If the glans and urethral meatus can be seen, no immediate treatment is required. On occasions, steroid ointment may be useful in preventing further scarring before urinary obstruction occurs.

Severe phimosis with urinary obstruction is an important diagnosis to make because surgical treatment (circumcision) is needed. The scarring of the foreskin has reduced the opening of the foreskin to a pin-hole. The scar surrounding the tiny opening appears as pale, unyielding tissue which cracks and fissures readily. The glans cannot be visualized at all, and there is a history of marked ballooning of the foreskin which persists after micturition has ceased (Fig. 5.4). This is the cardinal sign of phimosis because it indicates urinary obstruction requiring immediate treatment. The bladder should be palpated, since distension may indicate significant subacute, or even chronic, urinary retention.

THE RED, SWOLLEN PENIS

The penis becomes swollen and red in response to either inflammation (balanitis) or venous congestion (paraphimosis). The dramatic onset and magnitude of the swelling reflects the rich blood supply and loose skin of the shaft and foreskin. Commonly, balanitis and paraphimosis are confused with each other because their effect on the penis is similar (Fig. 5.5). An accurate diagnosis to distinguish these two conditions is important, because their treatment is different. A red, swollen penis may be produced also by local allergy (e.g. as part of idiopathic scrotal oedema).

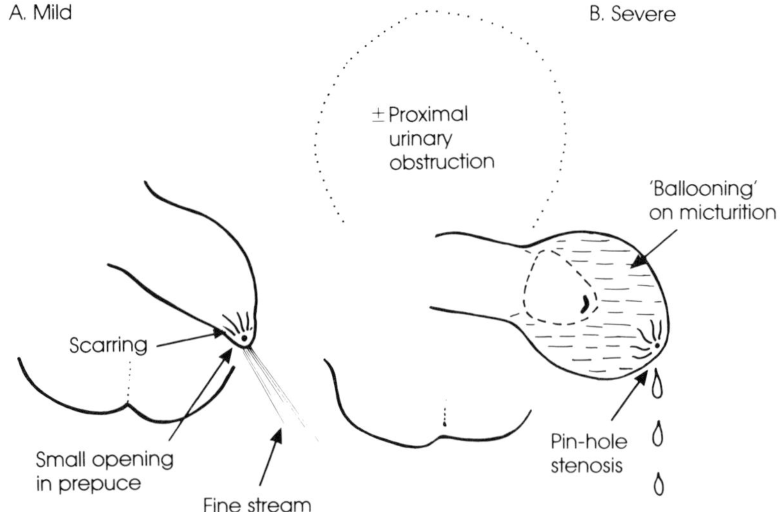

Fig. 5.4: *Comparison of the signs and symptoms of mild* (A) *and severe* (B) *phimosis. Ballooning of the foreskin on micturition is evidence of urinary obstruction and necessitates immediate treatment.*

Balanitis

This is a superficial infection of the foreskin occurring in response to infected, pooled urine or retained secretions (smegma) between the glans and the inner prepuce (Fig. 5.6). Therefore, balanitis cannot occur in correctly circumcised boys. The foreskin has very loose stroma, ensuring that even minor superficial infection, such as balanitis, causes marked swelling. In other words, the infection looks much worse than it really is! Moreover, not only is the degree of swelling dramatic, but also it can develop very quickly (i.e. within a few hours).

Prompt treatment results in rapid resolution of the superficial infection and avoids the progressive scarring which leads to phimosis. Where topical antibiotics cannot be applied (because of apprehension or pain), systemic antibiotic treatment is required.

Paraphimosis

Paraphimosis is purely mechanical in origin and not an inflammatory condition. The foreskin has been retracted proximal to the coronal groove and has not returned to its former position. If the opening in the distal foreskin is small, the retracted foreskin will compress the shaft of the penis at the coronal groove, and the arrow-head shape of the glans prevents replacement. Venous obstruction of the glans rapidly leads to engorge-

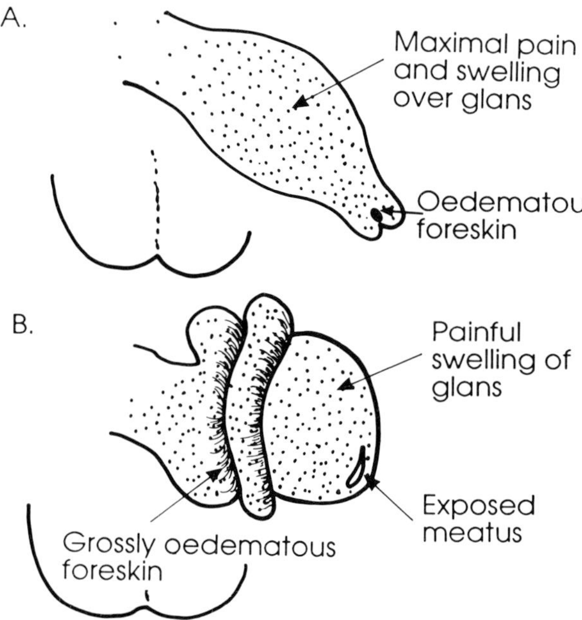

Fig. 5.5: *The two causes of the red, swollen penis.* A. *Balanitis.* B. *Paraphimosis.*

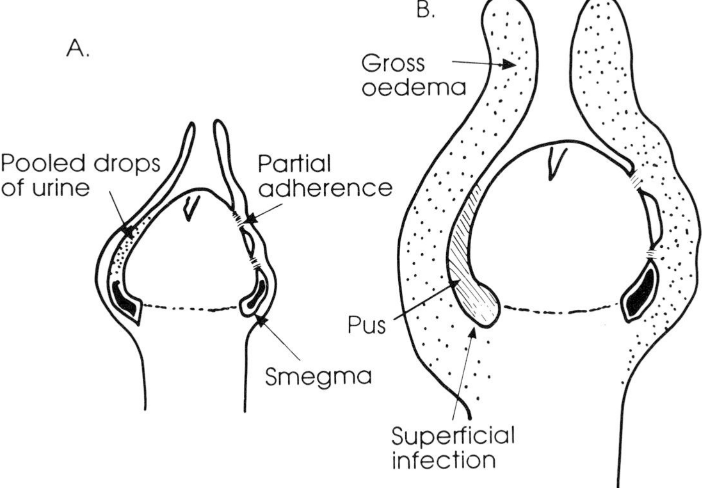

Fig. 5.6: *The pathogenesis of balanitis. Drops of contaminated urine remain under the partially adherent foreskin* (A), *leading to an infection with gross secondary inflammation* (B).

ment and oedema of the glans and foreskin, and at first glance, may mimic the ballooning seen in balanitis. When the oedema is severe, it causes distortion and deviation of the glans: the foreskin appears as a pale and eccentric 'tyre' immediately proximal to the glans. Sometimes, the oedematous swelling of the foreskin dwarfs the glans which is unable to swell to the same degree.

The clinical features which distinguish paraphimosis from balanitis are the painful, gross swelling of the glans with a visible urethral meatus, and the retracted swollen foreskin behind the corona of the glans (Fig. 5.5).

Venous congestion from compression of the penis at the coronal groove occurs when the size of the distal preputial opening is narrower than that of the penile shaft, while the greater width of the glans prevents easy replacement of the foreskin to its correct position (Fig. 5.7).

Diagnosis is important since delay allows progression of oedema and makes subsequent reduction more difficult. The oedema of the glans and foreskin is reduced by manual compression, and the foreskin is drawn forward over the glans to reassume its original position.

It must be remembered that: (1) paraphimosis only occurs in uncircumcised or incompletely circumcised boys; and (2) the swelling of paraphimosis is caused by venous obstruction, whereas in balanitis it is the inflammatory response, and in phimosis, the urinary distension.

MEATAL ULCER

This is caused by chemical and/or physical irritation at the tip of the glans around the urethral meatus in the circumcised child. Ammonia produced by micro-organisms in sodden cloth nap-

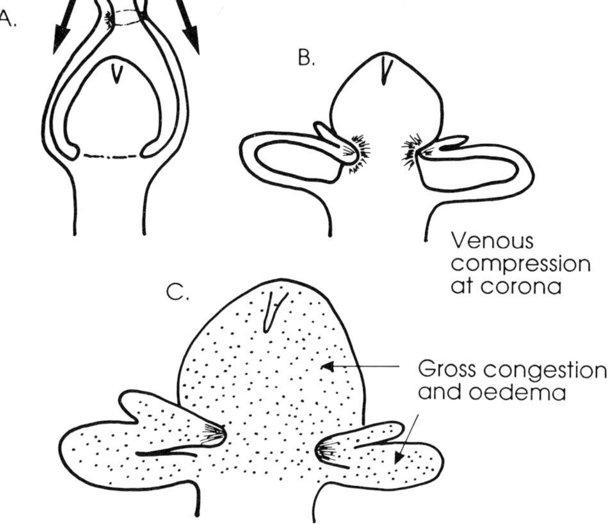

Fig. 5.7: *The pathogenesis of paraphimosis. A tight foreskin is retracted behind the coronal groove* (A), *leading to venous occlusion in the shaft* (B). *Gross congestion and oedema quickly ensue* (C).

pies causes a chemical dermatitis of the nappy area, including the glans where the mucosa at the urethral opening is particularly vulnerable. The sensitive tip of the recently circumcised penis also may be abraded by friction on hard, rough nappies. In uncircumcised babies, ammoniacal dermatitis may lead to a mild phimosis by inflammation of the foreskin, but does not cause a meatal ulcer.

A meatal ulcer is diagnosed by inspection of the tip of the (usually recently) circumcised penis of a boy who presents with pain on micturition (Fig. 5.8), or has a history of a poor stream which splays. The urethral meatus is inflamed and is acutely ulcerated. Where the ammoniacal dermatitis is severe, the ulceration may include the entire surface of the glans.

A meatal ulcer may be covered by a thin scab which partially occludes the meatus and hides the ulcer. The scab causes obstruction of the urinary stream, which may dribble, shoot out with a fine stream or deviate in one or more directions. Often, this is misdiagnosed as meatal stenosis, which is a chronic condition described below. Occasionally, a meatal ulcer with a scab causes complete urinary obstruction, with progressive distension of the bladder detected clinically by percussion and palpation of the lower abdomen. Correct diagnosis will allow quick resolution of the lesion: the scab is soaked off in the bath, vaseline or soothing cream is applied to the glans, and the nappies are left off or changed frequently.

MEATAL STENOSIS

Where a meatal ulcer is not treated quickly or is recurrent, healing occurs by fibrosis, rather than by epithelialization, and leads to meatal stenosis (Fig. 5.9). The slit-like meatus contracts down to a pin-hole, surrounded by obvious scarring.

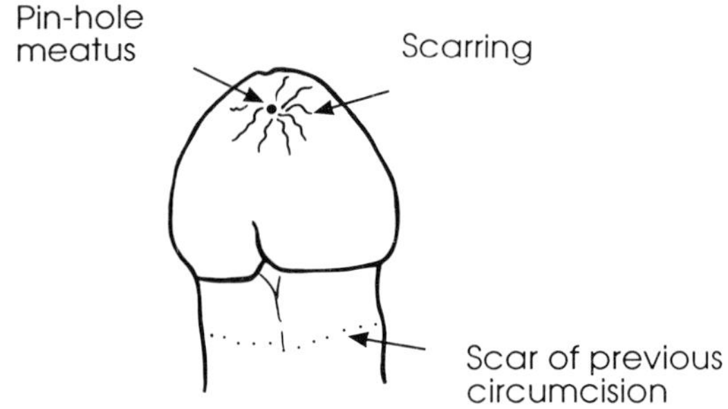

Fig. 5.9: *Meatal stenosis. The normal slit has been contracted by scarring to a pin-hole, producing urinary obstruction.*

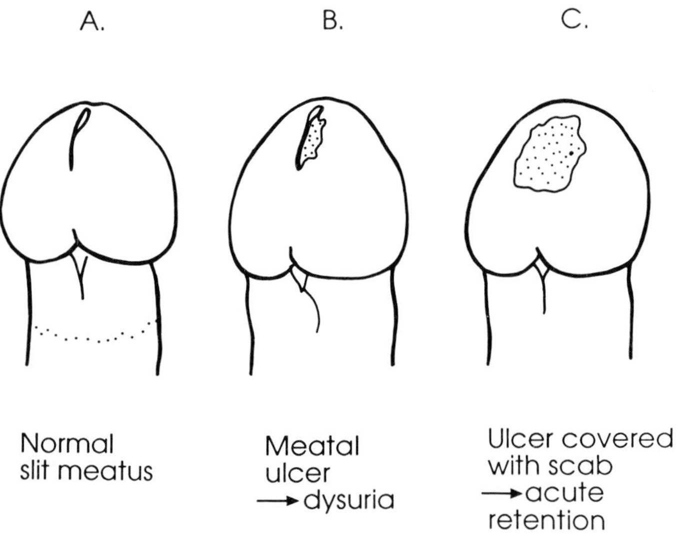

Fig. 5.8: *Meatal ulcer. A. The normal slit meatus. B. Ulceration of the edge of the meatus. C. A scab covering the meatus and ulcer, which may lead to acute retention.*

Difficulty in micturition, with or without a distended bladder, suggests that surgical treatment (meatotomy) is required urgently to relieve urinary tract obstruction.

HYPOSPADIAS

Hypospadias is caused by incomplete formation of the male urethra and its adjacent structures, including the corpus spongiosum and prepuce. In most boys the cause is unknown, although minor or temporary defects in the secretion or action of testosterone from the fetal testis is considered likely. Where genital development is severely deranged leading to ambiguous genitalia at birth, hypospadias invariably is present and commonly is severe.

There are three major abnormalities in a penis with hypospadias: (1) the dorsal hood; (2) a proximal urethral orifice; and (3) chordee, a ventral bend in the shaft of the penis (Table 5.2).

The end of the foreskin has a characteristic square end like a spade, unlike the cylindrical foreskin of the normal child (Fig. 5.10). When the examining fingers hold up the square corners of the dorsal hood of foreskin, the abnormalities on the ventral (anterior) surface of the penis are exposed. The foreskin is missing over the ventral part of the glans, which itself is splayed out and flattened rather than being conical. There is a variable groove where the urethral orifice should be situated, and a tiny blind pit in the floor of the groove is often visible.

The orifice of the urethra is commonly near the coronal edge of the glans, but can be anywhere along the ventral shaft of the penis, or even over the scrotum in the severest cases. The orifice is

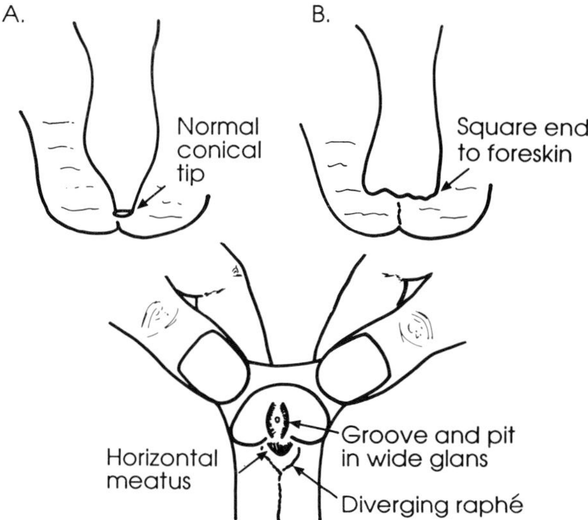

Fig. 5.10: *Hypospadias. The normal conical foreskin (A) is compared with the square-ended foreskin (dorsal hood) of hypospadias (B). In C, the dorsal hood is held up to reveal the splayed out glans with the groove and proximal meatus at the corona or on the shaft.*

marked by a horizontal slit, which can be difficult to see. The position of the urethral orifice can be determined by pulling out the ventral skin of the shaft, while holding the penis by the foreskin in the other hand. This opens up the orifice, confirming its position, and reveals whether stenosis of the opening is present (Fig. 5.11).

Around the orifice, the line of fusion of the urethral tube is deficient, and the skin immediately proximal to it is thin. Deficient ventral tissue, either proximal or distal to the urethral orifice, leads to a flexion deformity of the penile shaft (chordee). The bend may not be visible without manipulation or observation of the erect penis. The chordee is demonstrated by pulling the dorsal

Table 5.2 THE THREE ABNORMALITIES OF HYPOSPADIAS

Abnormality	Cause	Result
Proximal urethral orifice	Failure of fusion of inner genital folds up to the glans	Urinary stream at a right angle to the penile shaft
Chordee	Deficient corpus spongiosum and/or skin or fascia on the ventral surface	Ventral bend on erection precludes intercourse
Dorsal hood	Deficient ventral prepuce	Square-ended penis – a cosmetic defect

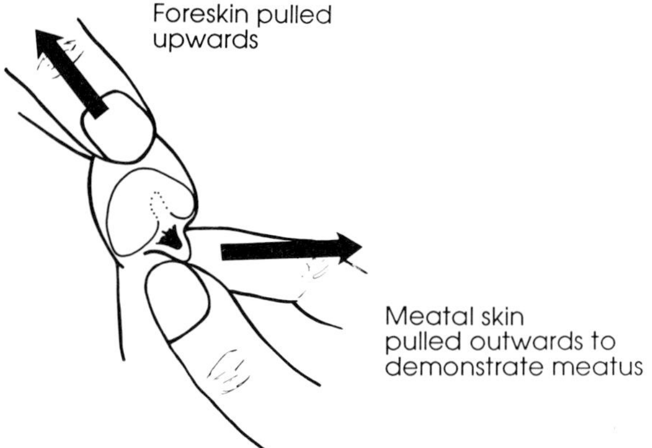

Fig. 5.11: *The technique of demonstrating patency of the meatus in hypospadias.*

hood upwards, or by retracting the skin of the shaft downwards (Fig. 5.12). The degree of chordee is shown by the angle between the glans and the shaft of the penis. This is a deformity which is crucial to recognize since, unless corrected, chordee will make intercourse painful or impossible after sexual maturity. The degree of chordee often becomes worse with growth of the penis, which means that it should not be assumed that neonates with little chordee will not need corrective surgery later. It is much safer to wait until three or four years of age before making a final decision.

If the urethral meatus is on the scrotum or at the penoscrotal junction, there is a high risk of abnormalities of sexual differentiation or urinary tract development. In severe hypospadias, therefore, the clinician must suspect intersex disorders and urinary anomalies. The absence of testes in the scrotum, with or without a bifid scrotum, is a cardinal sign of intersex such as congenital adrenal hyperplasia with severe virilization – the gonads may be ovaries and will not be palpable (Fig. 5.13). Females with complete virilization caused by adrenal hyperplasia can have a 'penis', which appears normal, although usually the phallus is obviously less well developed than that of a normal male. The degree of masculinity, therefore, does not of itself exclude intersex states. In babies with ambiguous genitalia, there may be a history of ingestion of androgens or even a family history of adrenal hyperplasia.

The two key physical signs to look for in neonates are the presence of palpable testes and a uterus on rectal examination. In neonates, the little finger introduced into the rectum can feel an infantile uterus and confirm the existence of an

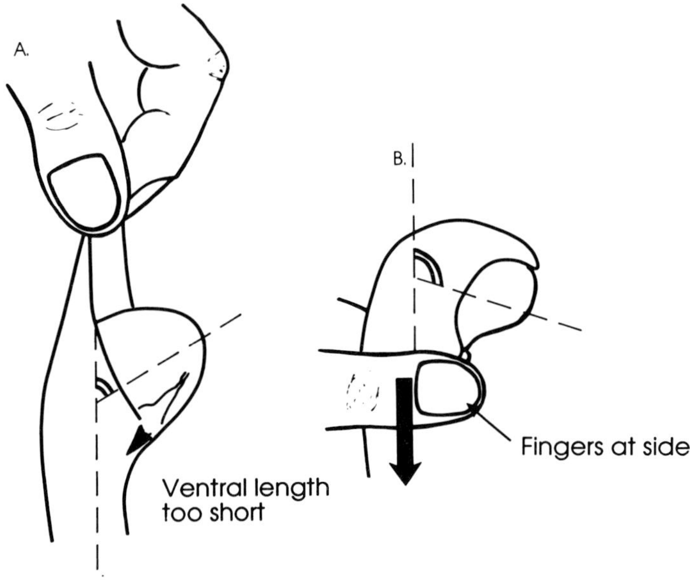

Fig. 5.12: *Chordee: demonstrating the bend caused by shortening of the ventral periurethral tissue planes compared with the dorsal corpora cavernosa. The dorsal hood may be pulled up* (A), *or the skin of the side of the shaft may be pulled down* (B).

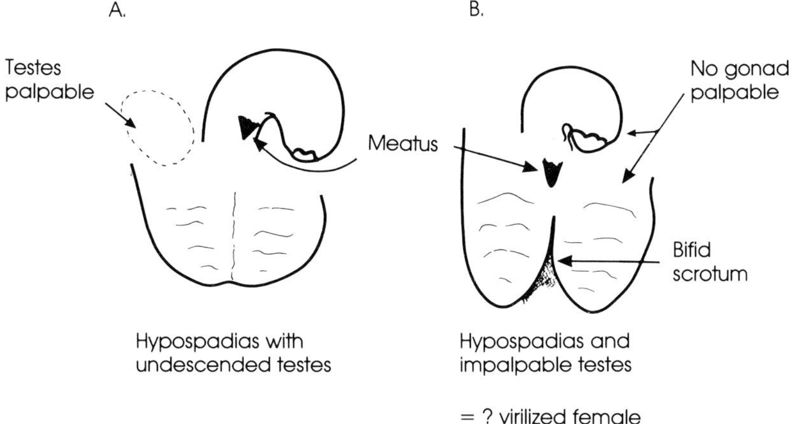

Fig. 5.13: *The comparison of hypospadias and undescended testes (A), with a virilized female with similar external appearance (B). The presence of two scrotal testes excludes most serious forms of intersex.*

intersex problem when 'hypospadias' and 'undescended testes' occur together. The clinical examination is discussed in greater detail in Chapter 22.

GOLDEN RULES

(1) Do not confuse the normal adherence of the foreskin with phimosis; both prevent retraction of the foreskin.
(2) Phimosis may cause severe urinary tract obstruction.
(3) Marked and persistent ballooning of the foreskin on micturition is pathognomonic of phimosis with urinary obstruction.
(4) Where the urethral meatus can be seen, severe phimosis cannot be present.
(5) The red, swollen penis is caused by infection (balanitis), venous congestion (paraphimosis) or, rarely, by allergic inflammation (idiopathic scrotal oedema).
(6) In balanitis, the maximum pain, redness and swelling is over the glans rather than the distal foreskin, which is oedematous but not sore.
(7) Paraphimosis can be recognized by the retracted oedematous foreskin behind the glans, which is identified by its meatus.
(8) Paraphimosis does not occur after adequate circumcision.
(9) Meatal ulcers may be covered by a scab, simulating meatal stenosis.
(10) Complete ulceration of the surface of the glans makes the meatus invisible.
(11) A baby with penoscrotal hypospadias with impalpable gonads should be managed as a case of intersex.
(12) Hypospadias, even when mild, needs early recognition to avoid unwitting circumcision (the skin of the dorsal hood is required for surgical correction).
(13) Acquired diseases of the penis produce parental anxiety, often out of proportion to the severity of pathology. The clinician should be wary of being pressured or panicked into a hasty or incorrect diagnosis, since most conditions are remedied easily once recognized.

6 The umbilicus

In the embryo, the primitive umbilical ring is a relatively large defect in the ventral abdominal wall transmitting a number of structures which connect the fetus to the cord and placenta (Fig. 6.1). In the five-week embryo, the mid-gut communicates with the yolk sac via the vitelline duct or yolk stalk. The yolk sac provides an early nutrient source for the embryo. In the next few weeks, the mid-gut develops more rapidly than the abdominal cavity and herniates through the umbilical ring into the extra-embryonic coelom (Fig. 6.2). By 10 weeks, the mid-gut has returned to the abdominal cavity and the vitelline duct subsequently degenerates (Fig. 6.3). If the vitelline duct does not involute, a vitello-intestinal fistula may result. Partial degeneration may result in a sinus, cyst or fibrous band connecting the ileum to the underside of the umbilicus. Continued growth of the duct at the intestinal wall produces a Meckel's diverticulum (Fig. 6.4). Failure of the mid-gut to re-enter the abdomen from the umbilical cord, or reherniation through the umbilical ring at a later stage, results in exomphalos. In this condition, the intestines and liver protrude through the abnormal umbilical ring into a thin avascular sac between the body wall and cord.

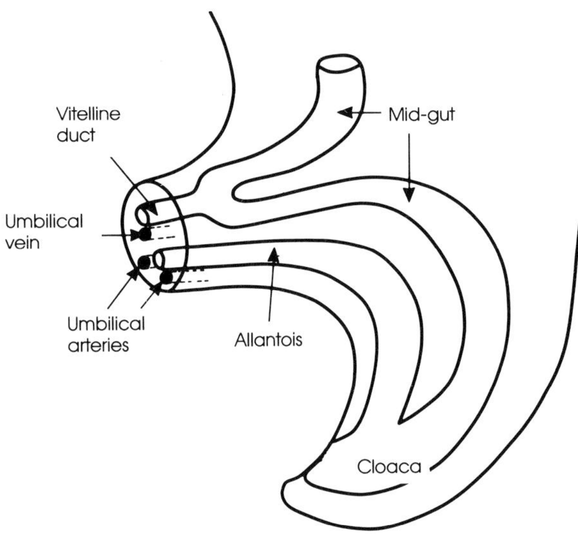

Fig. 6.1: *The structures which pass through the umbilical ring.*

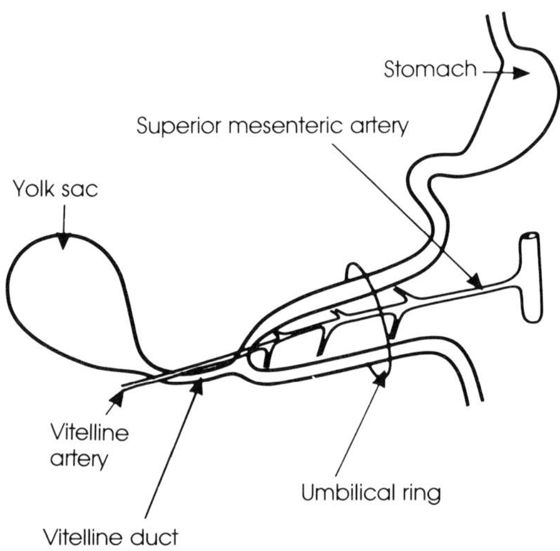

Fig. 6.2: *Herniation of the mid-gut through the primitive umbilical ring in the 6-week embryo.*

Another structure passing through the umbilical ring is the allantois, which contributes to the

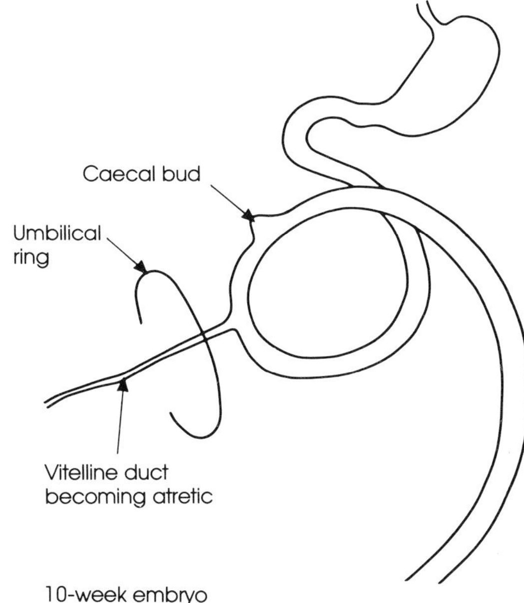

Fig. 6.3: *Return of the mid-gut to the abdominal cavity with rotation in the 10-week embryo.*

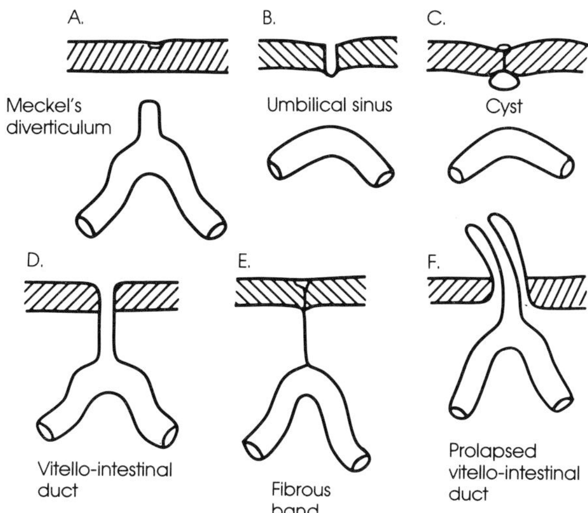

Fig. 6.4: *Malformations caused by a persistent vitelline duct.*

formation of the bladder after initial outgrowth from the hind-gut into the body stalk. The part of the allantois extending from the umbilicus to the bladder is called the urachus, but this structure is vestigial in man and its lumen closes before birth. The fibrous cord so formed persists into adult life as the median umbilical ligament, running between the peritoneum and transversalis fascia from the dome of the bladder to the umbilicus.

Failure of the urachus to obliterate results in urinary discharge from the umbilicus and is particularly associated with bladder outflow obstruction. Patency of one part of the urachus produces a urachal diverticulum, sinus or cyst (Fig. 6.5).

As the fetus grows, the umbilical ring remains constant, making it appear relatively smaller. At birth, the umbilical vessels are the only major structures in the cord, and when they involute, the umbilical ring becomes empty. If the ring does not constrict quickly, some of the contents of the abdomen may herniate through the skin-covered defect, a week or so after birth, as an umbilical hernia. These herniae tend to become smaller with time, such that 90% have disappeared by one year of age.

After separation of the umbilical cord, the exposed surface of the stump may become infected with the formation of sessile or pedunculated granulation tissue, the 'umbilical granuloma', which looks pink and moist. A similar appearance is produced by ectopic mucosa which represents persistence of the umbilical part of the vitelline tract.

In the uncommon condition of gastroschisis, the intestines protrude through a defect in the ventral abdominal wall immediately to the right of the umbilicus and are not covered by peritoneum or skin.

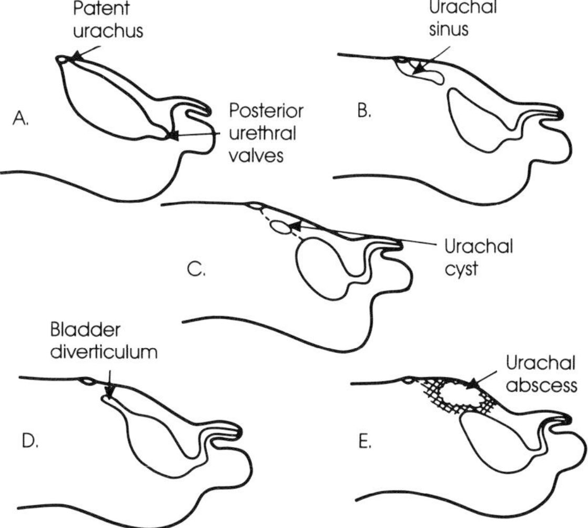

Fig. 6.5: *Urachal malformations.*

CLINICAL DIAGNOSIS

Is the umbilicus abnormal?

At birth, the umbilical cord is clamped and divided several centimetres from the umbilical ring. Over the next week, it dessicates and separates from the umbilicus. The umbilicus dries rapidly and appears as a corrugated dimple about 1 cm in diameter. Apart from an umbilical hernia, the commonest abnormality of the umbilicus is a persistent discharge which commences after detachment of the umbilical cord stump. More major umbilical abnormalities present as passage of urine or faeces from the umbilicus through a sinus opening, or as the obvious defects of exomphalos and gastroschisis.

The weeping umbilicus

The umbilicus dries within days of separation of the umbilical cord stump. If it remains moist, and there is a weeping discharge from granulation tissue at its base, an umbilical granuloma should be suspected. This condition is diagnosed on clinical grounds and requires no further investigation. However, several points must be considered before a diagnosis of umbilical granuloma is made. First, it should not have a urine or faecal discharge; if these are present, the umbilicus should be examined carefully for evidence of a sinus or fistula opening. This may lie at the base and may be in part concealed by the rest of the umbilicus. Secondly, age is of some significance in that an umbilical granuloma develops in the first month or two of life, whereas sinuses and cysts of urachal and vitelline origin usually appear at a later date. Thirdly, an umbilical granuloma is not associated with other congenital abnormalities, since it represents subacute infection of the necrotic cord stump.

An umbilical granuloma should be treated with local application of silver nitrate at weekly intervals for three weeks. If complete cure is not achieved within this time, it suggests that the diagnosis may be wrong and a paediatric surgical opinion should be sought.

Mucus discharge from the umbilicus

A sequestrated island of intestinal mucosa may occur at the umbilicus. This ectopic tissue produces mucus and appears as a small, red, shiny area at the base of the umbilical cicatrix. Exposure to the air may form crusting. This condition is often difficult to distinguish clinically from umbilical granuloma, but is of little importance as the management of both conditions is identical. Ectopic mucosa may be distinguished from granulation tissue because it is smooth, while a granuloma is nodular with visible capillary loops.

The umbilicus discharging faeces and air

Faeces and air discharging from the umbilicus is strongly suggestive of a patent vitello-intestinal tract. Careful examination of the umbilicus will reveal a small opening which can be probed with a No. 5 feeding tube. If the feeding tube is introduced as far as the ileum, larger quantities of faecal fluid can be aspirated. The treatment involves a small laparotomy with complete excision of the vitello-intestinal tract.

Rarely, intussusception of the patent vitello-intestinal tract may at first glance appear similar to that of gastroschisis. However, in most cases, the appearance is that of a double-horned protrusion, and it is the mucosal surface of the bowel which is protruding rather than the serosal surface. No

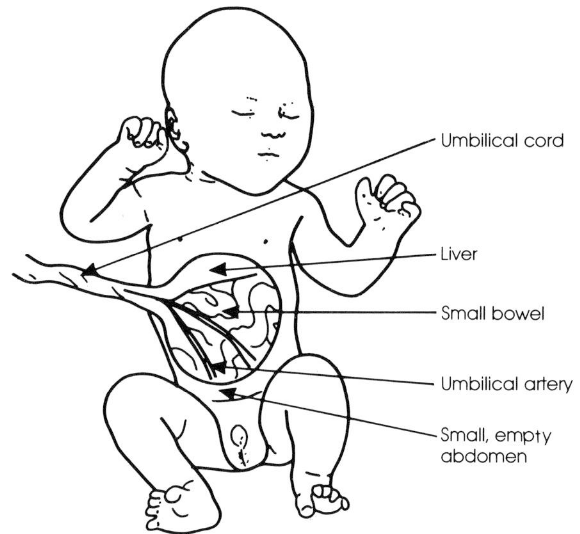

Fig. 6.6: *The appearance of an intact exomphalos at birth.*

mesentery is evident. Treatment of a prolapsed vitello-intestinal tract involves reduction of the prolapse with excision of the vitello-intestinal remnants.

Discharge of urine from the umbilicus

A patent urachus causes discharge of urine from the umbilicus. The urine may be infected, making it difficult to distinguish from faecal fluid. Again, with careful inspection of the umbilicus, a sinus opening will be evident. A patent urachus may indicate obstruction of urine outflow from the bladder, e.g. posterior urethral valves or an anorectal malformation. Injection of x-ray contrast material into the opening will delineate the anatomy. Treatment involves the management of the cause of bladder outflow obstruction, if present, and excision of the urachus.

The large umbilical defect covered by a thin membrane

In exomphalos, there is a large abdominal wall defect at the umbilicus with protrusion of abdominal viscera into a thin membranous sac formed by the amniotic membrane and peritoneum (Fig. 6.6). In most cases, the sac is intact, and for several hours after birth, the contents can be clearly seen through the translucent membrane, which becomes increasingly opaque with drying. The size and shape of the defect vary considerably – those with a relatively small neck appear pedunculated and poorly supported, whereas in others the greater diameter of the defect is at the neck (Fig. 6.7). Likewise, the skin of the ventral abdominal

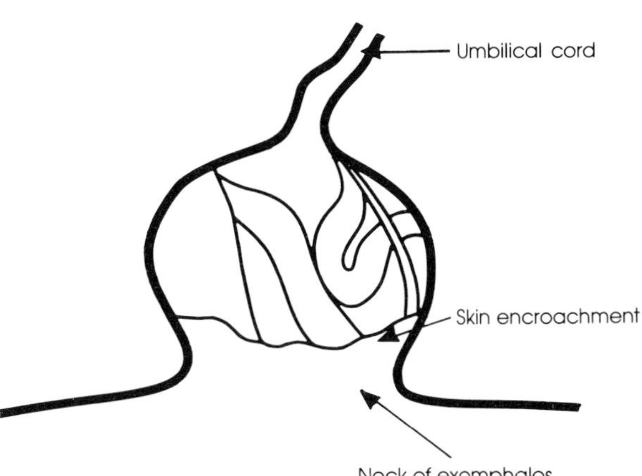

Fig. 6.8: *A lateral view of exomphalos, showing skin encroachment.*

wall extends up the side of the sac to a variable degree (Fig. 6.8). The umbilical cord is expanded over the dome of the defect, and the umbilical vessels can be seen coursing across its surface. The contents of the sac include small bowel, liver, stomach and colon.

Exomphalos is often associated with other major congenital abnormalities, particularly cardiac and renal anomalies. A less common but important association is Beckwith-Wiedemann syndrome, where there is hemihypertrophy (asymmetrical overgrowth of limbs), macroglossia, visceromegaly and abnormal facies with grooving of the ear lobes. The organomegaly is believed to be caused by excessive insulin production by the fetus. The exomphalos occurs because viscera are too large to fit inside the fetal abdomen. The importance of this lesion relates to profound neonatal hypoglycaemia secondary to

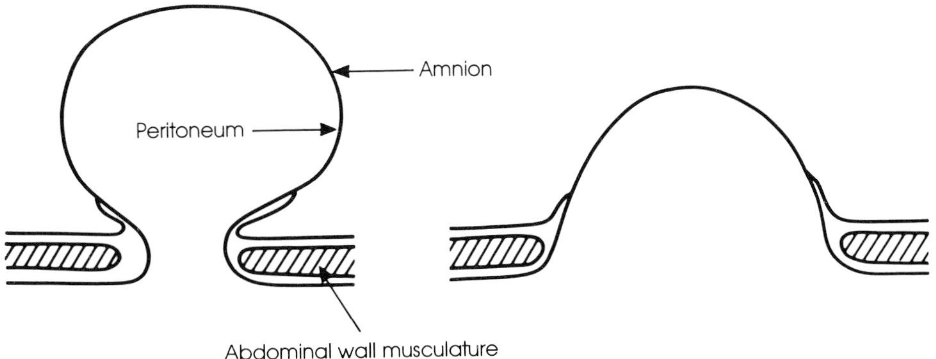

Fig. 6.7: *Variations in the cross-sectional shape of exomphalos.*

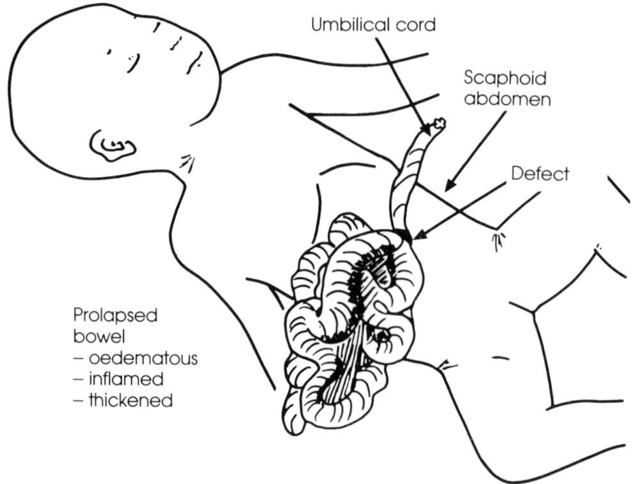

Fig. 6.9: *Gastroschisis.*

hyperinsulinaemia, and necessitates immediate clinical recognition, blood glucose estimation and the commencement of a glucose infusion.

As soon as the diagnosis of exomphalos is made, immediate measures must be undertaken to avoid heat and water loss. The large moist surface of the exomphalos sac allows rapid evaporation, leading to hypothermia. Therefore, the infant should be placed in an incubator with the whole abdomen wrapped in aluminium or plastic kitchen sheeting; this also reduces the likelihood of trauma or infection to the sac. The infant then should be transferred to a major paediatric hospital, where the subsequent management is dependent on the size of the defect and the presence of other abnormalities.

Bowel protruding from an umbilical defect

In gastroschisis, there is a small defect of the anterior abdominal wall immediately adjacent to the umbilicus. The vessels of the umbilicus are unaffected and leave the abdomen to the left of the extruded bowel. There is no covering membrane. The defect is much smaller than that seen in exomphalos and rarely exceeds 3 cm in diameter. The herniated bowel and its mesentery are thickened, congested and oedematous, bleed on contact and are covered by exudate and fibrin (Fig. 6.9). Gangrene of the bowel may occur where the blood supply to the bowel is occluded as a result of volvulus of the herniated loops or compression at the site of the defect. Where gangrene has occurred well before birth, the bowel disappears leaving an atresia. Again, heat loss is a major problem because of evaporation from the exposed moist surface of the bowel. Consequently, the contents should be wrapped in transparent plastic sheeting, and during transfer to a major paediatric hospital, the appearance of the exposed bowel should be monitored to ensure that traction on the mesentery or twisting is not causing bowel ischaemia. These infants require surgery on the first day of life, and a prolonged period of total parenteral nutrition until bowel function returns to normal.

The skin-covered umbilical swelling

Umbilical herniae are extremely common in infancy, particularly in premature children. The umbilical vessels involute during the first week after birth, leaving a potential defect in the abdominal wall. This fibromuscular hole, known as the umbilical ring, should close within a few weeks. When the bowel protrudes through it under the skin, an umbilical hernia is produced. The basic abnormality is a minor delay in contraction of the ring, a trivial developmental derangement, and not one associated with other major anomalies. When the infant lies at rest, no abnormality may be apparent other than some redundancy of the skin of the umbilicus. On any manoeuvre that increases intra-abdominal pressure, e.g. crying, straining or squeezing the abdomen, the hernia fills and becomes clinically apparent. Complete filling of the sac may produce a tense swelling which appears slightly blue beneath the skin in the neonate. The swelling is non-tender and can be reduced easily. By placing the index finger over the defect and pushing dorsally, an assessment can be made of the size of the defect in the linea alba (Fig. 6.10). It is common to find a surprisingly small defect in relation to the size of the hernia itself. The diameter of the umbilical ring gives a much better guide to the likely resolution of the hernia than the size of the sac which protrudes. The natural history is for the umbilical ring to decrease with time such that, in 90% of infants, the umbilical hernia has disappeared by the age of one year. As umbilical herniae virtually never strangulate or cause symptoms, the only indications for surgical intervention are: (1) where the umbilical hernia has persisted beyond two or three years of age; or (2) where the defect in the linea alba is large and apparently increasing in size. The practice of placing strapping across the hernia has not been shown to have any beneficial effect.

The swelling above the umbilicus (epigastric hernia)

A defect in the linea alba between the umbilicus and the xiphisternum may present as a painful lump in the midline when herniation of a small amount of extraperitoneal fat from the falciform ligament occurs through the small defect (Fig. 6.11). Usually, this becomes evident in the child

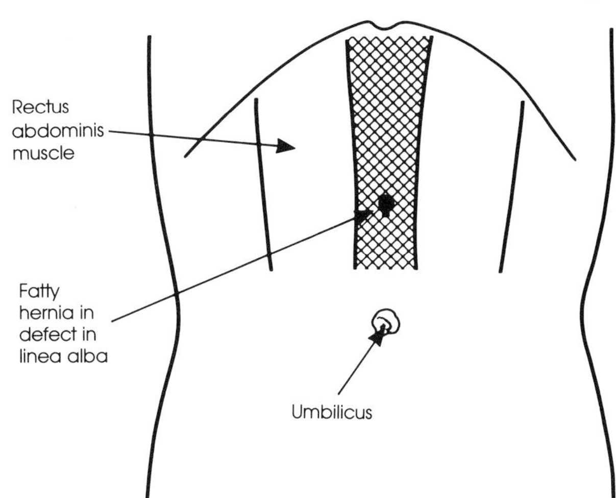

Fig. 6.11: *Epigastric hernia.*

beyond infancy and presents in two ways: first, a small, localized swelling may be observed; or secondly, an older child may complain of localized discomfort and draw attention to a hard tender swelling, which may not be visible externally but is palpable on careful examination. On occasions, epigastric herniae may be multiple. Treatment involves surgical repair as an elective procedure.

Spreading cellulitis around the umbilicus

Infection of the stump of the cord may produce spreading umbilical sepsis (omphalitis) and is caused by *Staphylococcus, Escherichia coli* or *Streptococcus*. The area becomes erythematous and swollen, and a small amount of pus may appear at the umbilicus. The danger of infection in this region is that it may extend up the umbilical vein

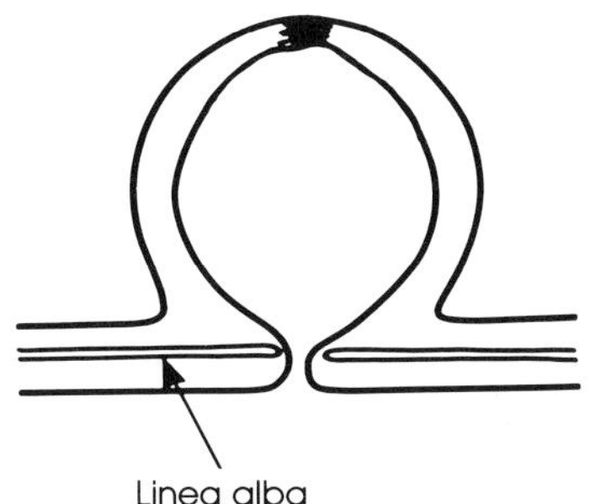

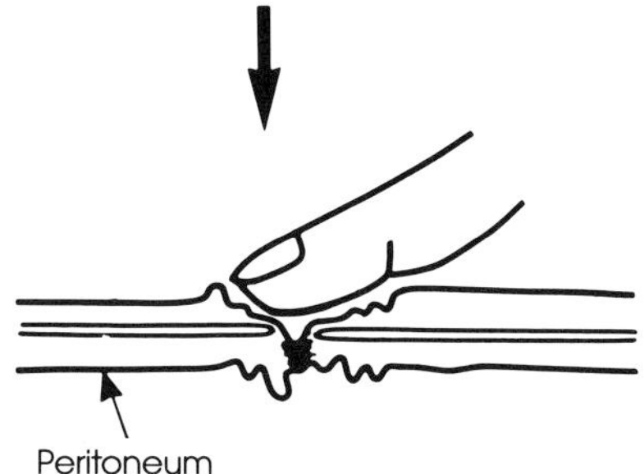

Fig. 6.10: A *method of reducing an umbilical hernia and assessing the size of the defect in the linea alba.*

into the portal vein and liver, or produce septicaemia. Thrombophlebitis of the portal vein was a common cause of portal hypertension before the seriousness of omphalitis was appreciated. Involvement of the superficial lymphatics which extend radially from the umbilicus, is evident as pink streaks along the surface of the skin. Umbilical sepsis, because of its potential complications, should be treated aggressively once culture swabs have been obtained.

Peritonitis in the neonate may also produce redness and swelling in the tissues immediately surrounding the umbilicus. In this situation, there is other evidence of peritonitis, with a distended tender abdomen in an extremely ill infant.

Rarely, infection of urachal or vitello-intestinal remnants produces a purulent discharge from the umbilicus.

GOLDEN RULES

(1) Look for a sinus opening in a weeping umbilicus: there may be persistence of urachal or vitello-intestinal elements.
(2) A weeping cherry-red swelling of the umbilicus appearing between one and six weeks of age is likely to be an umbilical granuloma which can be treated with local application of silver nitrate.
(3) Beware a granuloma which appears at the umbilicus after two months of age, or which fails to resolve with silver nitrate: this suggests a persistent, infected sinus.
(4) Beware urine discharge from the umbilicus: there may be lower urinary tract obstruction.
(5) The umbilicus discharging faeces is likely to be a patent vitello-intestinal tract.
(6) Beware heat loss in exomphalos and gastroschisis: evaporative loss from the moist membrane or directly from the bowel, results in rapid and major loss of heat – the sac and bowel should be wrapped in plastic sheeting.
(7) Beware Beckwith-Wiedemann syndrome in exomphalos: severe hypoglycaemia may cause brain damage.
(8) Beware associated anomalies in exomphalos: about half have major cardiac or renal anomalies.
(9) Umbilical herniae do not strangulate and have a natural tendency to cure themselves in the first few years of life.

7 Non bile-stained vomiting in infancy

The mechanical causes of non bile-stained vomiting in children are correlated closely with age (Fig. 7.1). Hypertrophic pyloric stenosis occurs between three and 12 weeks of age (most commonly between four and seven weeks), while intussusception is most frequent in older infants between three months and two years. Gastro-oesophageal reflux, which is extremely common in the first few weeks of life, becomes progressively less so with time.

In pyloric stenosis, there is postnatal thickening of the circular muscle of the pylorus which results in gastric outlet obstruction. As the narrowing progresses, the stomach becomes hypertrophied, producing visible gastric peristalsis. The vomitus contains no bile because the obstruction is proximal to the bile duct opening (Fig. 7.2).

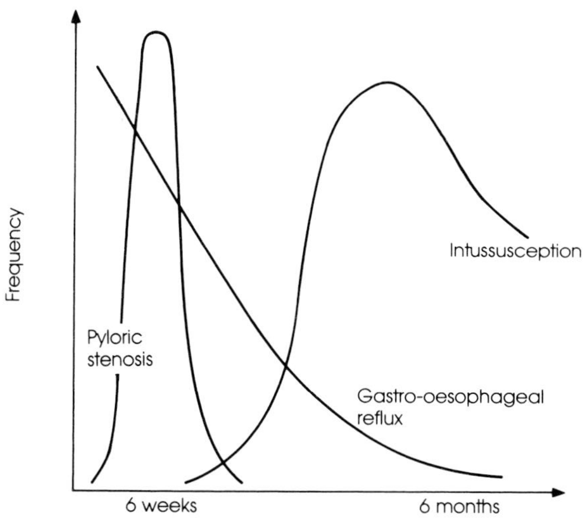

Fig. 7.1: *Surgical causes of non bile-stained vomiting.*

The cardia of the normal child acts as a sphincter to prevent retrograde flow of stomach contents up the oesophagus. In children with gastro-oesophageal reflux, there is no barrier to prevent this flow, with consequent free regurgitation of feeds.

CLINICAL FEATURES

Non bile-stained vomiting in an infant is caused most commonly by a feeding problem (Table 7.1). Where the mother is inexperienced or the baby is greedy, excessive feeding leads to gastric distension and vomiting. This problem is diagnosed by a careful history and observation of the feeding technique. The major challenge to the physician, however, is separating the trivial causes of vomiting (like excessive feeding) from more sinister diseases, such as systemic infection or mechanical obstruction and reflux. One simple way to approach the diagnosis is to follow the algorithm outlined in Fig. 7.3.

The history

Knowledge of the patient's age and a careful history usually will provide clues as to the correct diagnosis before the physical examination is commenced, since the commonest causes are strongly age-dependent (Fig. 7.1). The history should be aimed at answering the following questions:

(1) Is the infant well and active, and keen to take

Table 7.1 CAUSES OF NON BILE-STAINED VOMITING IN INFANCY

Feeding problem	Greedy, 'healthy' baby Inexperienced mother
'Hidden' infection – meningitis – urinary tract infection – gastro-enteritis	Systemic illness – vague systemic symptoms and signs in an 'unwell' baby
Gastro-oesophageal reflux	Mechanical problem – 'healthy' baby with or without failure to thrive
Pyloric stenosis	Mechanical problem – 'healthy' baby with or without failure to thrive
Inguinal hernia	Intermittent pain and/or mechanical obstruction

feeds? Reason: to separate mechanical or feeding problems from septic causes of vomiting.

(2) What is the duration, nature and timing of the vomiting? Reason: to separate gastro-oesophageal reflux from pyloric stenosis.

(3) Is the vomiting forceful? Reason: strongly projectile vomiting is suggestive of pyloric stenosis.

Overfeeding is seen in the most robust (or frankly obese) and greedy infant, who in all other respects appears healthy and well nourished. There is no weight loss, and careful history will reveal that the infant is receiving a more than adequate volume of feed. Many of these infants have coexisting gastro-oesophageal reflux, the symptoms of which settle with reduction of milk volume.

When sepsis is the cause of vomiting, the infant is usually unwell, lethargic and feeds poorly. In contrast, in pyloric stenosis, the infant is hungry, restless, crying and will feed with enthusiasm, but is simply unable to empty his stomach except by vomiting. The vomiting is characteristically forceful or projectile, and occurs after every feed. As soon as vomiting has occurred, the infant is ready to resume feeding. Most infants with pyloric stenosis present with symptoms of less than one week's duration. Where the duration is longer, blood (coffee-ground material) may be mixed with the vomitus, reflecting gastritis. The infant may also become severely dehydrated with a

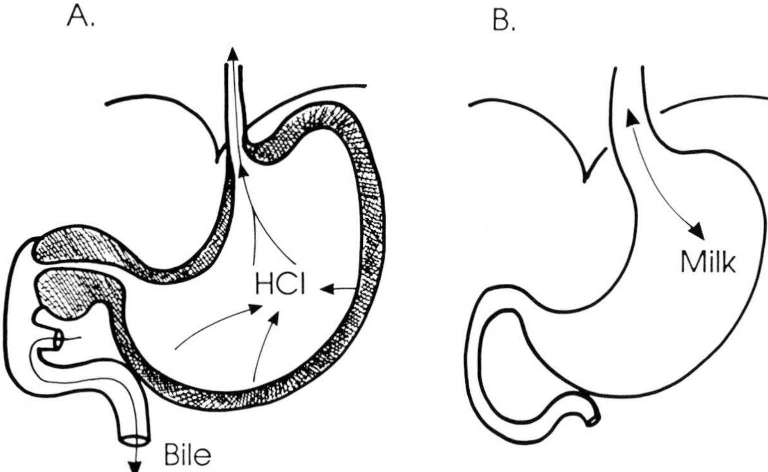

Fig. 7.2: *The pathology of pyloric stenosis* (A) *compared with gastro-oesophageal reflux* (B)*. The hypertrophied pylorus causes outlet obstruction of the stomach and prevents bile from reaching the stomach.*

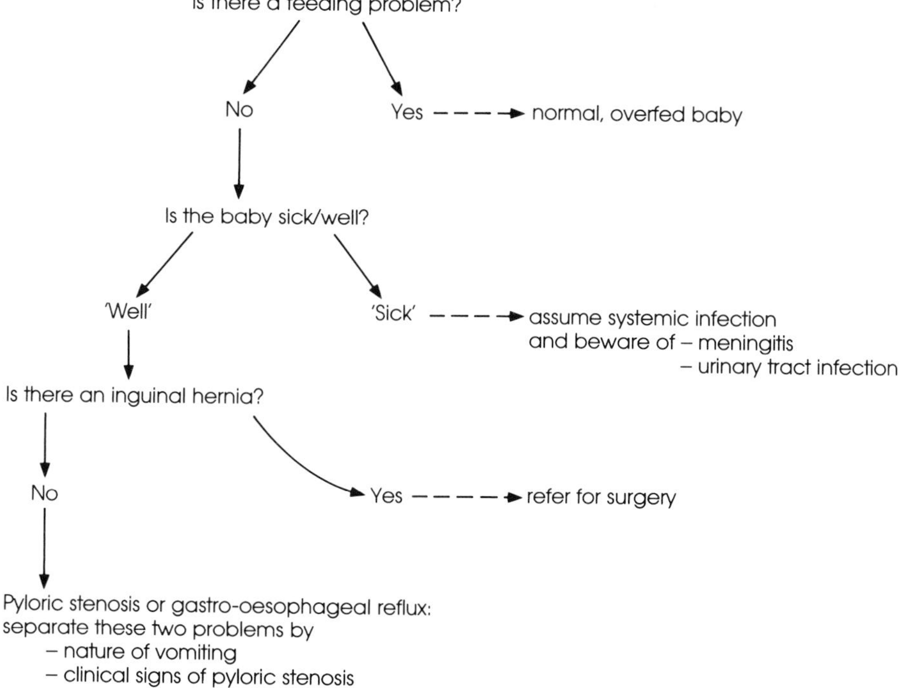

Fig. 7.3: A *simple algorithm which is useful in assessing any infant with non bile-stained vomiting.*

metabolic alkalosis from loss of water and hydrochloric acid in the vomitus. There is weight loss, the nappies are rarely wet or dirty, and there is no diarrhoea, as might be found in gastro-enteritis. There are no clinical signs pathognomonic of gastro-oesophageal reflux. Effortless vomiting of small or large volumes of non bile-stained material before, during or after feeds, in an otherwise healthy child is suggestive, but frequently the characteristics of the vomiting are nondescript and variable. The vomiting usually commences at birth, but becomes less pronounced with age. Minor intercurrent infection often exacerbates the symptoms.

The examination

Although specific symptoms and signs may indicate a site of infection, unwell babies should have a urine test and a lumbar puncture if there is any doubt about underlying urinary or meningeal infection. Commonly, there are no localizing signs of these infections in young infants.

Physical signs in gastro-oesophageal reflux are those of the complications rather than the reflux itself. Severe oesophagitis may cause haematemesis (usually coffee-ground vomitus) or pallor from chronic anaemia. Development of an oesophageal stricture may result in food sticking in the oesophagus, with retrosternal discomfort, choking and excessive salivation. Aspiration into the respiratory tract may result in recurrent chest infections with clinical signs of pneumonia. Weight loss and failure to thrive may be present.

In children under three months of age, the diagnosis should be made following the exclusion of sepsis and pyloric stenosis. In gastro-oesophageal reflux without complications, empirical improvement in symptoms with attention to posturing and food thickening, assists in the diagnosis. Dehydration commonly is evident in pyloric stenosis: the anterior fontanelle is depressed, the eyes sunken, the mouth dry and skin turgor reduced. Loss of subcutaneous fat produces a scrawny-looking and thin infant, and is the result of malnutrition (Fig. 7.4). The diagnosis of

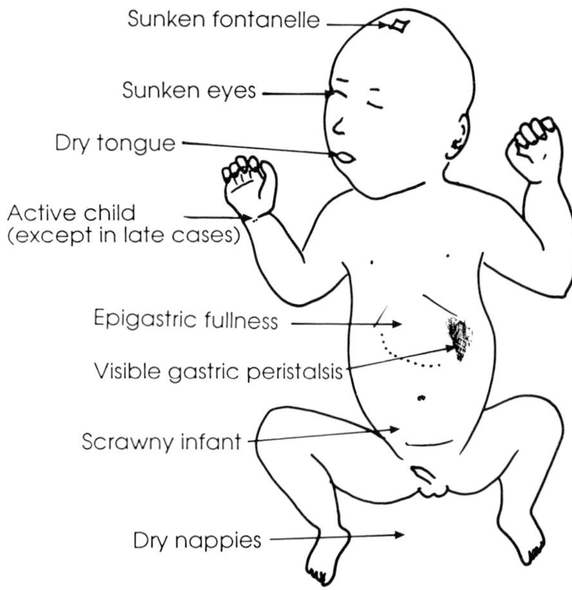

Fig. 7.4: *General features of pyloric stenosis.*

pyloric stenosis is made on clinical grounds and it is rarely that other investigations are required.

The clinical features of pyloric stenosis include:

(1) epigastric fullness
(2) visible gastric peristalsis
(3) palpable pyloric 'tumour'.

All babies have epigastric fullness after feeds as a result of a full stomach, but in pyloric stenosis, the stomach remains full between feeds and becomes hypertrophied. Waves of peristalsis, commencing under the left costal margin and directed to the right, can be seen when the abdomen is illuminated from the side (Fig. 7.5). The waves take 5–10 seconds to move across the abdomen and occur every 30 seconds. They are easier to see after a test feed, but caution must be taken to avoid overfeeding the infant until the pyloric 'tumour' has been palpated. The palpation of an enlarged pylorus or pyloric 'tumour' provides absolute confirmation of the diagnosis of pyloric stenosis.

The pylorus is a relatively mobile structure connected on the right to the less mobile first part of the duodenum. In pyloric stenosis, the hypertrophied pylorus can be felt as a hard but mobile mass, a little to the right of the midline in the upper abdomen. Traditionally, it has been described as 'feeling like an olive'.

In the calm, cooperative infant, the pylorus may be easily palpable, but in many it is discernible only with careful and patient examination. Both the child and examiner must be comfortable. The child may be positioned in the mother's left arm (Fig. 7.6) or supine in bed. The examining doctor should be seated on the infant's left side, and palpation is best achieved with the index, middle and ring fingers of the left hand. The examining fingers must be warm. Examination begins gently, to avoid frightening the infant and to avoid reflex contraction of the abdominal wall musculature. In the relaxed infant, where it is easy to feel through the rectus abdominis, the pylorus may be palpable near the midline. In most infants, the rectus abdominis presents a barrier to palpation such that the best area to palpate the 'tumour' is either in the midline itself or in the angle formed

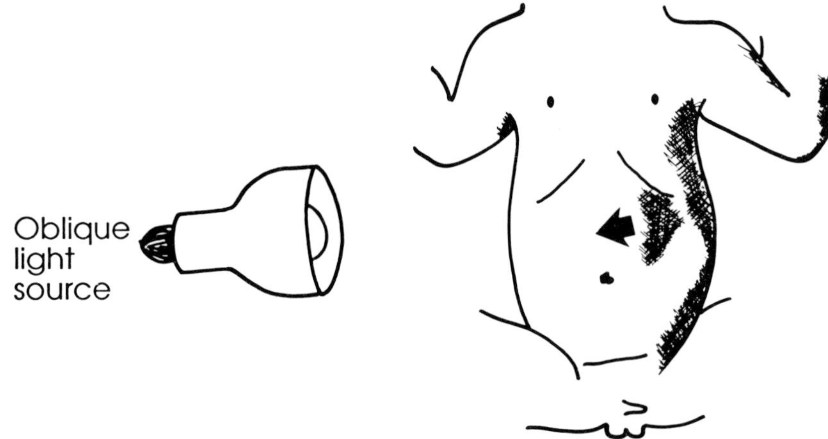

Fig. 7.5: *The direction of visible gastric peristalsis.*

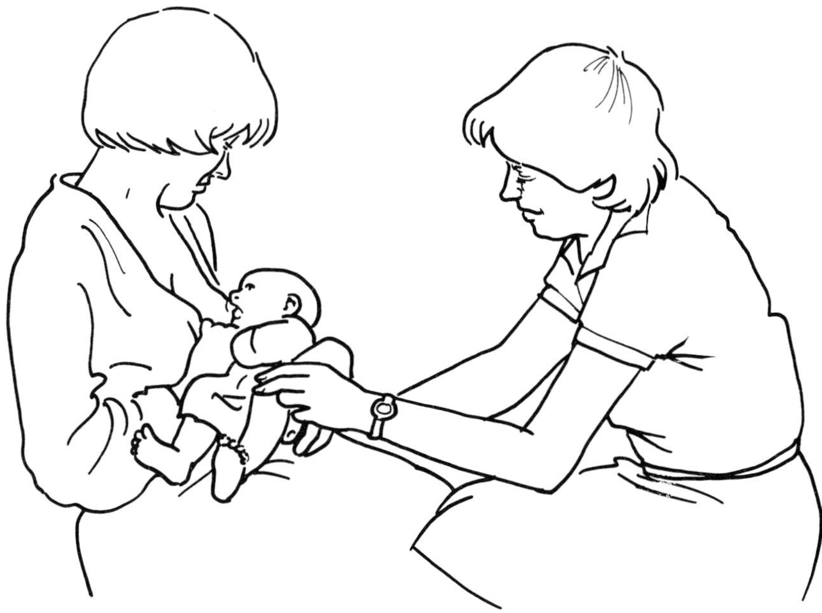

Fig. 7.6: *The examination is conducted with the clinician on the baby's left side, and with the baby kept calm by feeding.*

between the liver edge and the lateral margin of the right rectus abdominis (Fig. 7.7). The pylorus can be palpated against the anterolateral aspect of the vertebral bodies (Fig. 7.8).

Where the child is uncooperative, or there is difficulty in feeling the 'tumour', four manoeuvres may be performed:

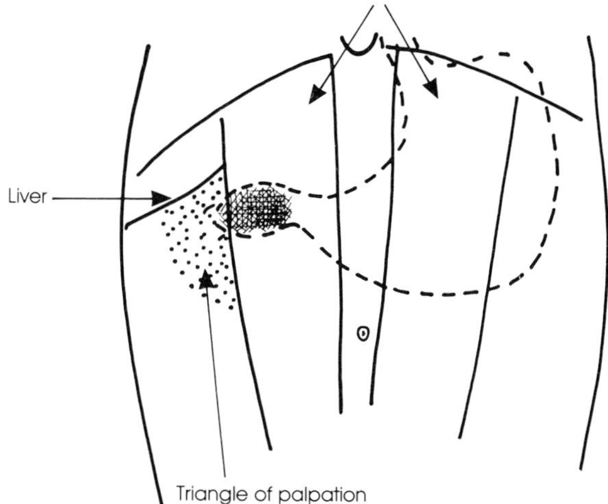

Fig. 7.7: *The triangle of palpation between the rectus abdominis muscle and liver edge. The enlarged pylorus is under the edge of the right rectus, half way between the xiphisternum and umbilicus. Alternatively, it is palpable in the midline through the linea alba.*

(1) The legs can be raised, flexing the hips and lower lumbar spine to reduce anterior abdominal wall resistance.
(2) The child can be fed, either with a bottle or from the mother's left breast, whilst being cradled in the left arm (Fig. 7.6). The purpose of this so-called 'test-feed' is to relax the infant and to distract him from the examination. It does not make the 'tumour' harder, and excessive feeding causes the over-distended stomach to obscure the 'tumour' and will almost certainly cause vomiting. Often, the 'tumour' can be felt most easily just after a vomit, when the overlying antrum is emptied.
(3) The infant can be balanced prone, with the examiner's finger-tips carefully positioned to palpate the pylorus against the vertebral column (Fig. 7.9).
(4) The infant can be re-examined after he has fallen asleep.

It is reasonable to spend 15–20 minutes palpating the upper abdomen for a 'tumour'. If the first attempt is unsuccessful, and the history is still suggestive of pyloric stenosis, a second (and if necessary a third) attempt to feel the 'tumour' should be made at a later stage. In the interim, any fluid depletion and electrolyte imbalance should be corrected.

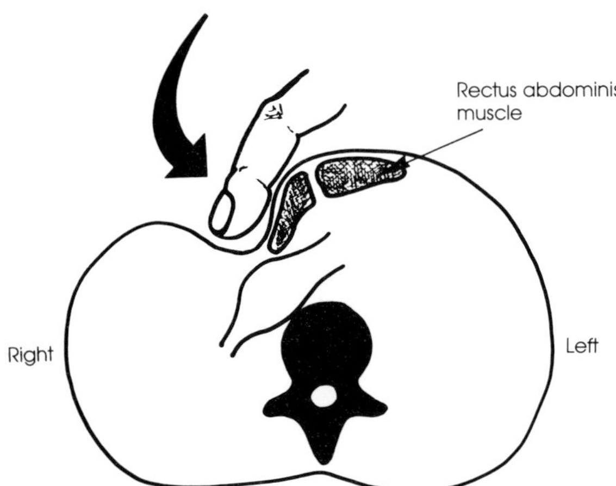

Fig. 7.8: *Palpation of the pylorus: the 'tumour' is palpated lateral to the right rectus abdominis muscle by pressing it against the vertebral column.*

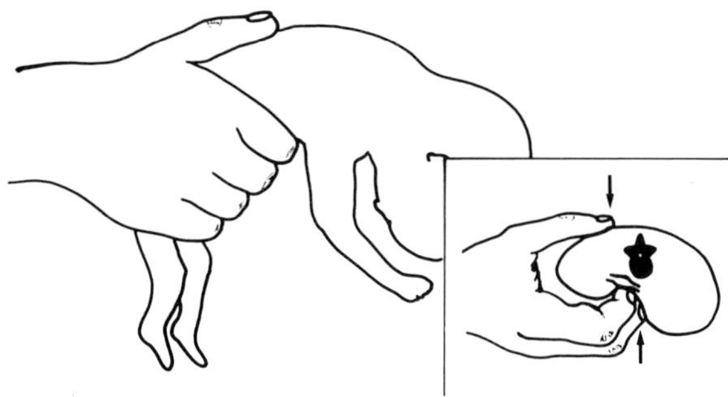

Fig. 7.9: *An alternative method of palpating the pyloric 'tumour' by compression against the right side of the lumbar vertebrae.*

GOLDEN RULES

(1) Likely causes of non bile-stained vomiting are closely dictated by age.
(2) Pyloric stenosis occurs between three and 12 weeks of age, usually between four and six weeks.
(3) The most useful feature distinguishing sepsis from mechanical causes of non bile-stained vomiting, is that in the latter, the child is otherwise well, active and keen to feed.
(4) The pathognomonic sign of pyloric stenosis is palpation of a pyloric 'tumour'.
(5) To palpate a pyloric 'tumour', both the infant and clinician must be comfortable and relaxed.
(6) If pyloric stenosis is suspected but a 'tumour' cannot be felt, the examination should be repeated after an interval, or when the infant is asleep.
(7) Surgery for pyloric stenosis must be delayed until the electrolyte and acid/base disturbance is fully corrected.

8 Colic

Colicky abdominal pain, with or without vomiting, is seen often in infants and in most instances does not reflect significant pathology. (Table 8.1). The most common colic is the so-called 'colic of infancy' or 'wind colic', a condition of little significance but one whose cause is unknown. It may result from air swallowing, constipation or immaturity of gut motility, but these theories are unproven. It is seen in the first three months of life and is characterized by episodes of uncontrollable crying or screaming which may occur at any time during the day but usually are one to two hours after feeds. It is not progressive, is not associated with vomiting, and the infant remains well.

Table 8.1 COLIC IN INFANTS AND CHILDREN

'Wind colic'
Gastro-enteritis
Constipation
Intussusception
Appendicitis (faecolith)
Bowel obstruction – congenital – acquired (adhesions)
Henoch-Schönlein purpura

Constipation is rare in breast-fed babies, but may develop in children receiving other feeds. Sometimes, the left colon contains palpable faeces, or there are hard lumps of faeces distending the rectum and anal canal.

A more serious cause of colic is intussusception which occurs most commonly in the child aged 3-12 months. Other causes of congenital or acquired bowel obstruction are rare and may be indistinguishable clinically from intussusception, but will become apparent at laparotomy. Bowel obstruction caused by adhesions should be considered where there has been previous abdominal surgery. Systemic diseases such as Henoch-Schönlein purpura, may simulate intussusception, probably because the allergic vasculitis produces submucosal haemorrhages which lead to intermittent intestinal obstruction, and occasionally even intussusception.

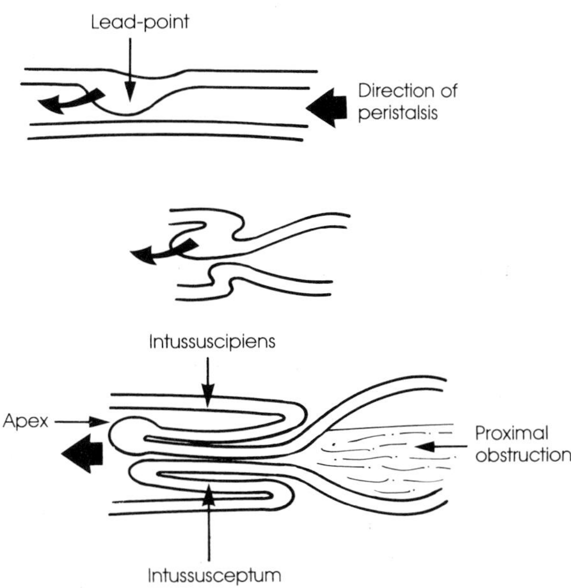

Fig. 8.1: *The process of intussusception. One part of the bowel (intussusceptum) is pushed by peristalsis inside the lumen of adjacent distal bowel (intussuscipiens).*

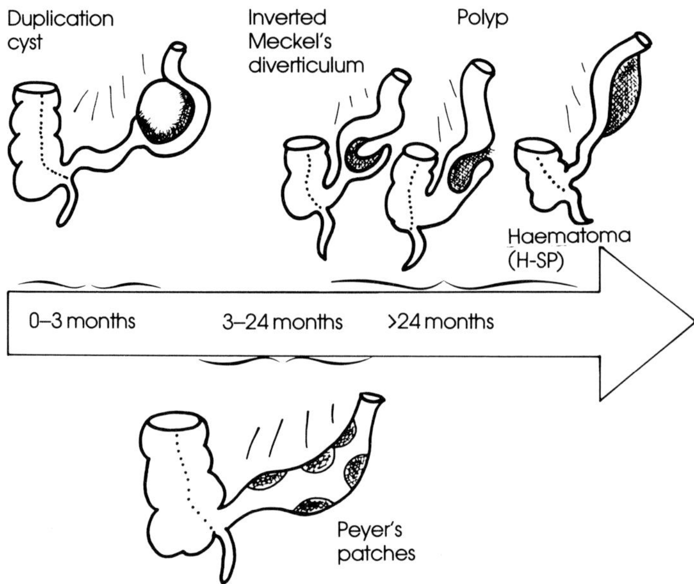

Fig. 8.2: *The causes of intussusception related to the age of the child. In the first three months, duplication cyst is a possible cause, while after 24 months of age, inverted Meckel's diverticulum, polyposis or a submucosal haematoma (Henoch-Schönlein purpura, H-SP) are more frequent. From 3–24 months of age, enlargement of Peyer's patches causes intussusception.*

In most infants with colic and vomiting, the differential diagnosis lies between gastro-enteritis and intussusception. Appendicitis is exceedingly rare in children under three years of age.

INTUSSUSCEPTION

Intussesception is an acquired form of bowel obstruction in which one part of the bowel is drawn inside the lumen of adjacent distal bowel (Fig. 8.1). Compression of the vessels in the mesentery leads to lymphatic and venous obstruction with secondary oedema. The lumen of the intussuscepted bowel is occluded by the intussusceptum and leads to dilatation of proximal bowel and colic. The bowel at the commencement of the intussusceptum is called the lead-point. The common lead-points in intussusception are shown in Fig. 8.2. Pathological causes of intussusception account for only 10% but include an inverted Meckel's diverticulum, intestinal polyps or, occasionally, duplication cysts of the small bowel or submucosal haemorrhage with Henoch-Schönlein purpura. 'Idiopathic intussusception' is most likely to occur between three months and two years of age, whereas pathological lead-points present at any age (Fig. 8.3). One possible explanation why intussusception occurs most commonly between four and seven months is shown

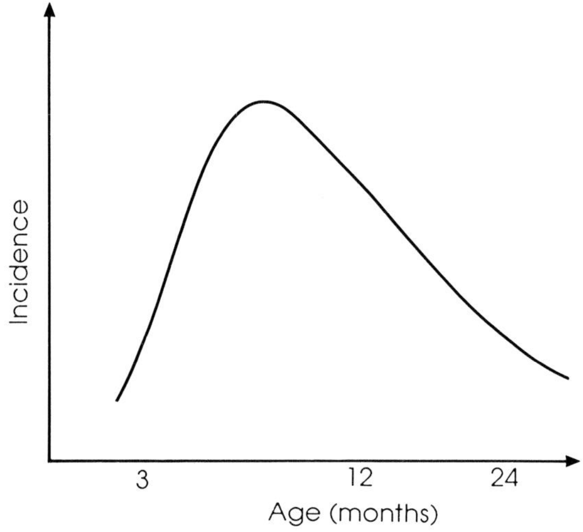

Fig. 8.3: *The incidence of intussusception in relation to age.*

in Table 8.2. The hyperplastic Peyer's patch is propelled by peristalsis through the ileocaecal valve and drags the rest of the ileum with it.

Table 8.2 WHY DOES INTUSSUSCEPTION OCCUR AT SIX MONTHS?

1. Passive immunity from the mother or breast milk is waning
2. Exposure to infective agents is increasing
3. The immune system is very reactive, leading to marked enlargement of Peyer's patches with infection.
4. The terminal ileum is relatively narrow in infants, predisposing to occlusion.

THE CLINICAL PRESENTATION

When any infant presents with vomiting and general malaise, intussusception must be considered as a possible diagnosis. In fact, vomiting is the most frequent symptom of intussusception, since colic is not always recognized as such in some small infants. The reasons for this are shown in Table 8.3. Small infants are unable to interpret fully the subjective sensation, have an incompletely developed body image and lack speech. Therefore, recognition of the pain by the clinician depends on the reflex response it induces in the infant – this includes vomiting, pallor, sweating, screaming and pulling up the knees. In some, there appears to be no pain at all. In a typical situation, the colic is moderate to severe, lasts a minute or two and is followed by a pain-free interval of up to 10-20 minutes. If the child screams or pulls up the knees, the parent has no difficulty in recognizing the underlying severe pain. Where the pain is so severe that the child does not want to scream, it may be recognized only by non-specific symptoms such as vomiting, pallor and sweating.

Table 8.3 CHARACTERISTICS OF PAIN IN INFANCY

1. *Subjective* sensation, immature interpretation
2. Lack of body image – pain not well localized to anatomical site
3. Lack of speech – pain not described
4. Pain recognized by its reflex autonomic effects – vomiting
   - pallor
   - screaming
   - pulling up the knees
   - sweating
5. Pain may not be present in some infants with intussusception

The relative frequency of the various symptoms of intussusception is shown in Table 8.4. Vomiting has a bimodal distribution in time relative to the onset of intussusception, with early reflex vomiting occurring until the stomach is empty, followed by an interval when vomiting is less frequent. Subsequently, if the diagnosis is delayed, there is a resurgence of vomiting, secondary to the bowel obstruction caused by the intussusception which usually commences in the terminal ileum (Fig. 8.4).

Table 8.4 SYMPTOMS OF INTUSSUSCEPTION

Vomiting	90%
Colicky abdominal pain	80–90%
Lethargy	70%
Pallor	65%
Blood in the stools (late)	55%
'Diarrhoea' (early)	30%
Recent upper respiratory tract infection	25%

The passage of loose motions may make the distinction between gastro-enteritis and intussusception difficult. In intussusception, there is a brisk, early evacuation of the distal colon which ceases when the colon is empty unless persisting blood in the bowel continues to irritate the colon. Initially, this has the appearance of diarrhoea since several stools may be passed in quick succession (Fig. 8.5). The presence of blood in the stools is a relatively late sign (Fig. 8.6). Mucosal congestion of the intussusceptum leads to blood and mucus being squeezed out, producing the so-called 'red current jelly' stool. Blood in the stools is not seen in the early phases because, initially, the intussusceptum is not haemorrhagic. As time progresses, it becomes a more frequent sign as the congestion becomes increasingly severe and gangrene ensues.

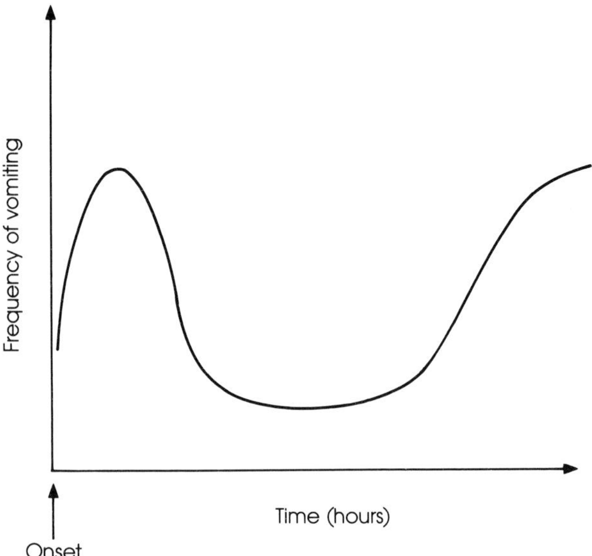

Fig. 8.4: *The presence of vomiting in relation to the onset of intussusception. Early reflex vomiting from pain occurs until the stomach is empty. After a variable interval, late vomiting develops with progressive bowel obstruction.*

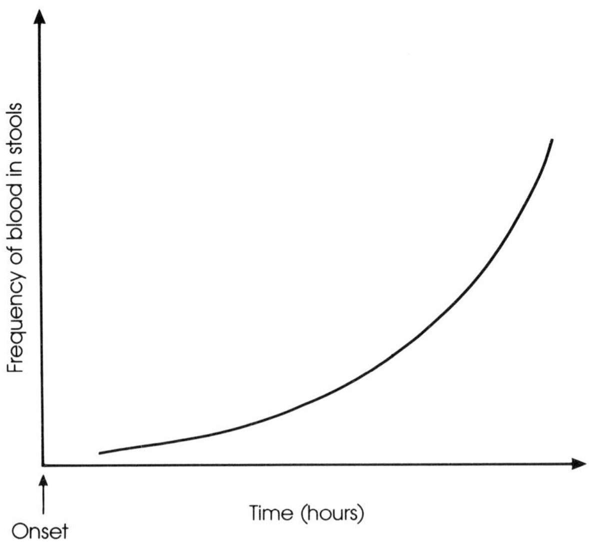

Fig. 8.5: *The relationship of blood in the stools to the onset of intussusception. Initially it is rare, but as oedema and vascular congestion progress, it becomes more common. Mucosal congestion leads to blood and mucus being squeezed out, which produces 'red current jelly' stools.*

The overall picture of a child with intussusception is shown in Fig. 8.7. There is often a history of a recent upper respiratory tract infection (which may be the origin of the micro-organism causing Peyer's patch enlargement). Colicky pain may be present with screaming and pallor, with the legs pulled up and fists clenched. The restless movement of the child during the episode of pain provides good evidence that there is no peritonitis, as once the peritoneum becomes inflamed the child will lie still. Between episodes of pain, the infant is pale and lethargic. Late signs, such as dehydration, bowel obstruction or circulatory collapse, become evident with progression of the intussusception.

The key to clinical diagnosis relies on the suspicion of intussusception in a pale, lethargic infant with vomiting and colic; the diagnosis is confirmed by the demonstration of a mass in the abdomen (Table 8.5). A useful general approach is shown in Fig. 8.8. The child should be examined for signs of dehydration or circulatory insufficiency, evidence of a concurrent or recent upper respiratory tract infection, or stigmata of other conditions which may predispose to intussusception. The examination of the abdomen should await the cessation of the episode of pain: the colic of intussusception lasts only a few minutes so the abdomen is examined once the colic has ceased. Evidence of constipation should be sought by palpation for hard faeces in the left colon and sigmoid. The abdomen should be examined for

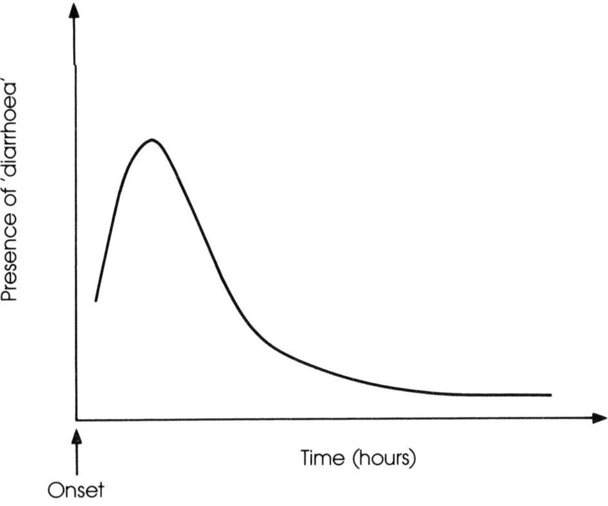

Fig. 8.6: *The relationship of 'diarrhoea' to the onset of intussusception. Reflex peristalsis from the mass, or blood in the proximal colon, causes early and rapid evacuation of the distal colon.*

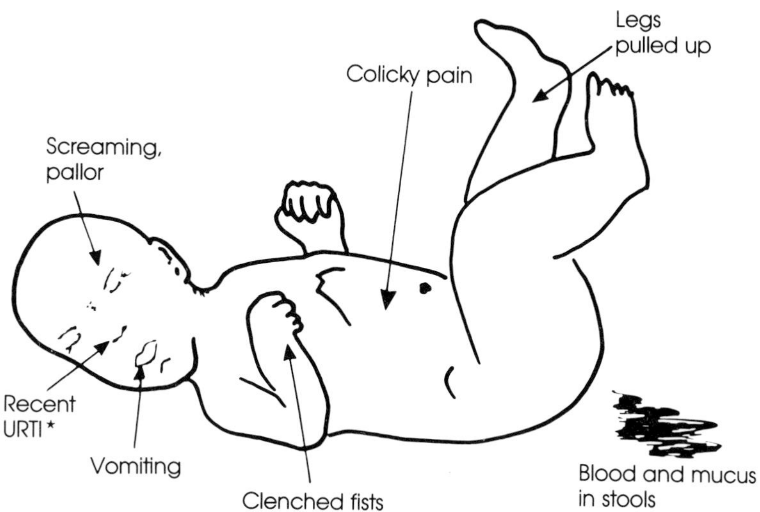

Fig. 8.7: *The general appearance of an infant with intussusception. Late signs include distended abdomen, dehydration, shock and cardiovascular collapse.*

*Upper respiratory tract infection

tenderness and guarding indicating peritonitis. Appendicitis, although exceedingly rare in the normal age group for intussusception, must be considered always, particularly if the pain is not overtly colicky.

Palpation of an intussusception mass clinches the diagnosis. The mass is sausage-shaped and usually behind the right rectus abdominis muscle on the right side of the abdomen but may cross the midline just above the umbilicus (Fig. 8.9). The right iliac fossa often feels 'empty'. The mass may be difficult to feel, particularly in the presence of abdominal distension or tenderness, and is nearly always more medial in the abdomen than the inexperienced examiner expects, slightly within the line of the normal surface markings of the

Table 8.5 SIGNS OF INTUSSUSCEPTION

Abdominal mass	70%
Rectal blood	53%
Tenderness	40%
Dehydration (greater than 5%)	15%
Rectal mass	10%
Peritonitis	5%
Shock	5%

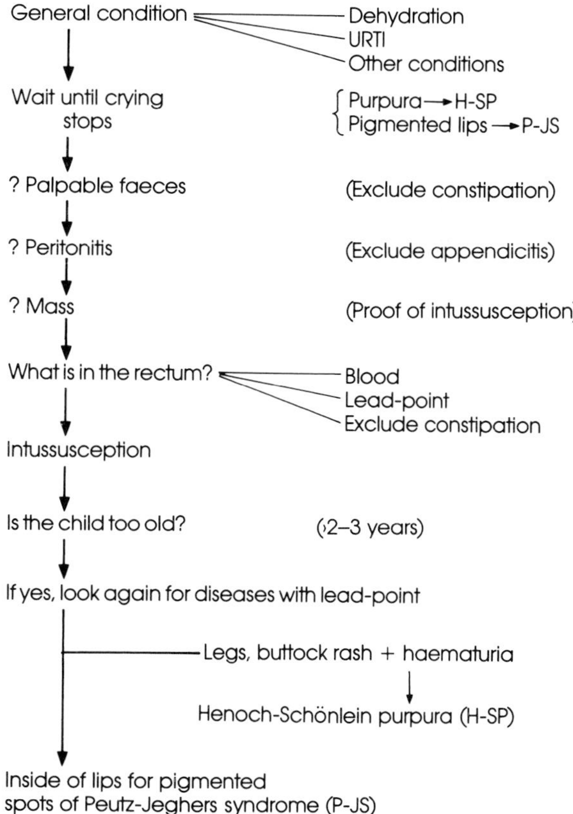

Fig. 8.8: *An algorithm for the clinical examination of a child with suspected intussusception.*

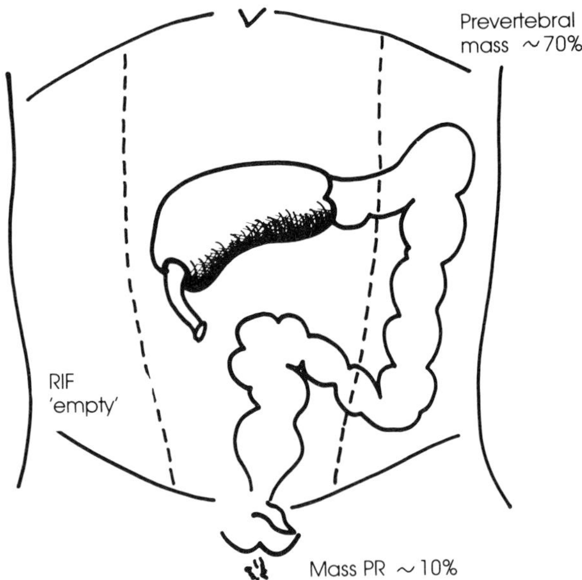

Fig. 8.9: *The intussusception is usually palpable as a prevertebral mass behind the rectus abdominis muscle.*

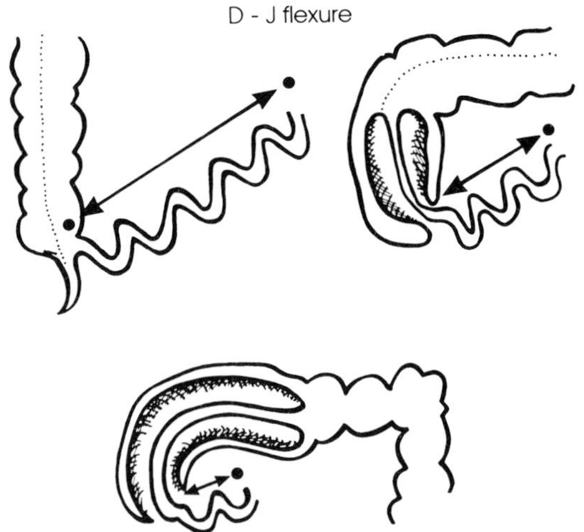

Fig. 8.11: *The explanation for the central position of an intussusception mass in the transverse colon. As the ileum intussuscepts, the mesentery is shortened, with the effect that the colon is pulled closer to the duodenojejunal (D-J) flexure. Intussusception beyond the transverse colon is rare because the mesentery is not of infinite length.*

colon (Fig. 8.10). As the intussusception progresses, it draws its mesentery with it, which has the effect of pulling the colon towards the root of the bowel mesentery, behind the rectus abdominis muscles (Fig. 8.11). The mass can be palpated beneath the lateral edge of the right rectus muscle, but is usually best felt in the midline above the

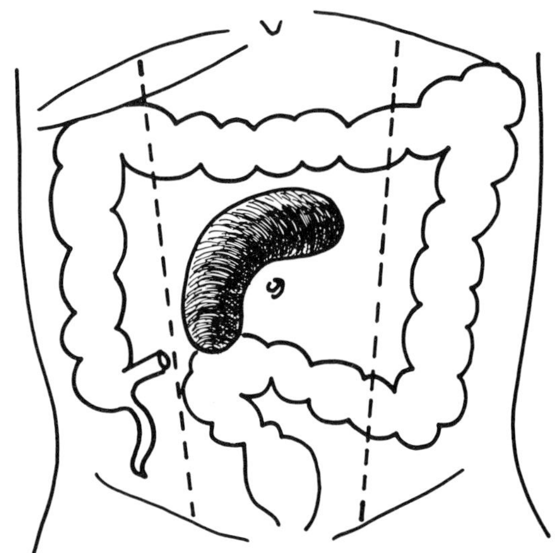

Fig. 8.10: *The common position of the intussusception mass compared with the normal position of the colon.*

umbilicus (Fig. 8.12). At this point, the colon is maintained close to the anterior abdominal wall by the spine and great vessels. The hand of the examiner should be placed lightly on the epigastrium until the child is relaxed. The finger-tips can then be rolled forwards and backwards over the surface of the horizontally placed sausage-shaped mass. The palpation of an intussusception mass is most difficult when it is behind the rectus abdominis muscles or when the abdomen is distended or tender.

Examination of the rectum will usually reveal it to be empty. The appearance of blood on the glove or a palpable lead-point would be further evidence of intussusception. Rectal examination is also useful to exclude constipation where diagnostic difficulty exists. In 10% of patients, the apex of the intussusception is palpable in the rectum and occasionally may protrude from the anus, in which situation it needs to be distinguished from prolapse of the rectum (Fig. 8.13). This is readily achieved by digital examination of the sulcus between the protruding mucosa and the anal margin. If there is a prolapsed intussusception there is no fornix on digital examination, whereas if the protruding mucosa is caused by prolapse of the rectum there is a short, blind-ending fornix.

Once the diagnosis of intussusception is confirmed in a child outside the usual age range of intussusception, clinical examination is directed at looking for a possible cause. In practice, the only conditions causing intussusception which have external manifestations are Henoch-Schönlein purpura and some forms of polyposis. Therefore, the legs and buttocks of older children should be examined for the haemorrhagic rash of Henoch-Schönlein purpura. The urine should be examined for proteinuria or haematuria. Inherited forms of polyposis rarely cause intussusception in small children, because the polyps take years to grow to a size that causes intussusception, but do cause intussusception in the child over five years of age. In Peutz-Jeghers syndrome there is pigmentation around the mucocutaneous junctions of the mouth and the anus.

GOLDEN RULES

(1) The peak incidence of intussusception is between four and seven months, but the condition may occur at any age.
(2) Intussusception in children greater than three years of age suggests an underlying lesion of the bowel, e.g. polyposis in Peutz-Jeghers syndrome.
(3) 'Pain' is a *subjective* symptom and may not be recognized in intussusception, particularly where the child is too young to describe the sensation.
(4) Intermittent screaming is easily recognized as colic, but intermittent pallor without screaming may also represent colic.
(5) Beware vomiting and colic in an infant without diarrhoea: it is hazardous to diagnose

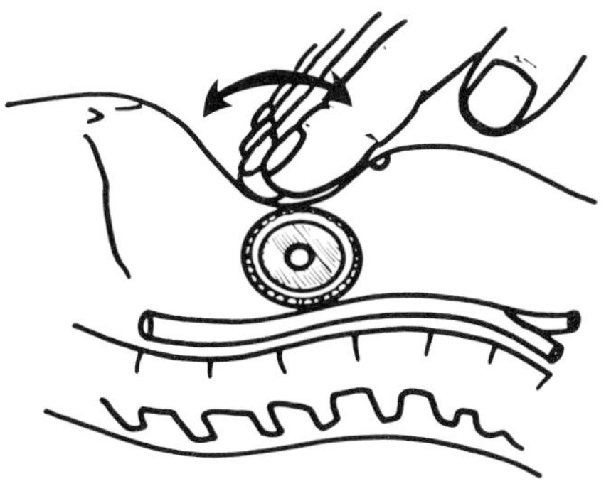
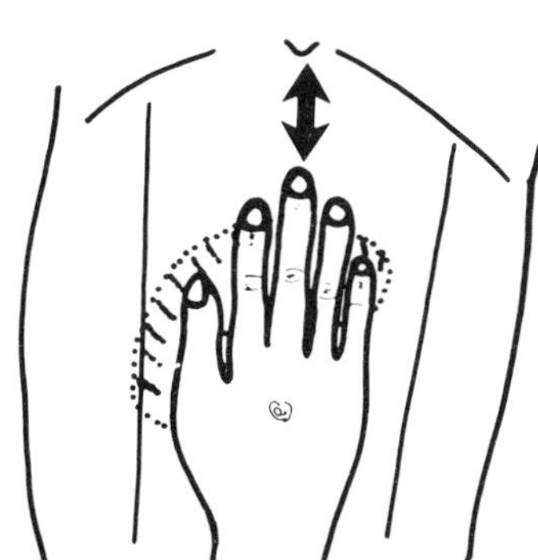

Fig. 8.12: *Palpation of the sausage-shaped mass where it crosses the midline above the umbilicus. The fingers roll over the horizontally oriented sausage.*

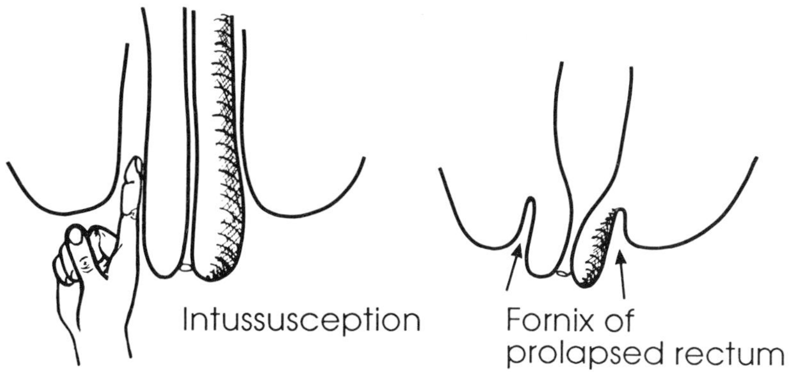

Fig. 8.13: *The distinction between rectal prolapse and the rare anal presentation of intussusception relies on the demonstration of a fornix on digital examination.*

gastro-enteritis if vomiting persists for more than 24 hours.

(6) Beware the infant with severe malaise and lethargy after prolonged vomiting: dehydration and shock may simulate meningitis.

(7) Beware the infant with vomiting and 'diarrhoea' which ceases spontaneously: ileocolic intussusception causes reflux evacuation of the distal colon and may simulate gastro-enteritis in its early stages.

(8) Blood (red currant jelly – blood and mucus) in the stools is a *late* sign of intussusception: the diagnosis should not be delayed until it is present.

(9) The mass of intussusception may be difficult to feel because it is *behind* the rectus abdominis muscles, is tender or is in a distended abdomen.

(10) If severe abdominal colic continues for more than two hours in an infant, intussusception should be considered.

(11) A diagnostic enema should be performed if there is difficulty distinguishing gastro-enteritis from intussusception.

9 The neck

The surgical lesions affecting the neck are numerous and common, with enlarged lymph nodes being responsible for most examinations. To enable discussion of the various presentations of neck abnormalities, has been divided the chapter into postural deformities (i.e. wry-neck) and lesions laterally or in the midline of the neck.

TORTICOLLIS

The common cause of torticollis or wry-neck is tightness of one sternomastoid muscle following an idiopathic inflammatory process in the perinatal period. At two to three weeks of age, a visible or palpable swelling develops in the sternomastoid muscle (the so-called 'sternomastoid tumour'), which may persist for some months. Older children may present with a fibrotic, short sternomastoid which is presumed to be the legacy of previous inflammation.

The appearance of head tilt varies with age. Small infants have their heads turned to one side and a little tilted, but make no correction for this. Since they do not need to stand up, there is no need for them to maintain the plane of their eyes horizontally. Children able to walk compensate for the more pronounced tilt by elevating one shoulder to keep the eyes as level as possible. Furthermore, they do not turn their heads to the contralateral side, but instead compensate by twisting the neck to keep the eyes pointing forwards. The first question in torticollis is to establish whether the wry-neck is caused by shortness of one sternomastoid muscle or not (Table 9.1). It is important to realize that alternative diagnoses *must* be sought if the sternomastoid muscle is not short and tight (Fig. 9.1).

Table 9.1 CAUSES OF WRY-NECK

1. Sternomastoid tumour/fibrosis
2. Ocular imbalance
3. Cervical hemivertebrae
4. Posterior fossa tumours

Differential diagnosis

Is the sternomastoid tight?

The anterior border of the muscle stands out as a tight band, except in small infants where the neck may be so short that the muscle cannot be seen readily. It is important, therefore, to palpate the full length of the muscle to define whether an inflammatory 'tumour' or area of fibrosis is present. Where the sternomastoid is abnormal, further abnormalities of growth tend to occur (see below). Where the torticollis is not caused by an abnormality of the sternomastoid, the muscle is neither prominent nor shortened.

Is a squint present?

A squint is a common cause of head tilt which results from an imbalance in the rotation of the eyes. The tilt compensates for the abnormal position of the eyes, such that the squint may not be obvious at first. By straightening the head passively, the squint will become apparent.

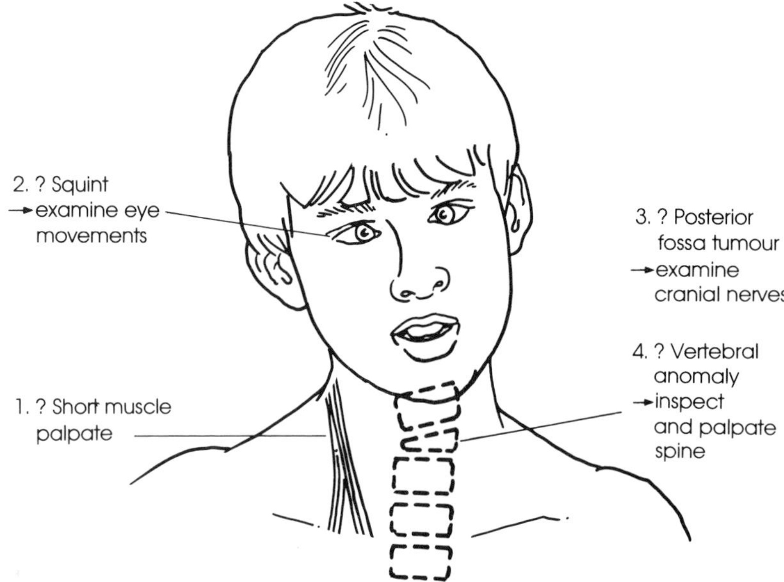

Fig. 9.1: *The clinical questions in the differential diagnosis of torticollis.*

Is there a brain tumour?

Posterior fossa tumours, which are not uncommon in children, may compress the brain stem at the foramen magnum to produce acute stiffness of the neck and cause the head to be held to one side. The neck is 'frozen' in this position and is difficult to move actively or passively. The presence of a central nervous system tumour may be known already, but occasionally, acute torticollis is the first presentation. A careful, neurological examination should be performed with emphasis on the lower cranial nerves and cerebellar function.

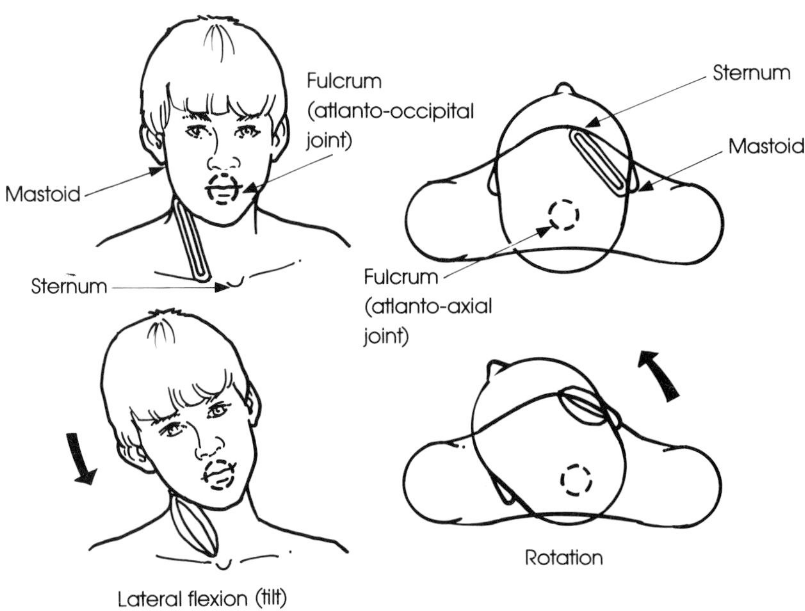

Fig. 9.2: *Sternomastoid muscle action causes tilting and rotation of the head.*

Is there a vertebral anomaly?

Structural lesions in the cervical vertebrae will produce a tilt of the head which may be confused with that of other causes. Congenital anomalies such as hemivertebrae will produce torticollis from birth without progression. Vertebral lesions can be identified clinically by inspection and palpation of the dorsal cervical spines, and confirmed on x-ray.

Sternomastoid torticollis

A sound clinical understanding of this abnormality depends on a knowledge of how the sternomastoid muscle works (Fig. 9.2). It has a complicated action which combines lateral flexion with rotation towards the opposite shoulder. The mastoid is not only above the sternum, but also significantly posterior to it. The rotation towards the contralateral side on contraction of the sternomastoid is important to appreciate because it is the primary effect of shortening in infancy (Fig. 9.3). Ipsilateral head flexion occurs as well, but is less noticeable in a tiny infant bundled up in a rug!

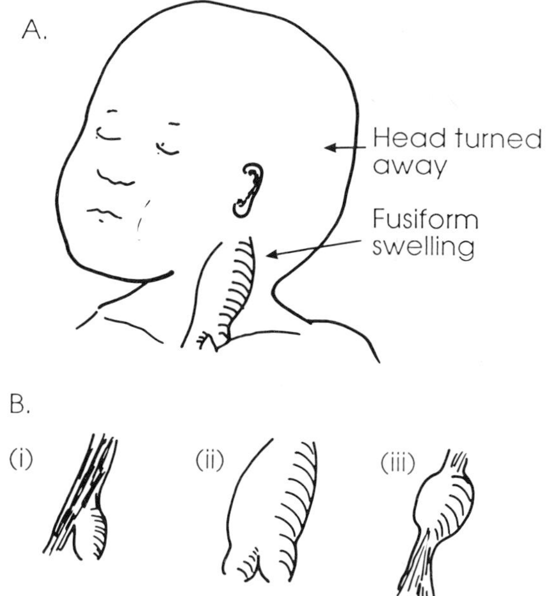

Fig. 9.3: *Infantile sternomastoid 'tumour'. A. The head is turned away from the fusiform cervical swelling. B. The inflammation may affect (i) the head, (ii) the entire muscle, or (iii) one part of the main muscle.*

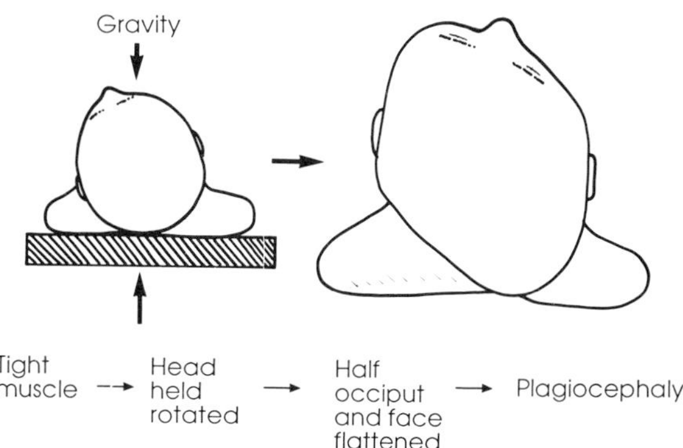

Fig. 9.4: *The cause of plagiocephaly.*

The sternomastoid tumour may affect all or part of the muscle, including its two inferior heads (Fig. 9.3). The resulting fibrosis likewise can affect a localized part of the muscle. Remember that not all 'tumours' lead to significant fibrosis and shortening later in life: the majority resolve after a few months with no sequelae. Furthermore, there are some older children who present with fibrosis without a history of a 'tumour' in infancy.

The mechanisms of secondary deformity

The effect of gravity

In small infants with torticollis and fixed rotation of the head, gravity deforms the head as it lies on the bed because it remains in the same position for a prolonged period. The baby's head is turned towards the contralateral side with the contralateral occiput pressing on the bed. Flattening of the occiput leads to secondary flattening of the ipsilateral forehead (Fig. 9.4). This asymmetrical skull deformity is called plagiocephaly, and is best observed from above the head.

Plagiocephaly can become marked if the child is not nursed prone with the head turned towards the affected side. The skull bones are very soft and pliable in the small baby and readily deform, but once the torticollis resolves, the plagiocephaly tends to resolve as well.

The effect of growth

Progressive deformity with growth is seen in older children when one tight sternomastoid muscle immobilizes the face for a long time. The

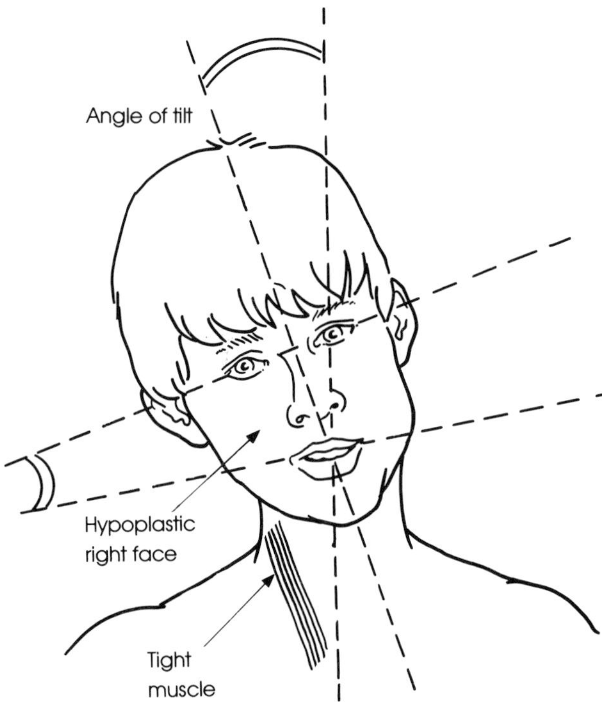

Fig. 9.5: *Estimating the degree of hemihypoplasia of the face by comparing the plane of the eyes with the plane of the mouth. When the shoulders are level, the head is tilted.*

side of the face that is limited by the fibrotic muscle grows more slowly than the normal side, and causes progressive asymmetry (Fig. 9.5). This inhibition of the growth of the mandible and maxilla embodies an important principle of paediatrics: *normal growth of the bones depends on normal muscular movement.*

The degree of hemihypoplasia of the face can be determined by the angle between the plane of the eyes and the plane of the mouth. Normally, these lines are parallel, but form an angle to each other when the face is asymmetrical. The larger the angle between these lines, the more severe is the asymmetry. Hemihypoplasia is a crucial sign to observe because it indicates that surgery is necessary to release the tight muscle.

The effect of postural compensation

When children are old enough to walk, the eyes are kept horizontal to facilitate balance and coping with gravity. If a short fibrous sternomastoid causes tilting and rotation of the head, the child will compensate for this by elevating the ipsilateral shoulder to keep the plane of vision horizontal (Fig. 9.6).

Examination of the child will show the eyes to be level and (possibly) hemihypoplasia of the face. The ipsilateral shoulder is lifted up to relieve tension on the sternomastoid. There is cervical and thoracic scoliosis to compensate further for this. Other adjacent muscles, such as the trapezius, may be wasted because of inactivity.

How to assess limitation of movement

The rotational component of the action of the sternomastoid is easy to measure. Rotation is assessed by standing behind the child's head and passively rotating the head while it is held between both hands. The aim is to rotate the head until the nose reaches each shoulder (180° total range) (Fig. 9.7). Note that the sternomastoid is stretched to its maximum length by lateral rotation to the side of the affected muscle. Where the muscle is fibrotic, it cannot be stretched to its full length and rotation to the ipsilateral side is restricted. The angle reached at the limit of movement is judged easily from above, and can be recorded for future reference.

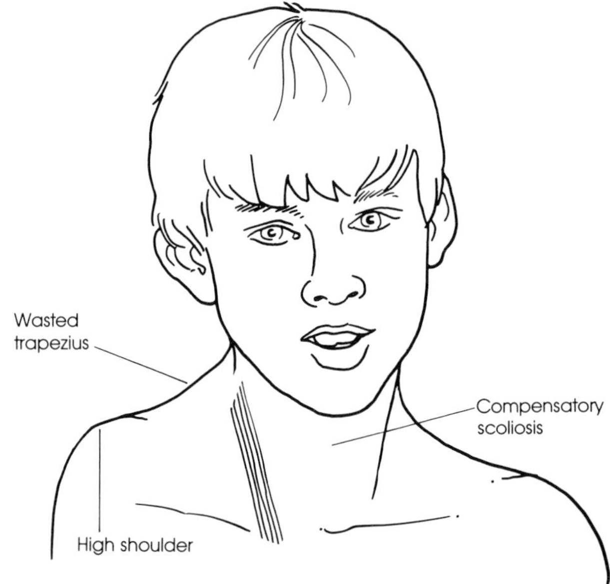

Fig. 9.6: *Torticollis compensated for by cervical scoliosis and a high shoulder to keep the eyes level with the horizon.*

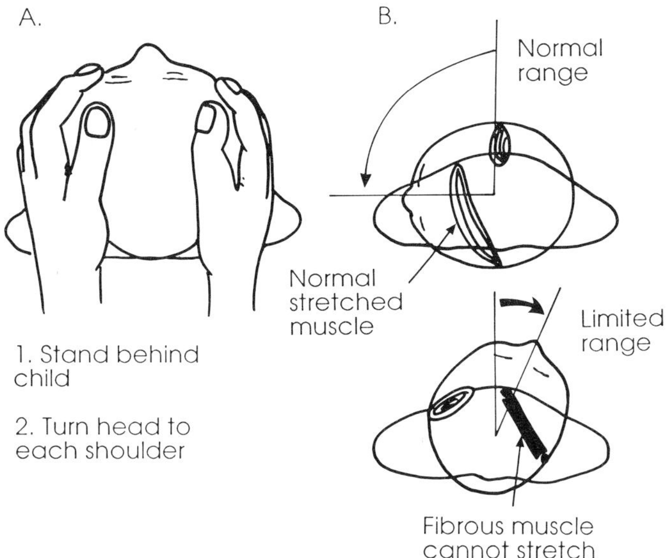

Fig. 9.7: *Determination of the degree of limitation of head rotation.* A. *Position of the hands to rotate the head passively.* B. *Normal versus limited rotation.*

THE SIDE OF THE NECK

Lumps in the side of the neck are caused most commonly by inflammation in lymph nodes. The mouth permits entry of pyogenic bacteria, viruses or rarer organisms (such as atypical mycobacteria), which colonize the surrounding lymphatic tissue. In addition, the sheer volume of lymphatic tissue in the neck means that often malignancies affecting lymph nodes will be found here first. Leukaemia, lymphoma and secondary neuroblastoma may present in this way (Table 9.2).

The embryological development of the neck is complicated by the large number of structures within it, including the branchial clefts and arches – the distant homologues of the gill slits. Various branchial cysts and sinuses may occur, although most are rare. Also, hamartomatous overgrowth of some tissues (e.g. jugular lymphatic spaces or blood vessels) is encountered.

Where is it?

The sternomastoid muscle is the essential landmark for all lesions in the lateral part of the neck, and often the key to diagnosis is localization of the lump in relation to this muscle (Fig. 9.8). Lesions (inflammatory or neoplastic) in the lymph nodes will be found along the jugular chain or other known sites (Fig. 9.9). Infected nodes are more likely to be in the submandibular and tonsillar regions (anterior border of the upper third of the sternomastoid) than elsewhere, since the commonest portals of entry drain through these nodes. Infections gaining entry through abrasions (particularly on the scalp) may involve less common sites, such as the occipital nodes (Fig. 9.9). Nodes at the base of the neck (supraclavicular nodes) may become involved from infections arising on the arm, axilla or chest wall (Fig. 9.9).

Remnants of the branchial system of clefts and arches are found most commonly near the anterior border of the lower third of the sternomastoid (second cleft) (Fig. 9.10) or, rarely, near the upper end of the sternomastoid (first cleft) (Fig. 9.11). Deep-seated lesions behind the lower third of the sternomastoid may be in the thyroid: neoplasms are rare but well documented in adolescents, especially in girls. Uniform enlargement of the thyroid is not difficult to separate from other lesions because of its characteristic shape.

The hamartomatous conditions, such as lymphangioma ('cystic hygroma'), occur along the

Table 9.2 LATERAL NECK SWELLINGS

1. *ACUTE LYMPHADENITIS*
   Short history (days)
   Signs of inflammation (unless exposed to antibiotics)
2. *ATYPICAL TUBERCULOUS (MAIS) LYMPHADENITIS*
   1–2 month history in a 1–2 year old
   Very low-grade inflammatory signs (= cold abscess)
   Purple discoloration of the skin (when near the surface)
   Collar-stud abscess
3. *MALIGNANT NODES*
   Child <5 years – leukaemia, neuroblastoma
   Child >5 years – lymphoma, leukaemia
   Non-tender, rubbery/stony
   + history/signs of disease elsewhere
4. *BRANCHIAL CYST* (2nd or 3rd clefts)
   Single cyst beneath the middle third of the sternomastoid
   Transilluminable (clear mucus)
   Branchial sinus opening at the anterior border of the lower part of the sternomastoid
5. *HAEMANGIOMA* (hamartoma)
   Sign of emptying (cavernous spaces)
   + overlying skin vessels/colour
   + bruit
   (+ excess flow – cardiac failure – enlarged liver)
   (+ platelet trapping – haemorrhage)
6. *LYMPHANGIOMA* (hamartoma) (= cystic hygroma)
   Brilliantly transilluminable
   Enlarges rapidly with infection or haemorrhage
   Single cyst/diffuse multilocular
   Soft, flabby, non-tender (except if secondary infection)
7. *STERNOMASTOID 'TUMOUR'*
   Fusiform swelling within the sternomastoid
   Neonate/infant
   No obvious signs of inflammation
   Torticollis
8. *SALIVARY GLAND SWELLINGS*
   (Parotid) pain and swelling worse with eating
   (Sialectasis) infected saliva massaged from Stensen's duct
   (Submandibular calculus) palpable/visible in the floor of the mouth

jugular lymph channels, in or around the partoid gland, or near the region of the thoracic duct at the base of the neck (Fig. 9.12).

If the swelling is in the sternomastoid muscle itself, then a sternomastoid 'tumour' is the likely diagnosis (see under Torticollis). The relationship of a mass to the sternomastoid is easier to determine when the muscle is made to contract (Fig. 9.13).

What are its characteristics?

Pyogenic infection in the tonsillar nodes, which is common in infancy, will demonstrate all the features of acute inflammation unless modified by antibiotic treatment. The duration of symptoms is short (a few days), but the symptoms progress rapidly. The systemic effect of pyrogens will cause fever, malaise and loss of appetite.

All the signs of acute inflammation will be present, namely (1) heat, (2) redness, (3) swelling, (4) tenderness, and (5) loss of function/lack of movement. The heat produced by the inflammation can be felt by the back of the examiner's fingers, and this should be sought first before the skin temperature is altered by the palpation process itself. When the infection is near the surface,

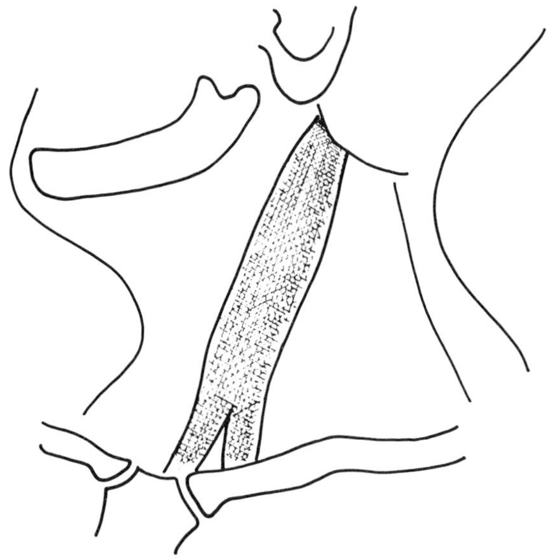

Fig. 9.8: *The sternomastoid muscle: the key to the localization and identification of cervical masses. It divides the neck into anterior and posterior triangles.*

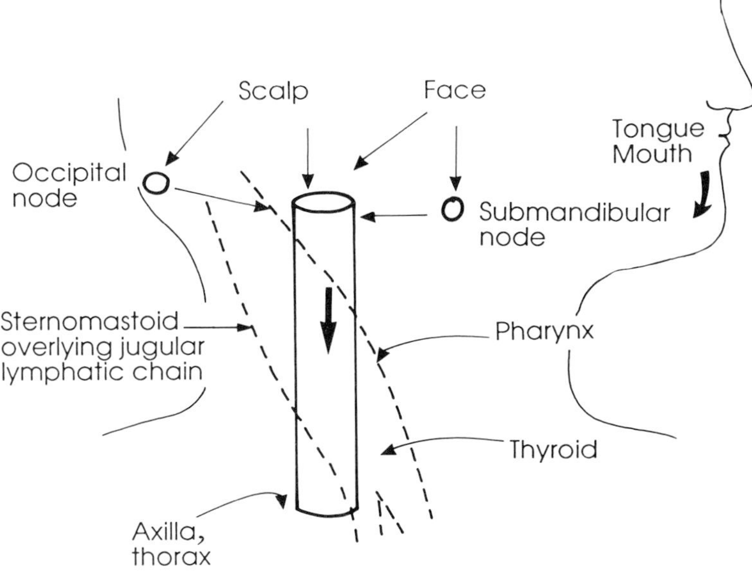

Fig. 9.9: *The lymphatic drainage of the head and neck channelling into the jugular lymphatic chain.*

the redness is obvious. However, infection in the deep jugular chain may not exhibit this sign because of the thick intervening sternomastoid muscle and investing deep cervical fascia.

Tenderness of a mass of inflamed nodes is determined on palpation, although it may not be evident if the inflammatory process has been modified by previous antibiotics. Reflex spasm of

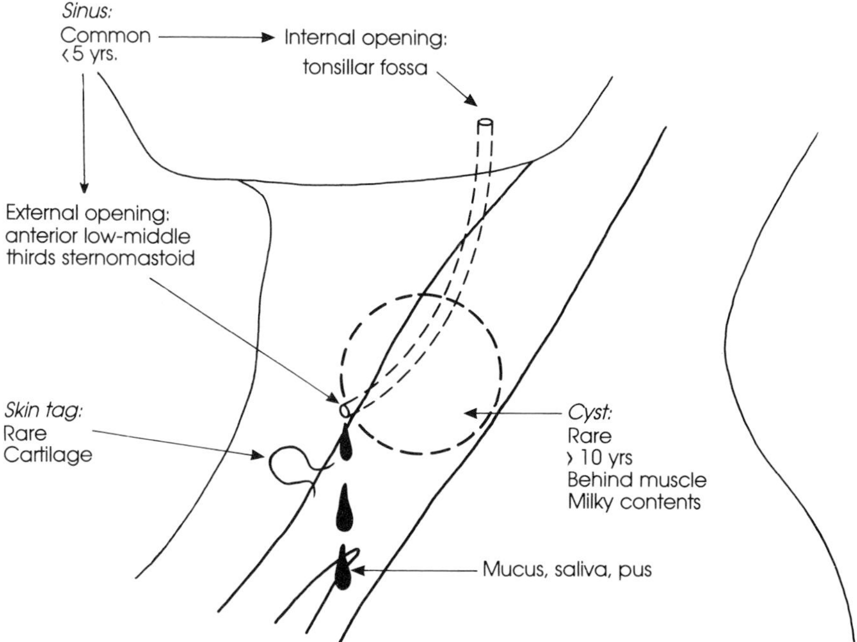

Fig. 9.10: *Second branchial cleft (sinus/cyst) and arch (skin tag) remnants.*

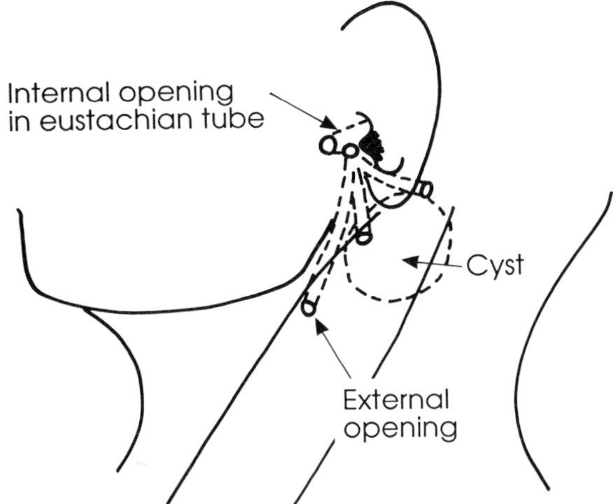

Fig. 9.11: *The rare first branchial cleft defects, producing a sinus or cyst near/behind the anterior border of the upper third of the sternomastoid.*

adjacent muscles may produce an acute stiff and wry-neck. Both active and passive movements will be limited and/or painful.

The relationship of inflammatory lesions to the sternomastoid muscle (Fig. 9.8) will determine the ease with which these signs are elicited: a thick overlying muscle provides effective 'camouflage' for even a large abscess.

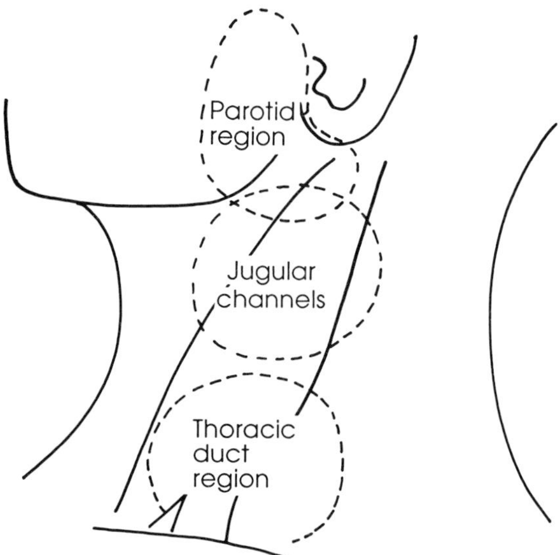

Fig. 9.12: *The three areas of primitive lymphatic development, being the common sites for lymphangioma (cystic hygroma).*

Fluctuation may indicate an abscess with a liquid centre. The tight, deep cervical fascia, however, may mask the softness of the lesion if it is deep-seated. The mass should be grasped between the fingers of one hand, and the other hand should compress the centre (Fig. 9.14). The proof of fluctuance can be obtained on some occasions by needle aspiration of pus. In small infants, where abscesses are common, aspiration of the fluid will confirm the diagnosis and, on occasions, may alleviate the need for further intervention, since the antibiotics will cause resolution once the avascular nidus has been evacuated.

Modified signs of inflammation

This is an important presentation for two common conditions:

(1) pyogenic infection suppressed by antibiotics;
(2) atypical mycobacterial infection.

Suppressed pyogenic infections are found in all the common drainage areas from the mouth and pharynx. The duration of symptoms is prolonged and inflammatory signs are less obvious, particularly if the focus is deep to the sternomastoid. One way to reveal the signs is to stop antibiotic treatment and repeat the examination several days later, at which stage the inflammatory signs may reappear. Mycobacteria from the '*MAIS*' complex (*Mycobacterium avium intracellulare scrofulaceum*) are common organisms in the soil in temperate climates. They will produce disease in populations not previously immunized or exposed to the human strain. The symptoms and signs of inflammation are less than with pyogenic infections: MAIS infection produces a diminished inflammatory response in 'slow motion' – the duration of the lump is more likely to be six weeks to two months, rather than two days. Pain, tenderness and heat are usually not severe enough to be noticed and a typical 'cold abscess' is produced. The natural history of MAIS infection is important because if untreated, it will form a chronic discharging sinus (Fig. 9.15). The aim is to diagnose the condition before eruption through the skin occurs, so that the lesion can be excised before an ugly scar develops. The characteristic sign of MAIS infection is purplish discoloration of the skin which precedes the skin breakdown. The

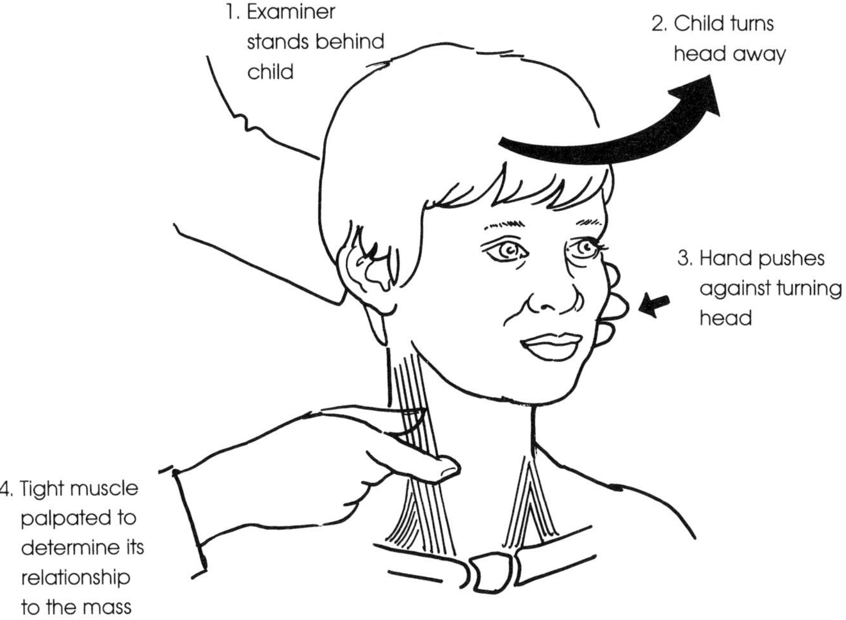

Fig. 9.13: *How to determine the relationship between a lateral cervical mass and the sternomastoid muscle.*

colour is caused by low grade inflammation in the skin as the infection spreads towards it through the subcutaneous tissue, and signifies progression of MAIS infection to form a 'collar-stud' abscess (Fig. 9.15). Recognition of the 'collar-stud' abscess stage is useful for distinguishing it from other lesions (Fig. 9.16).

Non-inflammatory masses

Neoplastic infiltration causes painless enlargement of the lymph nodes, which are firm and rubbery. Several nodes may be enlarged in one area. Some tumours make the nodes feel hard and stony (e.g. neuroblastoma). Asymptomatic nodes greater than 2 cm in diameter should arouse suspicion of malignancy and warrant biopsy.

Haemangiomas have several characteristic signs:

(1) The presence of abnormal overlying vessels or discoloration of the skin – a red/purple colour signifies surface capillaries, a dull blue hue indicates larger deep-seated vessels

(2) The sign of emptying – external compression will empty the blood and the mass will shrink,

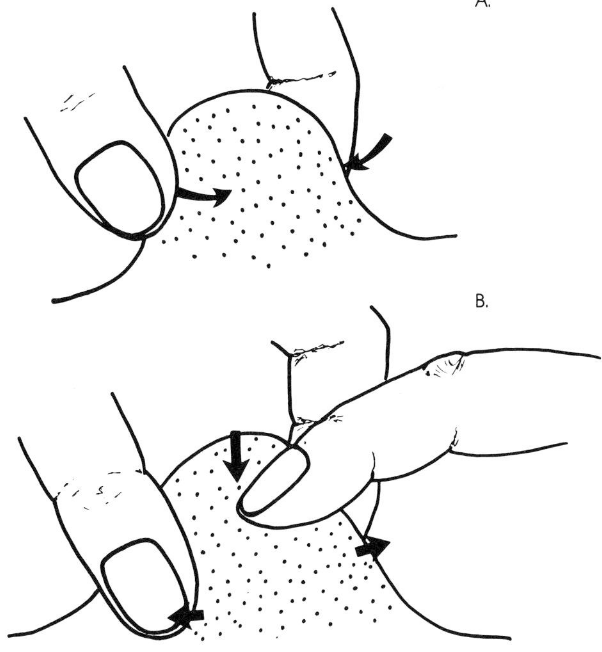

Fig. 9.14: *Testing for fluctuance.* A. *The mass is grasped between finger and thumb.* B. *The centre of the mass is prodded by the other hand; this produces a fluid thrill which is detected by the finger and thumb.*

refilling again once the compression is released (Fig.9.17)

(3) A bruit – which will be heard with a stethoscope if the blood flow is excessive.

Does the mass transilluminate?

This is the cardinal sign of a lymphangioma (or cystic hygroma) (Fig. 9.18), provided that there has not been secondary infection or haemorrhage into the cystic spaces (from contained haemangiomatous elements), both of which are common. The other signs supporting the diagnosis of lymphangioma are its multicystic nature and its tendency to infiltrate the entire area, rather than be confined by a capsule or anatomical planes.

Does the mass move?

Unlike masses in the midline of the neck, which move if attached to the tongue, hyoid or larynx, lateral cervical masses are usually immobile. One exception is a mass in the lateral lobe of the thyroid, which moves up and down with swallowing (Fig. 9.19). Inflammatory swellings tend to have reduced local mobility because cellulitis surrounding an abscess obliterates the normal tissue planes along which movement would normally occur (Fig. 9.20).

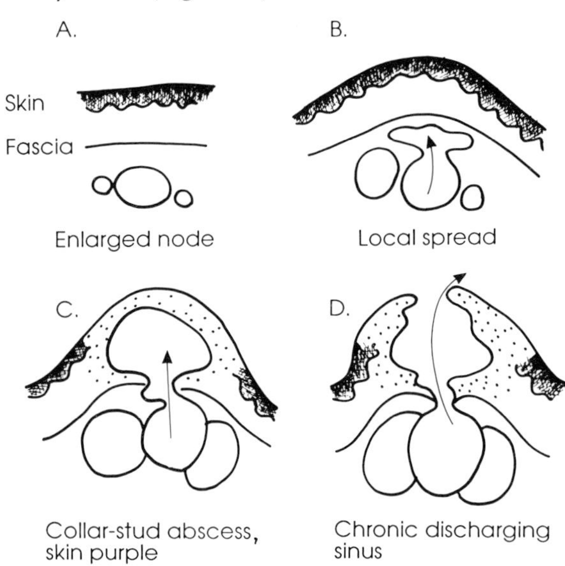

Fig. 9.15: *The four stages of Mycobacterium avium intracellulare scrofulaceum (MAIS) infection in a lymph node.*

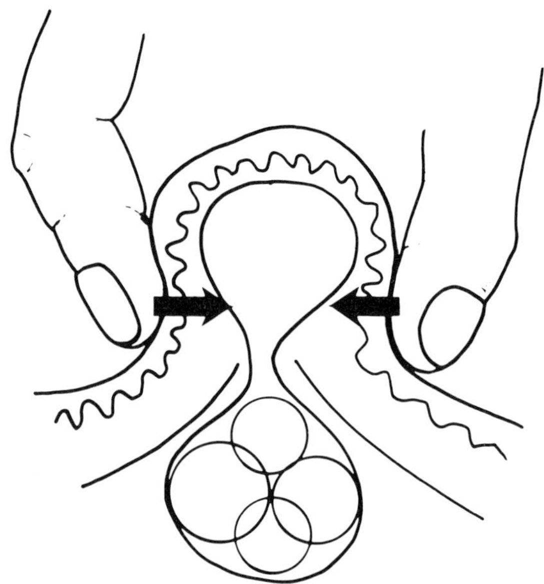

Fig. 9.16: *Palpation of a collar-stud abscess. The narrow 'waist' distinguishes this lump from other lesions. This is a difficult sign to elicit, but is useful if positive.*

Secondary effects of the lesion

When a swelling appears anywhere in the neck, the effects on adjacent normal structures need to be considered. Large lesions beneath the deep fascia and sternomastoid will compress not only the carotid sheath but also the central viscera (trachea and oesophagus). Rare lesions, such as retrosternal goitre, may compress the venous drainage of the head and upper limbs. Oropharyngeal displacement by a large mass (e.g. branchial cyst) is not a serious concern, but the small calibre of the trachea makes it vulnerable to lateral compression. An abscess in the lower jugular nodes or a thyroid nodule can compress and displace the trachea. Therefore, the position of the trachea should be determined accurately (Fig. 9.21); displacement suggests that x-rays are needed to confirm whether there is compression.

Haemartomata of lymph and blood vessels are not confined by tissue planes, and may undergo rapid enlargement (secondary to infection, haemorrhage or thrombosis) and compress the trachea. Haemangiomata may cause difficulties at birth by virtue of their enormous size resulting in

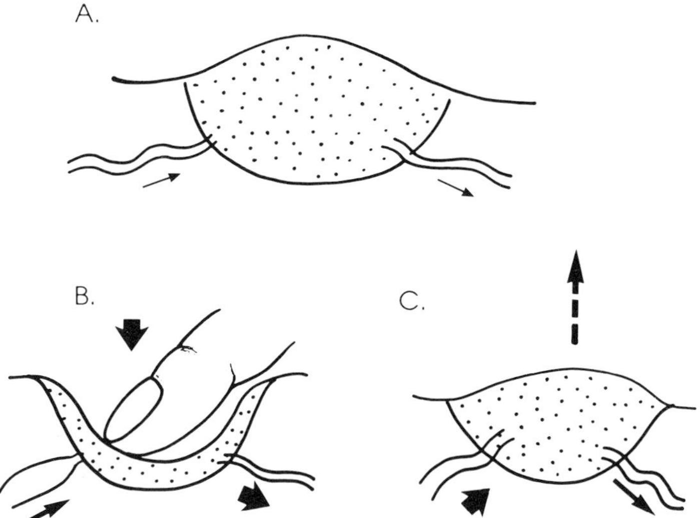

Fig. 9.17: *The sign of emptying. A. Cavernous sinuses remain expanded by blood flow. B. Digital pressure empties the lesion. C. Sinuses quickly refill with blood after removal of pressure.*

tracheal compression and displacement of the head to the contralateral side.

Examination of the neck is not complete until contiguous areas have been examined, since a pathological process (or its effects) has no regard for the arbitrary boundaries between the neck and the head, chest and axillae. Examination of the upper lobes of the lungs by percussion and auscultation will reveal whether a low cervical mass extends into the thorax. Particular lesions may have secondary effects which are the key to their diagnosis. A second branchial cleft defect may present as a small punctum at the junction of the middle and lower thirds of the anterior border of

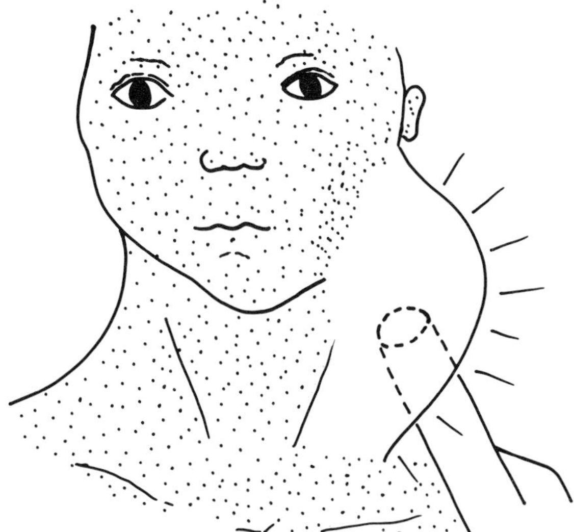

Fig. 9.18: *Transillumination of a lymphangioma (cystic hygroma).*

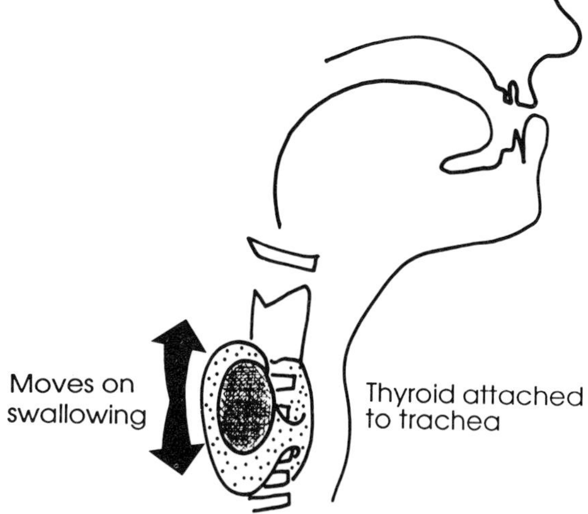

Fig. 9.19: *Movement of a lateral thyroid swelling on swallowing occurs because the thyroid is attached to the trachea.*

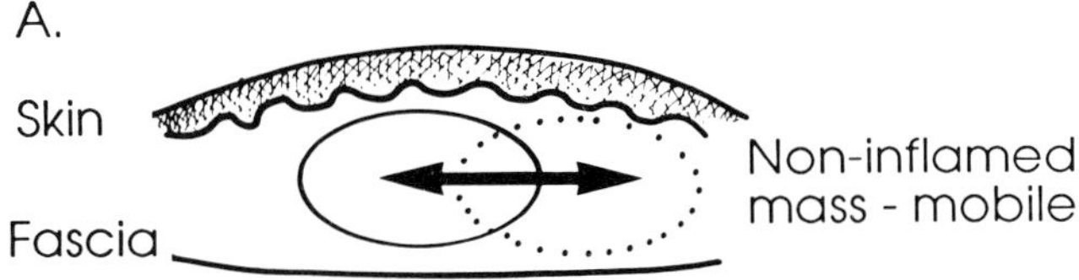

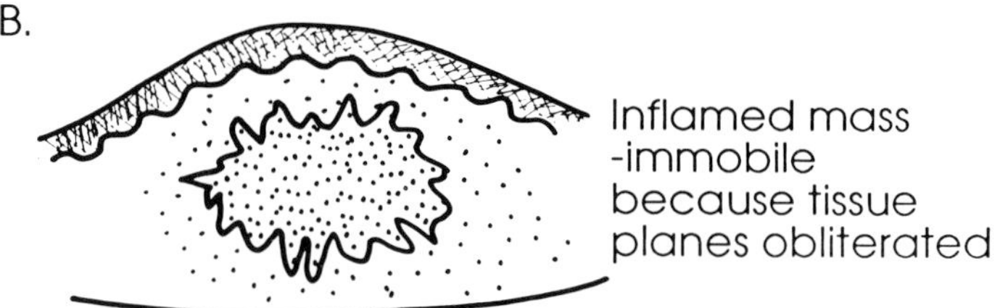

Fig. 9.20: *The different mobility of a non-inflamed mass (A), compared with that of an abscess with surrounding cellulitis (B).*

the sternomastoid. Recurrent infection is common but non-specific; however, dribbling of saliva/mucus when infection is absent is pathognomonic.

Large haemangiomata may produce two systemic effects of importance:

(1) Cardiac failure secondary to high blood flow – this manifests itself in infants as tachypnoea and an enlarged liver (easily diagnosed on percussion)

(2) Haemorrhagic disease secondary to platelet-trapping in the lesion, which produces thrombocytopenia.

Is there an underlying cause elsewhere?

In all swellings, the clinician must consider whether there is a distant cause, particularly if inflammatory or neoplastic origins are likely. For cervical swellings, therefore, this means that the

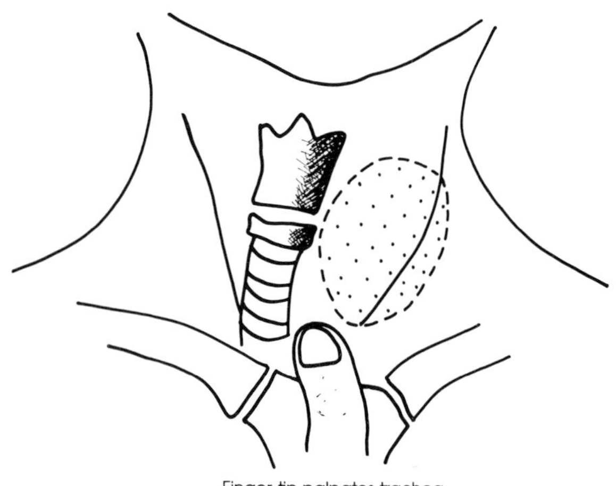

Fig. 9.21: *The assessment of tracheal position where there is a low cervical swelling. Compression of the trachea is a significant risk if the trachea is displaced.*

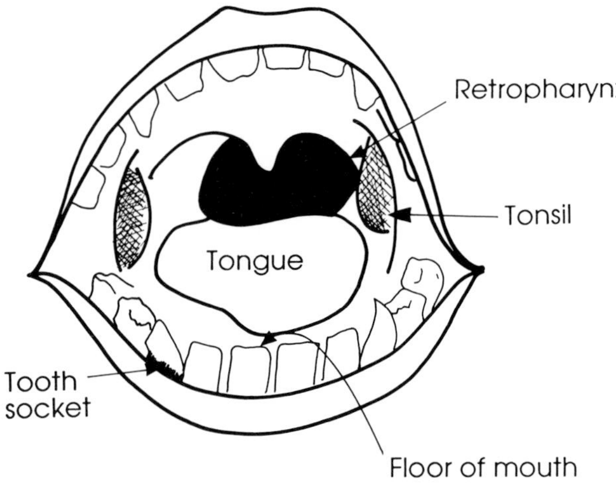

Fig. 9.22: *Intra-oral foci for cervical infections.*

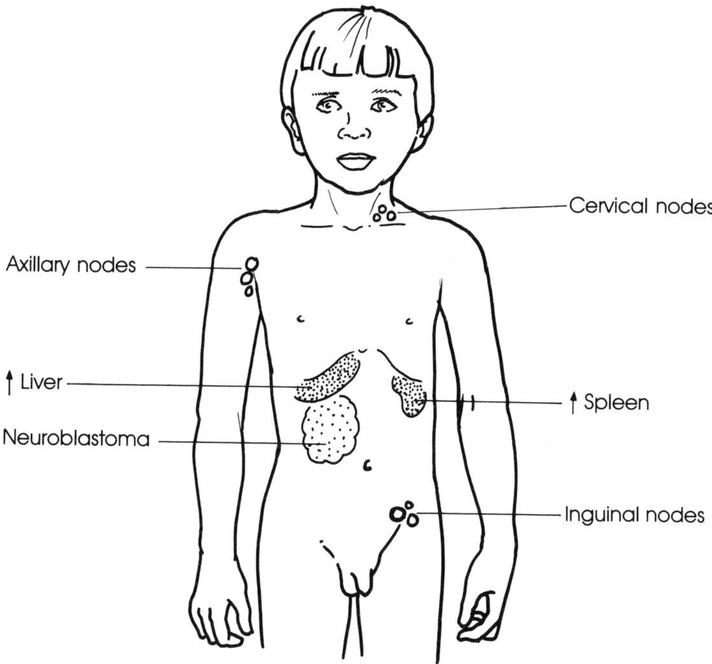

Fig. 9.23: *The places to look for a malignant focus when a cervical node is found.*

mouth should be searched for an inflammatory cause, e.g. infected tooth socket, tonsillitis, or retropharyngeal abscess (Fig. 9.22). Neoplastic causes should be investigated by a systematic search of all lymphatic tissues, including axillae, groins, liver and spleen (Fig. 9.23). Particular attention should be paid to examination of the abdomen to look for evidence of neuroblastoma, which arises from the adrenals or sympathetic ganglia, and commonly spreads to lymph nodes.

MIDLINE SWELLINGS OF THE NECK

While not as frequent as laterally placed neck lumps, midline neck lumps in children are not rare. They are usually one of three things: a submental lymph node, thyroglossal cyst or dermoid cyst. Ectopic thyroid tissue is seen less commonly. It is important to identify those swellings of thyroglossal origin as their treatment requires total excision of the thyroglossal duct system (Table 9.3).

Table 9.3 MIDLINE NECK SWELLINGS

LIKELY LESIONS

1. *SUBMENTAL LYMPH NODE*
   Immediately behind mandible
   Usually small, may be multiple
   Evidence of regional infection (usually inside the mouth)
2. *DERMOID CYST*
   Slow growing and spherical
   Does not transilluminate (contains sebaceous material)
   Painless
   Not attached to the hyoid – usually just behind the mandible or just above sternal notch
3. *THYROGLOSSAL CYST*
   Unilocular hemisphere
   May be large or enlarge rapidly
   Often transilluminable (contains clear mucus)
   Attached to the hyoid
   Commonly develops secondary infection
4. *ECTOPIC THYROID*
   Similar in site to thyroglossal cyst

Solid
Not translucent
Normal thyroid is absent

5. *GOITRE*
Neonate or pubertal girl
Diffuse
Lower neck

Where is the swelling?

The exact location of the lump must be established (Fig. 9.24). If it is immediately behind the mandible it is likely to be a submental node or dermoid cyst. If it is situated in relation to the hyoid bone, a thyroglossal cyst should be considered (Fig. 9.25). Submental lymph nodes often are small, and may be multiple and slightly to one side of the midline. Likewise, thyroglossal cysts close to the thyroid cartilage may be pushed to one side, whereas dermoid cysts almost always remain in the midline.

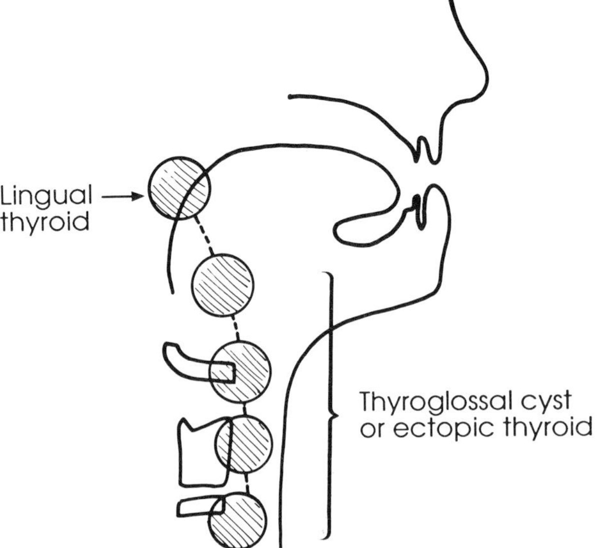

Fig. 9.25: *The line of descent of the embryonic thyroid may be the site of a maldescended thyroid gland or a thyroglossal cyst.*

Is it fluctuant?

It is uncommon for any of the lesions to be fluctuant, even when infected (except the very large infected thyroglossal cyst), mainly because of the tension within the cyst itself.

Is it inflamed?

Look for inflammation with redness overlying the swelling, and for tenderness on palpation. The rare suppurative submental lymphadenitis and the more common infected thyroglossal cyst may

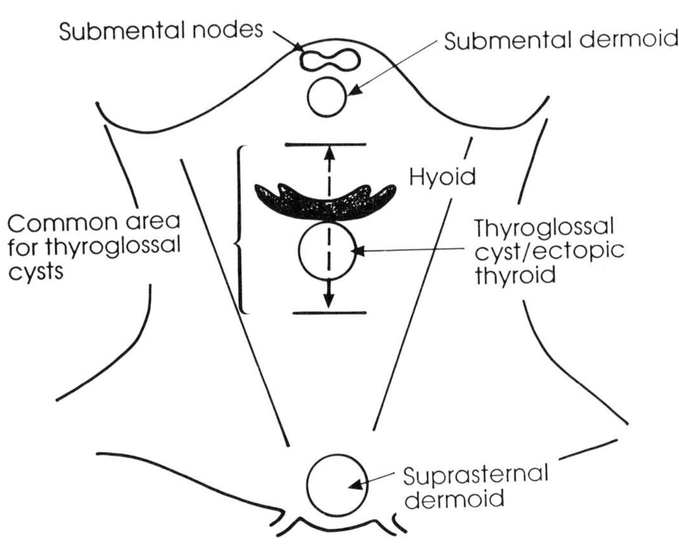

Fig. 9.24: *The common positions of midline cervical masses.*

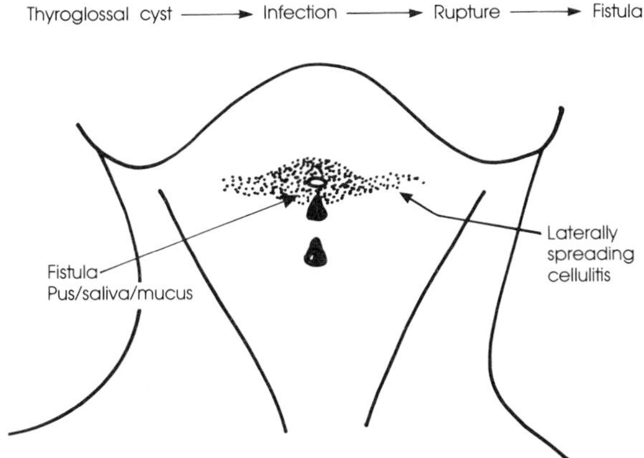

Fig. 9.26: *The mechanism of thyroglossal fistula formation. Note how cellulitis of a thyroglossal cyst/fistula spreads laterally.*

present in this way. The erythema surrounding an infected thyroglossal cyst extends laterally further than it does in the midline (i.e. it progresses transversely more than vertically). The swelling should be inspected for evidence of a fistula opening, through which a discharge may be intermittent or have occurred previously – this would be consistent with a thyroglossal fistula (Fig. 9.26).

Does it transilluminate?

This requires a strong torch and dark room. The dermoid cyst contains thick secretions and will not be translucent, whereas a thyroglossal cyst may transilluminate (Fig. 9.27). A thyroglossal cyst will not be translucent when it is infected, contains solid thyroid tissue, or is lying more deeply.

Does it move?

The dermoid cyst moves with the skin in all directions but moves little on swallowing or tongue protrusion. The thyroglossal cyst is attached to the hyoid bone, and so moves upwards on tongue protrusion and in both directions on swallowing (Figs. 9.28 and 9.29). One has to be aware that there is some movement of all midline cervical swellings but their movement is less pronounced than that of the thyroglossal cyst.

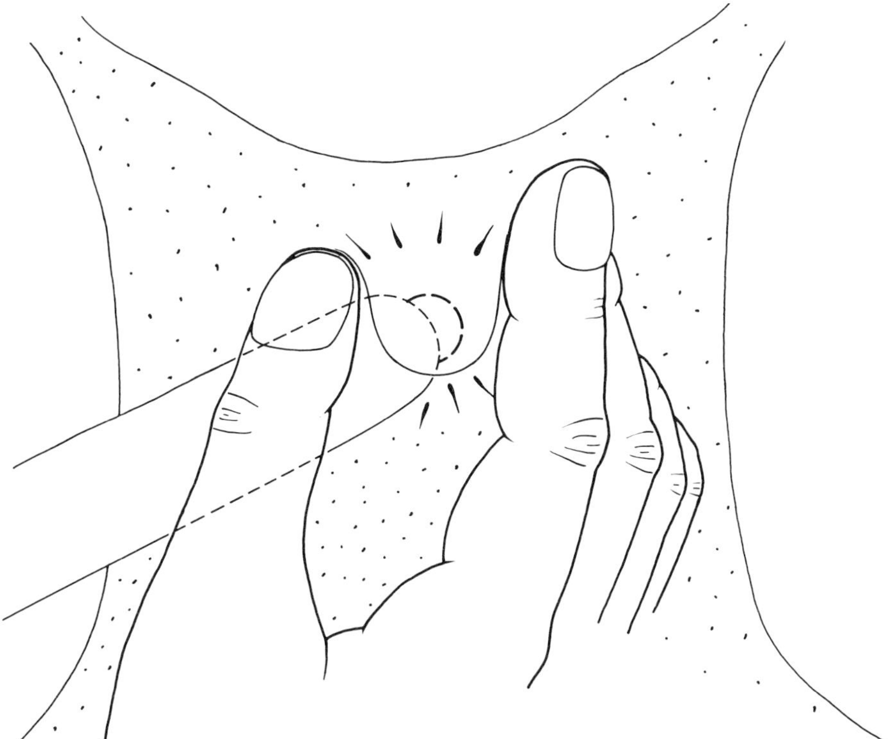

Fig. 9.27: *Transillumination of a thyroglossal cyst.*

Is there evidence of sepsis in the mouth?

Inspect the mouth, the lower gums and teeth, and the tongue for evidence of infection (Fig. 9.30). Examine the neck for other enlarged nodes.

Can the thyroid be palpated?

The thyroid gland can be palpated from in front or behind, but palpation is perhaps most easily performed from behind using the flat of both hands (Fig. 9.31). The fingers palpate the thyroid tissue on either side of the trachea in the space medial to the lower end of the sternomastoid muscle. Next, inspect the back of the tongue for ectopic thyroid tissue (lingual thyroid). Where, after full examination, doubt persists as to the exact location of the thyroid tissue, where a thyroglossal 'cyst' feels solid, or where there is a lingual thyroid, a thyroid scan is indicated to delineate the exact location of all functioning thyroid tissue.

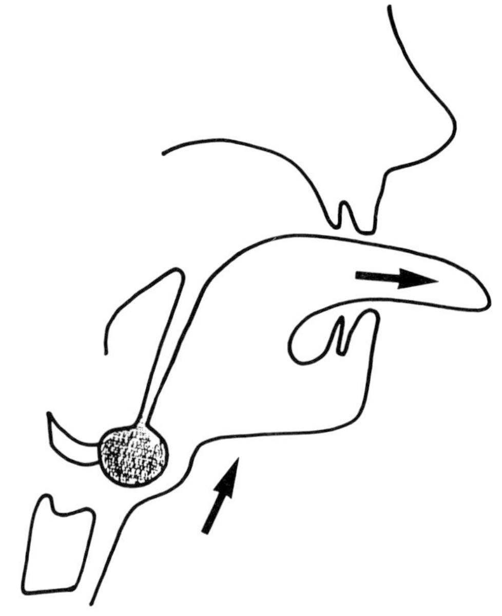

Fig. 9.28: *The movement of a thyroglossal cyst on protrusion of the tongue.*

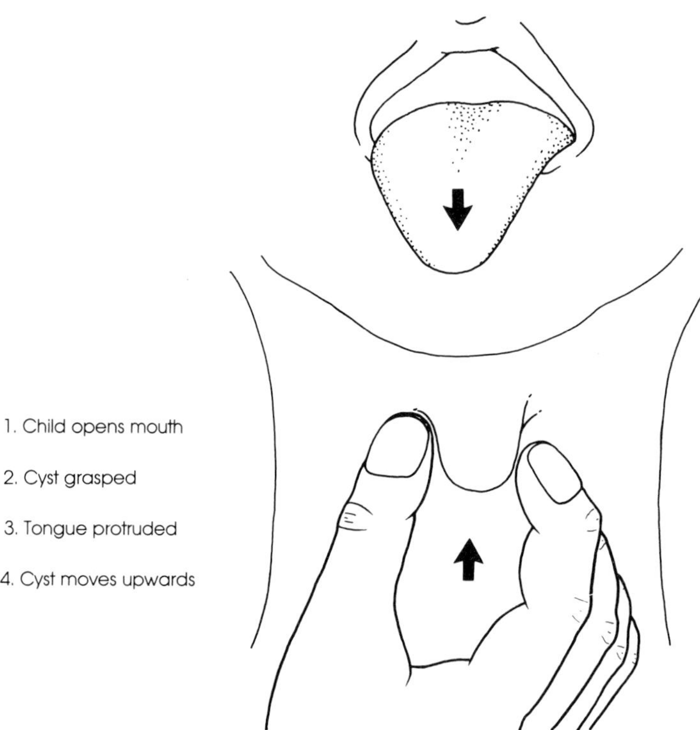

Fig. 9.29: *The way to demonstrate movement with the tongue protrusion test: the movement of the cyst is felt better than seen. The cyst can be grasped more easily when the child's mouth is open.*

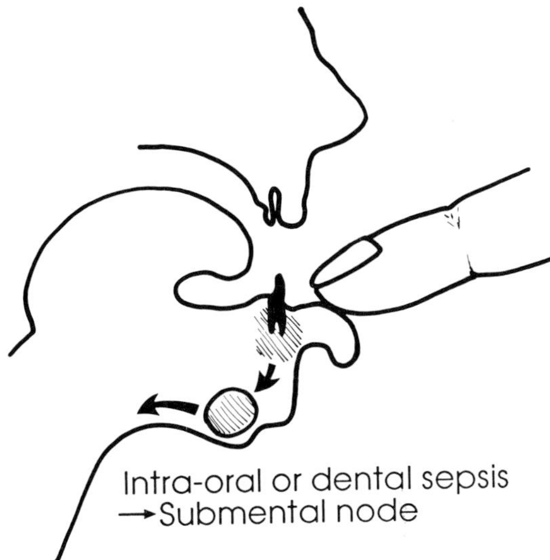

Fig. 9.30: *Examination of the teeth and floor of the mouth to look for a septic focus.*

GOLDEN RULES

Torticollis

(1) Bone growth is dependent on normal neuromuscular activity – therefore, immobilization of half of the face leads to hypoplasia of adjacent facial bones.
(2) Hemihypoplasia of the face is a crucial physical sign because it indicates the need for early surgery.
(3) Beware of torticollis where the sternomastoid is *not* tight – another cause *must* be found.
(4) A tight sternomastoid causes rotation of the head to the opposite side in infants (because they do not compensate consciously for eye tilt).
(5) In older children (after walking), the horizontal plane of the eyes is maintained at the expense of development of secondary deformity of the shoulders and spine.

The side of the neck

(1) Swellings present at birth are haemartomata (lymphangioma, cavernous haemangioma).
(2) The sternomastoid muscle provides the key to localization of lateral neck lumps.
(3) Beware the hidden focus: the entire head and neck is drained by the jugular lymph nodes – enlargement of these nodes necessitates a search for disease elsewhere.
(4) Beware low cervical swellings – they can displace or even compress the trachea.

Midline neck swellings

(1) Examination of a midline cervical swelling includes inspection of the mouth, palpation of the thyroid and lateral neck, and attempted transillumination of the lump.
(2) Thyroglossal cysts are attached to the hyoid bone, and therefore tend to move with the hyoid on swallowing or protrusion of the tongue.
(3) Beware the midline 'cervical abscess'! A mid-

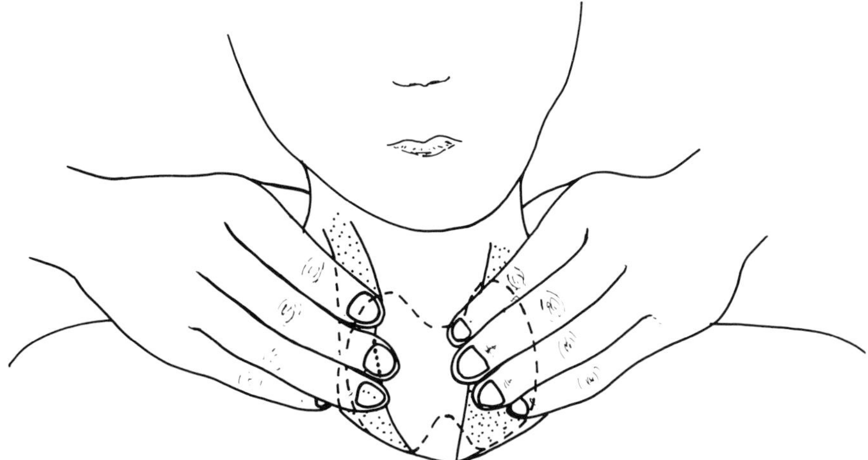

Fig. 9.31: *Thyroid palpation. 1. Stand behind the child. 2. Insinuate the tips of the fingers under the edges of the sternomastoid to feel each lobe. 3. Feel the gland while the child swallows to detect movement.*

line 'cervical abscess' is likely to be an infected thyroglossal cyst, and therefore simple incision and drainage will be inadequate treatment.

(4) A thyroglossal cyst may become infected and rupture through the skin to present as a discharging sinus.

(5) Beware the ectopic thyroid! Thyroid tissue can occur anywhere along the line of the thyroglossal tract.

(6) Where an ectopic thyroid is present, it should not be excised; it may be the only thyroid tissue.

(7) Where the identity and location of the thyroid is uncertain, a thyroid scan should be performed.

10 The head and face

THE HEAD

The rapidly growing postnatal brain must be accommodated by an increasingly large skull. The sutures allow adjacent bones of the vault to grow without compression of the brain. Abnormalities of the size and shape of the head are caused by neural tube defects, defects in cerebrospinal fluid (CSF) flow or brain growth, craniosynostosis, or deformity secondary to abnormalities of the neck (Table 10.1).

Is the head big?

The absolute size of the skull is not as important as its *relative size*, compared with the size of the rest of the body and the age of the child. Standard growth charts allow for these changes with age, but require the head to be measured accurately (Fig. 10.1). The maximum circumference is measured in the fronto-occipital plane, usually just above the ears. A non-elastic tape measure (e.g. paper) is used and serial measurements are plotted on a head circumference chart (Fig. 10.2). Two common patterns suggest an abnormally large head:

(1) a large circumference since birth, which remains relatively bigger than normal or may even increase with age, indicating a congenital or inherited abnormality;

(2) a circumference within the normal range but increasing faster than expected, indicating an acquired abnormality.

If the head is too big or enlarging too quickly, hydrocephalus is likely to be the diagnosis, but other uncommon conditions can produce a big head (Table 10.2) and need to be considered.

To determine if the big head is caused by

Table 10.1 ABNORMALITIES OF THE CRANIUM ACCORDING TO AETIOLOGY

Condition	Frequency	Aetiology
1. Hydrocephalus	Common	Intracranial haemorrhage Infection Tumour Congenital aqueduct stricture
2. Plagiocephaly	Common	Intra-uterine distortion Restricted neck movement (torticollis)
3. Microcephaly	Common	Primary brain anomaly Secondary brain injury Premature fusion of sutures
4. Encephalocele	Uncommon	Failure of neural tube fusion
5. Craniosynostosis	Uncommon	Premature closure of suture lines

Table 10.2 CAUSES OF A BIG HEAD

Common	Excess CSF (hydrocephalus) Cerebral haemorrhage in the premature baby Spina bifida Aqueduct stenosis
Uncommon	Large brain (macrocephaly) Thick skull bones (osteofibromatosis) Subdural haematoma Cyst Cystic neoplasm

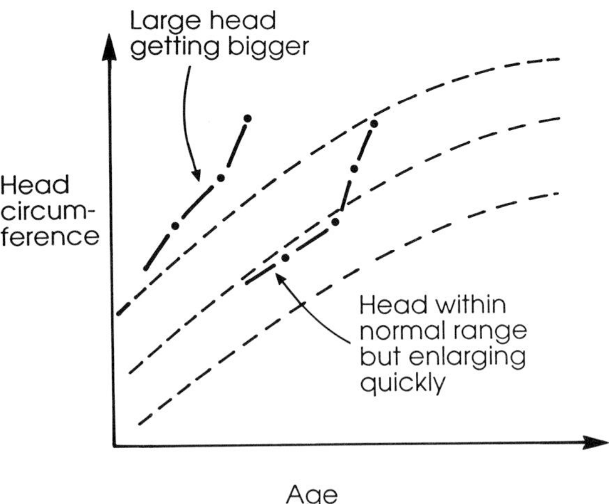

Fig. 10.2: *The head circumference chart, showing the two common patterns seen in a child with a large head. Increase in size at a rate faster than normal is suggestive of hydrocephalus.*

hydrocephalus, look for the following signs (Figs. 10.3 and 10.4). The anterior fontanelle can be seen and palpated, may be larger than normal and bulging with increased pressure from within. The sutures are widely placed, with a gap palpable between adjacent bones of the vault. The forehead tends to overhang the relatively smaller face, with the anterior horns of each dilated lateral ventricle pushing out the sides of the forehead to produce 'bossing'. Superficial, congested veins are visible under an attenuated and tight scalp. Sutures not commonly open, such as the metopic and lambdoid sutures, may be palpated. The eyes appear to deviate downwards to give the so-called 'setting-sun' appearance. The explanation for this is not completely understood but may be compression of brain stem oculomotor connections. Occasionally, the shape of the occiput is helpful since the size of the posterior fossa is determined by the type and site of the obstruction to CSF (Fig. 10.5). Percussion of the skull produces a higher-pitched, drum-like resonance compared with normal (Fig.

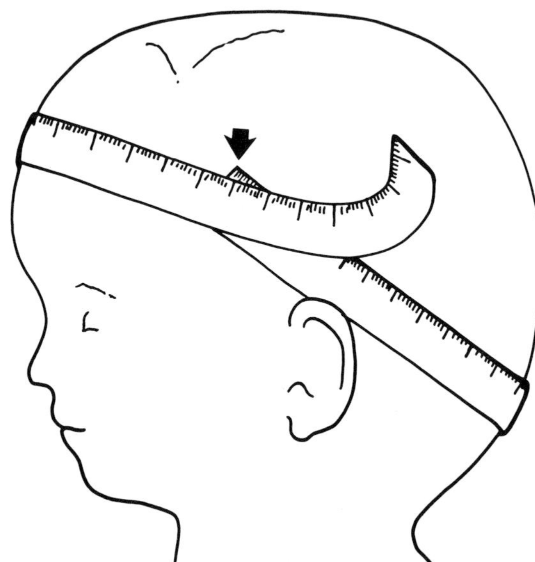

Fig. 10.1: *Measuring head circumference. 1. Record the maximum fronto-occipital length. 2. Use a non-elastic tape-measure. 3. Plot the result on a head circumference chart.*

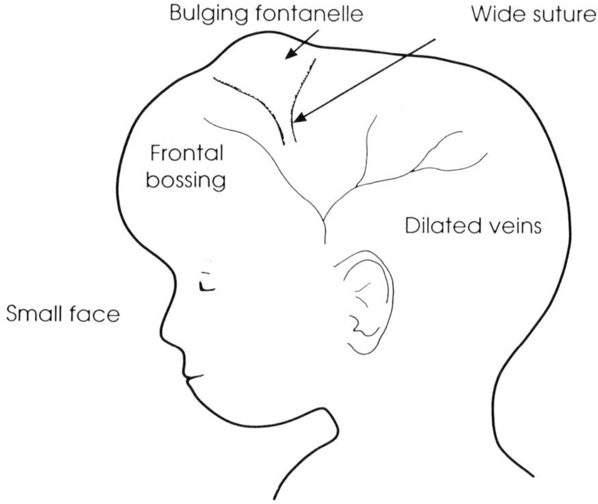

Fig. 10.3: *The clinical signs of hydrocephalus (lateral view).*

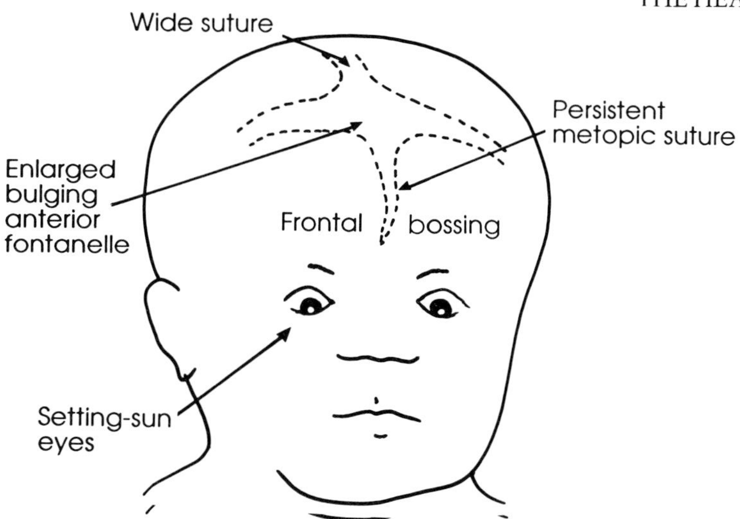

Fig. 10.4: *The clinical signs of hydrocephalus (anterior view).*

10.6), a sound which has been likened to that of a cracked earthenware pot in the older child where the sutures are interdigitating, and a more hollow percussion note in the infant.

The child should be taken to a dark room for transillumination of the skull (Fig. 10.7). A very bright torch is needed, and can provide useful information even before radiological investigation is undertaken. Extreme dilatation of all the ventricles with little brain present will make the entire vault transilluminate, whereas a localized cyst or subdural hygroma (haematoma which has been gradually replaced by CSF) will produce focal areas of transillumination.

All children with a proven or suspiciously large head should be referred to a paediatric centre for detailed investigation. Skull x-rays, ultrasound (if the fontanelles are open), computed tomography scan or radionuclide CSF dynamic scan may be performed. Magnetic resonance scanning may become used more widely in the future.

The classic signs and symptoms of hydro-

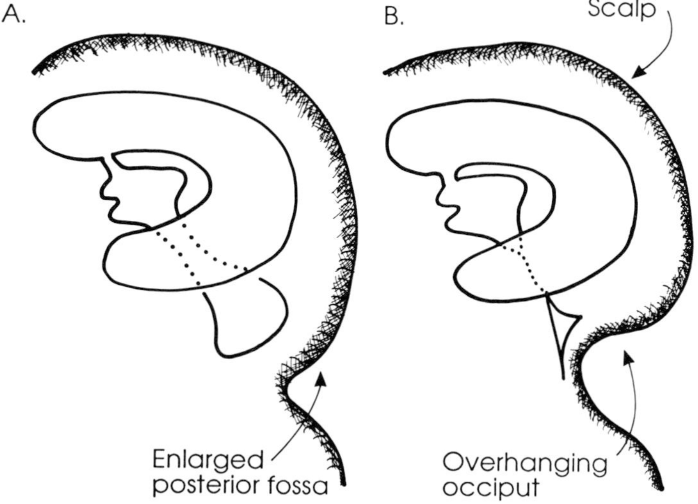

Fig. 10.5: *The effect of dilatation of the fourth ventricle on the shape of the back of the head in communicating hydrocephalus (A), and aqueduct stenosis (B).*

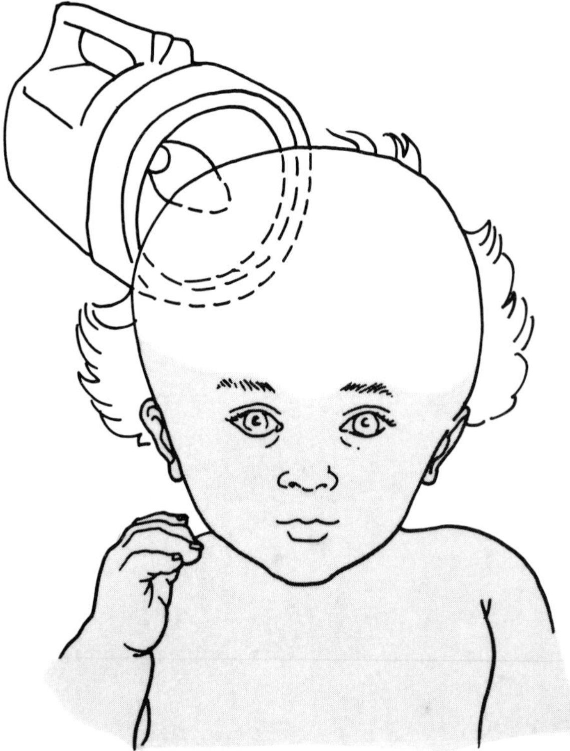

Fig. 10.7: *Transillumination of the skull for hydrocephalus. Water-filled, large ventricles transilluminate if the child is examined in a very dark room using a large, bright torch.*

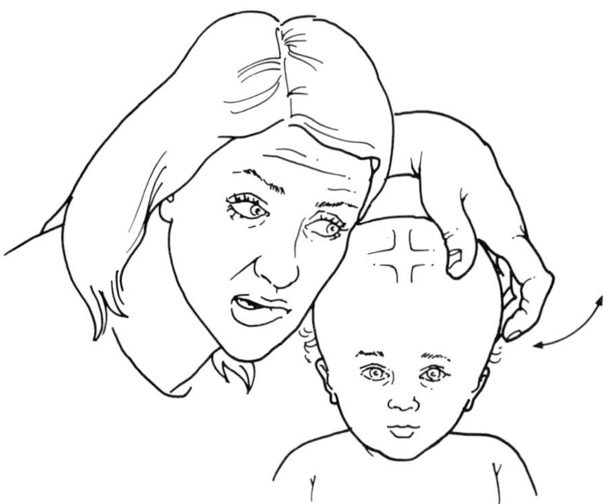

Fig. 10.6: *The 'cracked-pot' sign: the wide gap in the sutures changes the resonance of the skull on tapping and produces a dull thud.*

cephalus are seen only in the infant, before closure of the sutures (Fig. 10.8). After closure of the sutures, the cranium cannot expand readily, and an increase in its contents leads to an increase in intracranial pressure. The sutures close at about four years of age, or earlier if previous hydrocephalus has been treated with a ventricular shunt. This may have drained the CSF too well and allowed the bones to stick together before the brain tissue expanded to fill the space. The cardinal symptoms and signs of raised intracranial pressure are vomiting (often early in the morning), headache and papilloedema.

Assessment of possible raised intracranial pressure must take into account whether there is a CSF shunt already present (Fig. 10.9). If there is a shunt in situ, it is highly likely that malfunction of the shunt is the cause. If there is no shunt, the cause is likely to be a neoplasm, unless the child has had meningitis. Therefore, in taking a history of a child with headaches and vomiting, knowledge of previous shunt surgery is vital. It is also important to know whether there has been a delay or deterioration in milestones and mental development, or a change in behaviour, which suggest a slowly progressive lesion (e.g. tumour). Depression of the conscious state may be present, but often this is a late feature and a normal conscious state does not necessarily indicate that all is well. The pulse and blood pressure are classic signs of raised intracranial pressure. However, in childhood these parameters may remain normal until the intracranial pressure is so high that the patient is unconscious and close to death.

Examination of the retina will confirm the presence of papilloedema, the cardinal sign of raised intracranial pressure (see below). The sides of the head behind and above the ears should be palpated to find the ventriculoperitoneal shunt and test its function (see below). If there is no shunt present, a cerebral neoplasm is possible and localizing neurological signs should be sought.

Looking for papilloedema

Small children are not able to keep their eyes still which makes examination of the optic disc difficult. Since the disc and peripheral vessels are in the same focal plane, the ophthalmoscope is focused

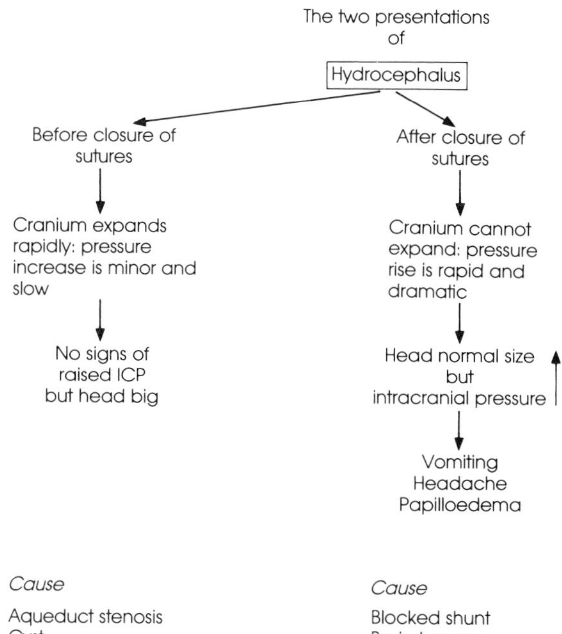

Fig. 10.8: *The two presentations of hydrocephalus in childhood, depending on whether the sutures are open or fused.*

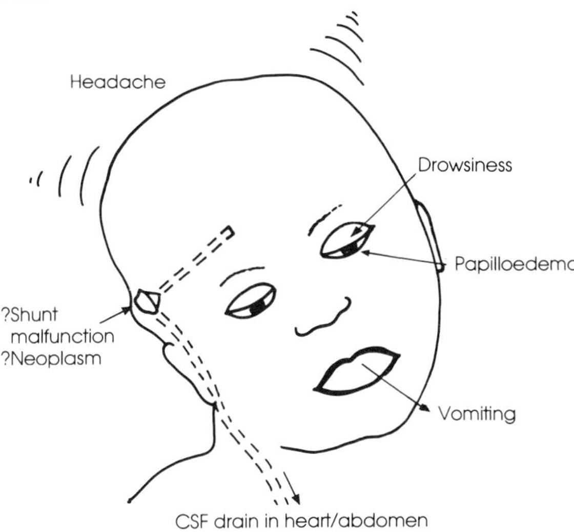

Fig. 10.9: *The presentation of hydrocephalus after fusion of the sutures: there may be a history of previous shunt surgery and/or mental impairment. Shunt blockage is the likely cause if hydrocephalus was treated previously. If there is no CSF shunt, localizing neurological signs should be sought to exclude a brain tumour.*

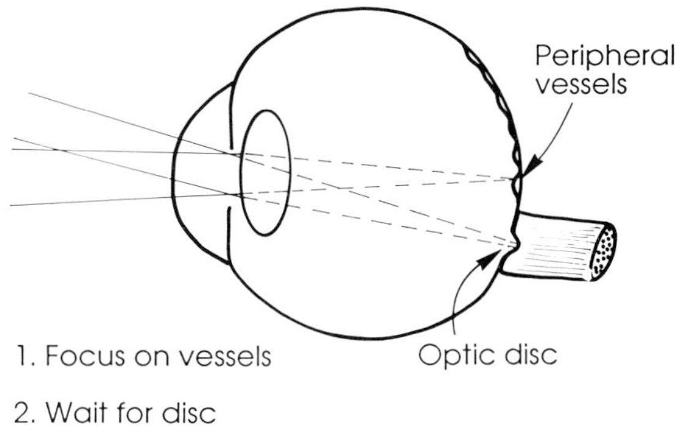

Fig. 10.10: *Examination of the eye in a child with possible papilloedema. Since the peripheral vessels and disc are in the same focal plane, get the vessels in focus first and wait for the disc to move into view. The child's eye moves frequently because of the low level of concentration.*

on the vessels first (Fig. 10.10). The examiner waits for the disc to move into the field of view as the child's eye moves.

When papilloedema is present, the disc is blurred at the normal focal length at which the peripheral vessels are clear (Fig. 10.11). The blurred image is easily mistaken for inadequate technique or an uncooperative child. If the peripheral retina is in focus, blurring in the region of the disc is a crucial sign and should not be ignored. Papilloedema can be confirmed by altering the focus to bring the top of the swollen disc into view, which allows the distended vessels and haemorrhages to be seen clearly (Fig. 10.12). Pharmacological dilatation of the pupil is useful if a clear view of the disc is not readily obtained.

Assessing a ventriculoperitoneal shunt

Most shunt devices used to drain CSF from the ventricles have three components (Fig. 10.13). There is a valvular pump, which is dome-shaped or tubular and is placed under the scalp. Attached to the pump are two catheters, one passing through a burr hole and the cerebrum into the dilated lateral ventricle, and the other passing subcutaneously from the parietal region via the neck and the chest wall (anteriorly or posteriorly) into the peritoneal cavity. Most modern catheters

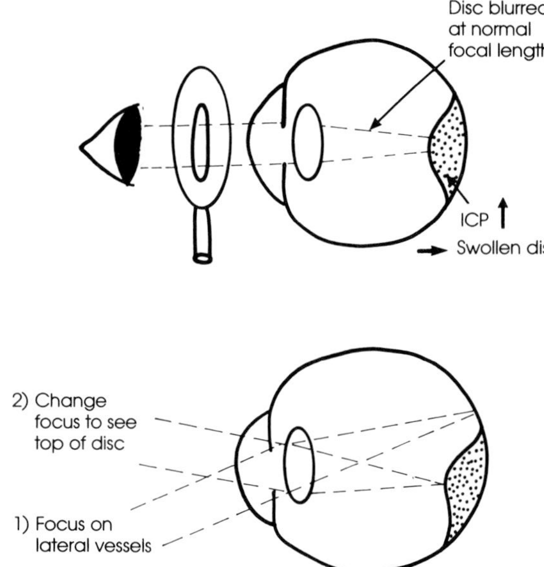

Fig. 10.11: *Papilloedema: a blurred image may be papilloedema or poor technique. Adjust the focus to the usual position (eye distortion is rare in young children). See the lateral vessels first, then alter the focus to see the swollen disc.*

contain a radio-opaque marker which enables the tubing to be seen on x-ray. The valvular pump allows CSF to flow in one direction only, and different models have valves which open at different pressures. Lower pressure valves are used in infants before closure of the sutures, since the intracranial pressure remains relatively lower.

The ventriculoperitoneal shunt is readily tested for normal function by compression of the reservoir with a finger (Fig. 10.14). CSF is forced down the exit catheter into the peritoneal cavity: it cannot re-enter the distal catheter because it has a slit valve at the end. When the finger is removed, the reservoir refills from the ventricular catheter within a few seconds or minutes, depending on the patency and pressure gradient across the ventricular catheter. Minor obstruction or valve dysfunction may be overcome by manual pumping – a procedure which is useful when the child is unwell from raised intracranial pressure.

Shunt malfunction may occur if either catheter becomes blocked (Fig. 10.15). Distal obstruction caused by debris or omental wrapping prevents the reservoir being emptied, while failure of the

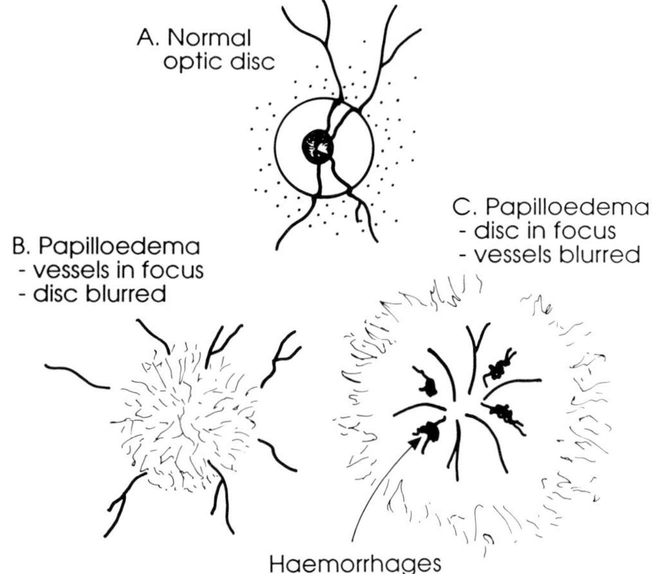

Fig. 10.12: *The optic disc as it appears normally (A), in papilloedema when the peripheral vessels are in focus (B), and in papilloedema when the disc itself is in focus (C).*

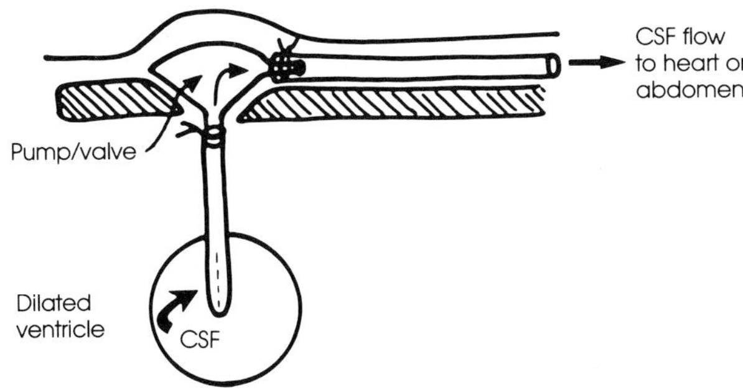

Fig. 10.13: *The components of the common ventriculoperitoneal shunt.*

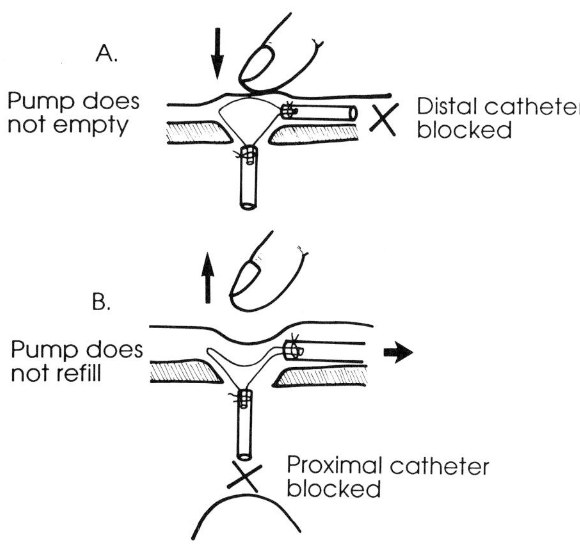

Fig. 10.15: *The effects of catheter blockage on shunt function.* A. *Distal obstruction, caused usually by omental wrapping secondary to infection, prevents emptying of the pump.* B. *Proximal obstruction, usually with choroid plexus or debris, or because the end is outside the ventricle, prevents the pump refilling after compression.*

reservoir to refill suggests proximal catheter blockage. Low-grade infection of the catheter causes inflammatory exudate to accumulate in the tubing, stimulates the omentum to wrap itself around its lower end, and may induce the formation of a pseudocyst around the peritoneal end. Proximal obstruction is produced by occlusion of the holes by choroid, brain, clots or inflammatory debris, but is less likely to indicate infection.

Leakage of CSF produces a different clinical picture (Fig. 10.16). The CSF may escape from the ventricle around the ventricular catheter, especially if this is blocked, and the reservoir will be covered by a cystic swelling of CSF. Leakage may occur at a loose connection or through a hole in the pump tubing. Disconnection of the distal catheter is common, and is caused by traction on the catheter through movement and growth. CSF accumulates within the fibrous tunnel which normally develops around the silastic catheter, and the catheter slides down the tunnel and curls up inside the peritoneum. The disconnection produces a partial obstruction to CSF drainage, but

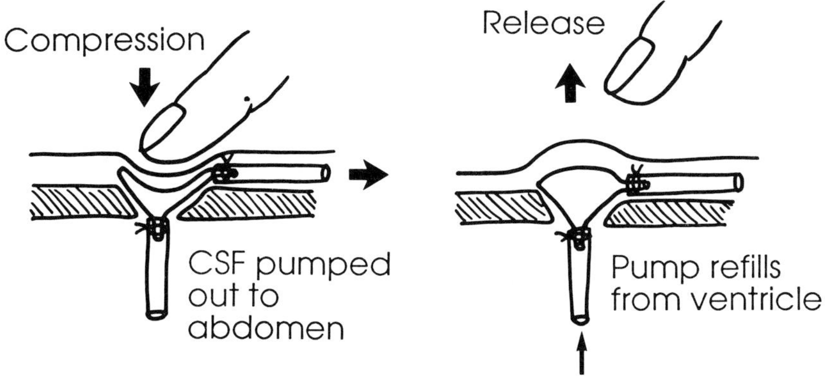

Fig. 10.14: *Testing for shunt patency by manual compression and release of the pump.*

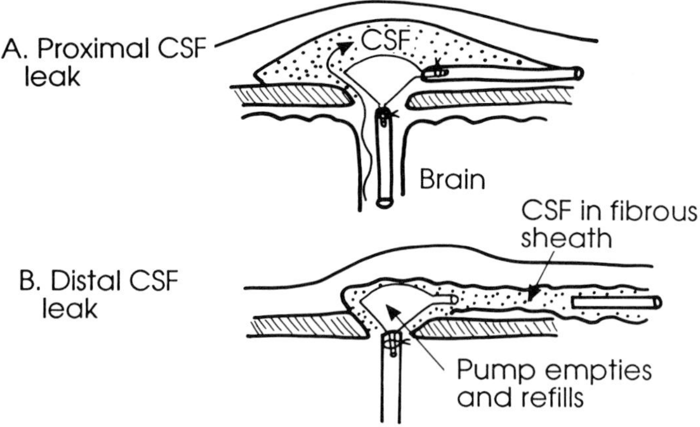

Fig. 10.16: *The effects of proximal (A) or distal (B) CSF leaks caused by disconnected tubing or puncture. When the distal catheter is loose, it slides down the fibrous tunnel and curls up in the heart or abdomen. The pump will empty and refill because the valve to prevent refilling is on the end of the distal catheter.*

the pump will feel normal, because CSF can re-enter the reservoir from the subcutaneous tunnel. This apparently normal function of the pump can occur even when there is complete obstruction proximally! Skull and abdominal x-rays will demonstrate that the shunt is disconnected or malpositioned.

Is the head too small?

A small head is not a condition which normally requires surgical investigation since the usual cause is primary failure of brain growth. The important surgical condition is premature fusion of the sutures, but this is rare. A clinical diagnosis is made readily on inspection of the shape of the cranium (Fig. 10.17). Signs of raised intracranial pressure, which may be present as well, must be actively sought.

Is the head the wrong shape?

Abnormal or premature fusion of the sutures (craniosynostosis) will distort the shape of the

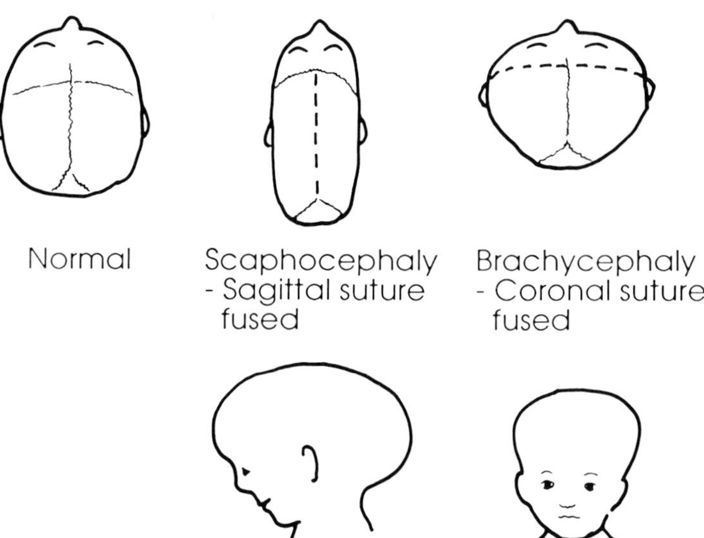

Fig. 10.17: *Skull shapes caused by craniosynostosis.*

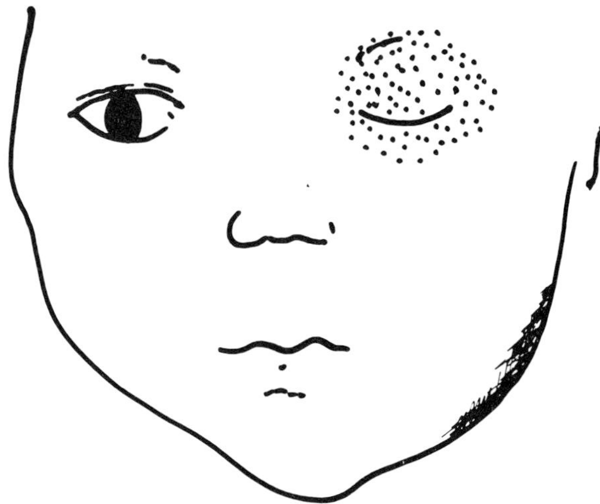

Fig. 10.18: *The red, swollen eyelids with orbital cellulitis.*

vault (Fig. 10.17), but the commonest anomaly is plagiocephaly, associated with torticollis (see Chapter 9).

Is there a lump on the head?

Lumps in the midline between the nose anteriorly and the foramen magnum posteriorly may be manifestations of incomplete fusion of the neural tube or its overlying ectoderm. Dermoid cysts, similar to the common external angular dermoid, are found occasionally and have the same clinical features (see below). Neural tube defects on the head produce an encephalocele or, occasionally, a meningocele. These abnormalities are described in detail in Chapter 18.

FACIAL LUMPS AND ANOMALIES

The common lesions around the face which require 'surgical' opinion are related to the eyes, ears and parotid gland. (Table 10.3)

The orbital region

Orbital cellulitis is a potentially dangerous infection because of the risk of intracranial extension. Erythema and oedema of the lids are obvious. The erythema is bright red and, if untreated, rapidly extends beyond the orbit. The swelling causes loss of the upper lid skin crease at an early stage and, with increasing involvement of both lids, causes complete closure of the palpebral fissure (Fig. 10.18). A pustular discharge will confirm the diagnosis and provide material for culture. Allergic reactions around the orbit may produce a similar appearance, but in most cases the less severe inflammatory reaction produces a less fiery appearance and there is absence of fever and systemic signs of sepsis. Allergic inflammation, depending on the cause, affects both eyes more evenly than does orbital cellulitis, where the process commences as a unilateral infection which

Table 10.3 CAUSES OF ABNORMALITIES OF THE FACE

Anatomical region	Condition	Frequency
Orbit	Cellulitis	Common
	External angular dermoid	Common
	Internal angular dermoid	Rare
	Anterior encephalocele	Rare
Ears	Pre-auricular sinus (helix)	Common
	Pre-auricular tag (tragus)	Common
	Bat ears	Common
	Microtia	Uncommon
	Low-set ears	Common
Parotid	Lymphadenitis	Common
	Parotid infection – mumps	Common
	– sialectasis	
	Lymphangioma (cystic hygroma)	Uncommon

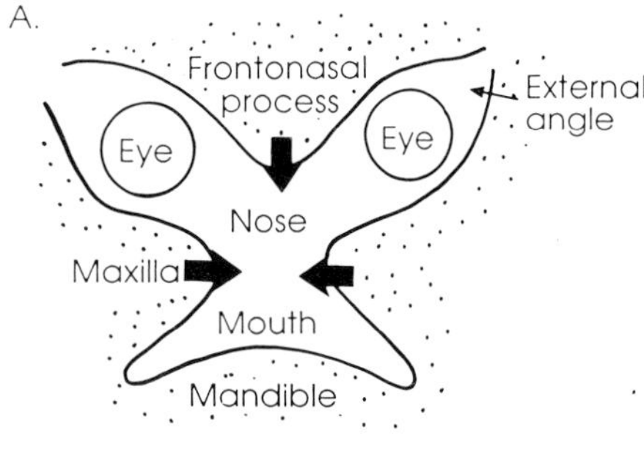

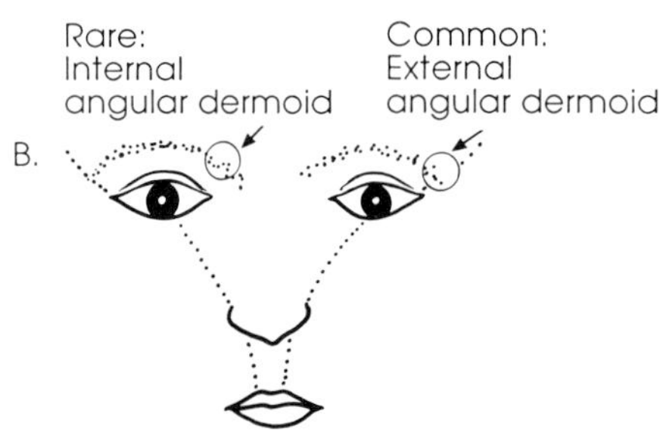

Fig. 10.19: A. *The early development of the face showing the fusion line at the external angle of the eye.* B. *Sites of angular dermoids. The internal angular dermoid is rare because this is not a line of fusion. Angular dermoids are usually tense (under the pericranium), dent the outer table of the skull and contain yellow/white sebaceous material.*

only in its later stages spreads to the contralateral side. The infecting organisms are usually *Streptococcus* and *Staphylococcus*. Treatment should be aggressive and instituted early. If the cellulitis is advanced or does not respond rapidly to oral antibiotics, the child should be admitted to hospital to receive high-dose intravenous antibiotics.

The commonest and simplest anomaly near the eye is a congenital dermoid cyst which occurs at the external angle of the orbit. The face develops from fusion of the frontonasal and maxillary processes around the eye (Fig. 10.19). The line of fusion above and lateral to the optic placode is the commonest site for a dermoid to form: a nest of skin cells becomes separated from the surface and develops into a cyst which is found on the rim of the bony orbit under the lateral end of the eyebrow (Fig. 10.19). Rarely, a dermoid may occur at the internal angle. Angular dermoids contain desquamated epithelium and skin secretions, and may have a faint white/yellow colour because of the high cholesterol content.

The cyst is firm (almost hard) and relatively immobile because it lies under the pericranium in a shallow cavity in the skull (Fig. 10.20). The outer table may be attenuated or absent. There is rarely a communication through the skull to produce the

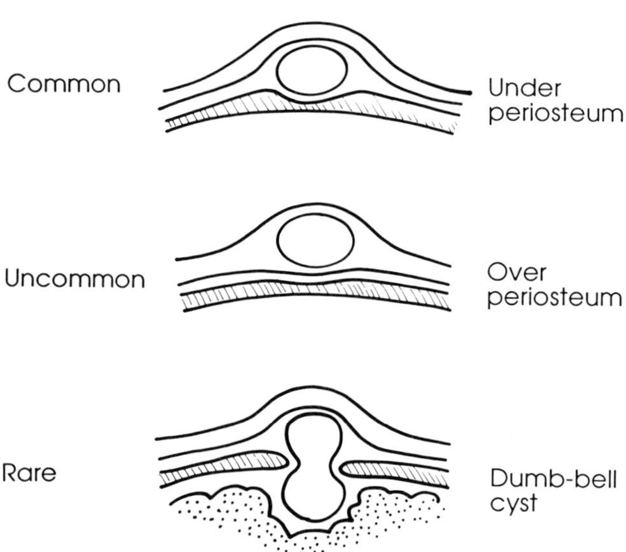

Fig. 10.20: *The different relationships of the external angular dermoid to the pericranium and skull bones.*

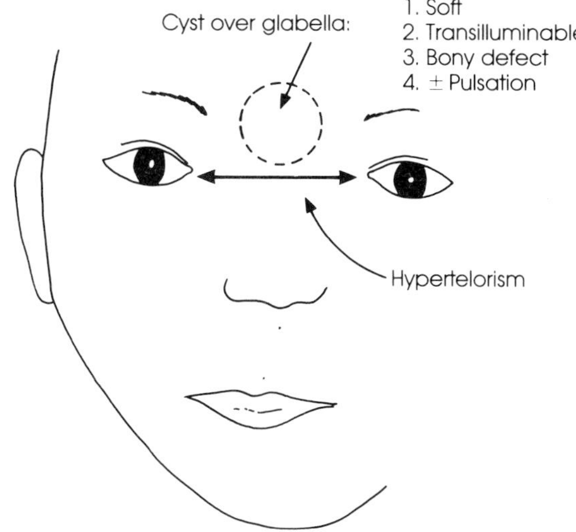

Fig. 10.21: *The site and characteristics of an anterior encephalocele secondary to anterior fusion deficiency of the neural tube.*

dangerous 'dumb-bell' cyst. Sometimes, the dermoid may be above the pericranium, in which situation it is softer, more mobile and may demonstrate fluctuance. There are no signs of inflammation.

Rarely, there are lumps between the eyes or over the bridge of the nose. The midline is a primitive site of fusion on the head during closure of the neural tube, hence encephaloceles can occur in this location. (Fig. 10.21). The mass feels soft and cystic, because of contained CSF, and may transilluminate if there is little brain tissue within it. Careful palpation of the base of the lesion will reveal a defect in the frontal bones. The cyst may conduct pressure waves and arterial pulsation from the subarachnoid space. Deficient fusion of the anterior neural tube will be associated with orbital displacement laterally, causing hypertelorism, where the distance between the palpebral fissures is abnormally large. Dermoid cysts may occur rarely in the midline (internal angular dermoids) but can be distinguished from encephaloceles because their characteristics are similar to external angular dermoids.

The ears

The pinna develops as an outgrowth of epithelium around the otic placode, which forms the tympanic membrane. The process is complex and prone to minor aberrations of development, many of which are common e.g. 'bat ears', pre-auricular sinus and skin tags (pre-auricular accessory ear) (Figs. 10.22–10.24)

Bat ear is a simple deformity of the pinna which is common and often requires no treatment. The antihelical fold is diminished or absent, causing the outer helix to be projected too far from the side of the head (Fig. 10.22).

Pre-auricular sinuses are extremely common and are found at the anterior end of the outer helix. Their only feature may be a tiny inconspicuous punctum which is often hidden by hair. If secondary infection occurs in the blind-ending sinus (which may be surrounded by cartilage), the side of the face near the upper helix will be inflamed (Fig. 10.23). The centre of the abscess is anterior to the punctum because the sinus track runs forwards away from the ear. This means that infection arising at the base is distant from the opening. The swelling needs to be distinguished from parotid swellings anterior to the tragus (see below).

Skin tags near the pinna are found anterior to the tragus and are forms of duplication of the pinna (Fig. 10.24). They may be floppy tags with a narrow stalk (and therefore readily removed by ligation of the base), or have a wide base contain-

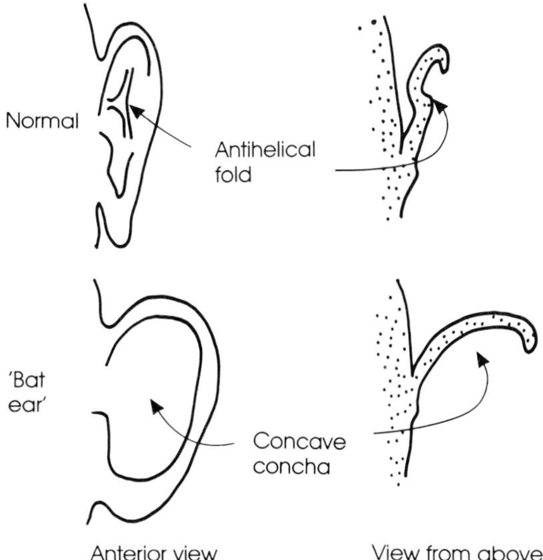

Fig. 10.22: *The features of bat ears compared with the normal ear.*

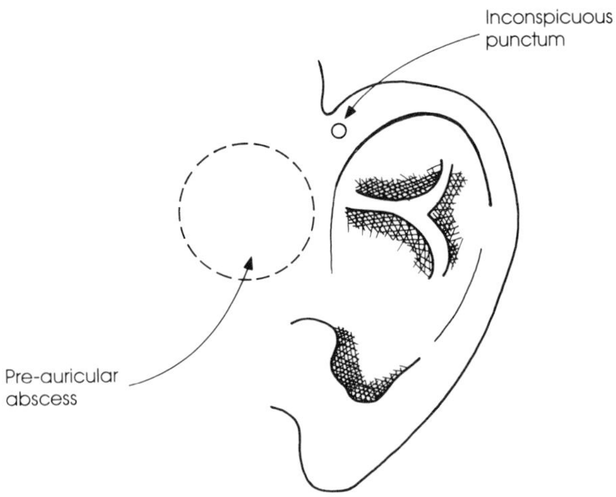

Fig. 10.23: *The infected pre-auricular sinus presents with an abscess anterior to the helix.*

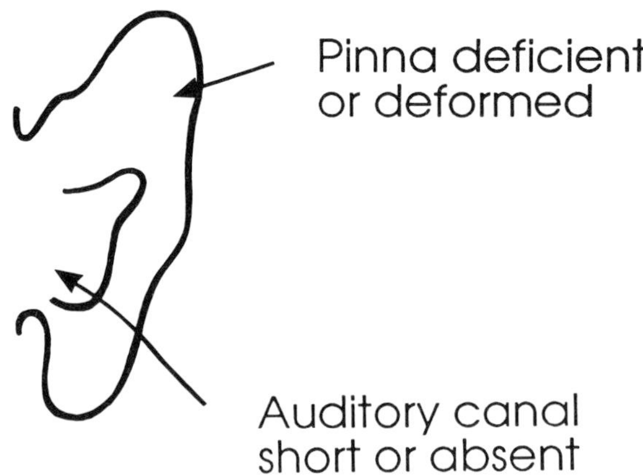

Fig. 10.25: *The characteristics of microtia.*

ing cartilage, more closely resembling an accessory ear. Palpable cartilage is important to identify because it indicates that a more formal surgical approach is required for removal.

More severe deformity or deficiency of the pinna is associated commonly with agenesis of the external auditory canal (Fig. 10.25). Presumably, the pinna requires a normal otic placode to develop normally, and in its absence remains hypoplastic. This association is confirmed by examining the auditory canal for patency. Where the canal is absent, the presence of an inner ear should be determined, because the hearing defect may be overcome. Weber's test is the easiest to perform in small children as they need only determine whether the sound is louder in the normal ear or evenly heard by both sides (Fig. 10.26 and 10.27).

One rather non-specific, yet common, anomaly of the ears is low position (Fig. 10.28). Normally, the top of the pinna is above a horizontal line through the eyes: in low-set ears, the pinna is lower than this plane. It is an important sign to observe because of its association with multiple anomalies in the baby.

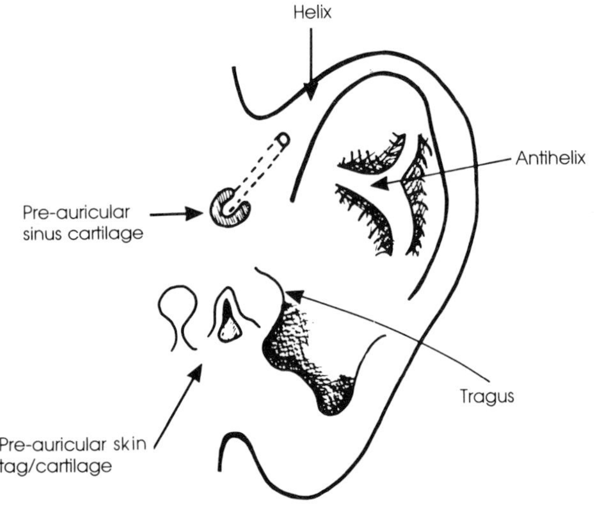

Fig. 10.24: *Pre-auricular sinuses and skin tags occur in different locations: the sinus is on the anterior edge of the helix, while the tag is adjacent to the tragus.*

The parotid region

The rarity of parotid tumours in childhood means that they are not considered in the differential diagnosis, except in rare circumstances. Most commonly, the parotid is swollen because of mumps, and this must be excluded in any patient with a parotid lump before other diagnoses are considered. Usually, mumps affects both parotid glands, and unilateral involvement should arouse suspicion of an alternative diagnosis. The history of contact one to three weeks previously, and the signs and symptoms of viraemia, usually rule out a surgical cause for the swollen parotid. Orchitis and pancreatitis may occur as complications of mumps, but they are rare in the prepubertal child.

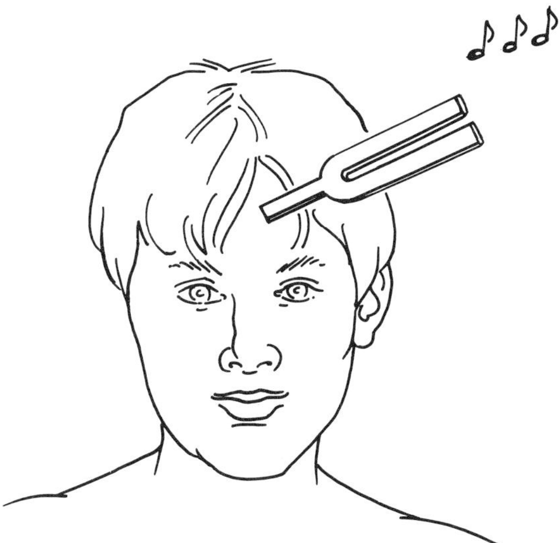

Fig. 10.26: *Testing for the inner ear in microtia. 1. Strike the fork and place it on the forehead. 2. The sound is heard in both ears if the inner ears are normal. 3. The sound is heard only in the normal ear if the inner ear is absent on the side of microtia.*

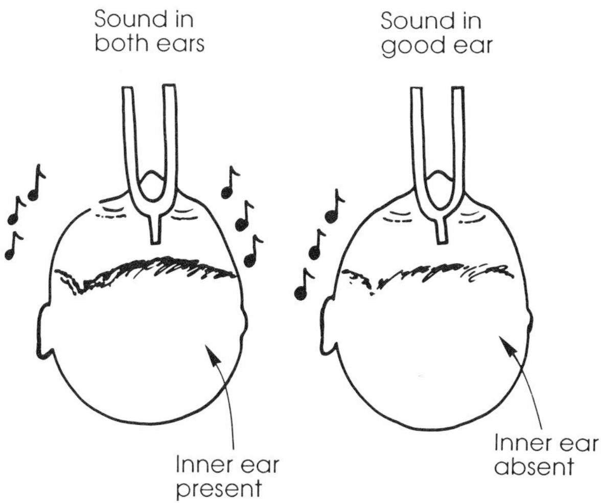

Fig. 10.27: *The effect of absence of the inner ear on sound: sound from the forehead tuning fork reaches the inner ear by bone conduction.*

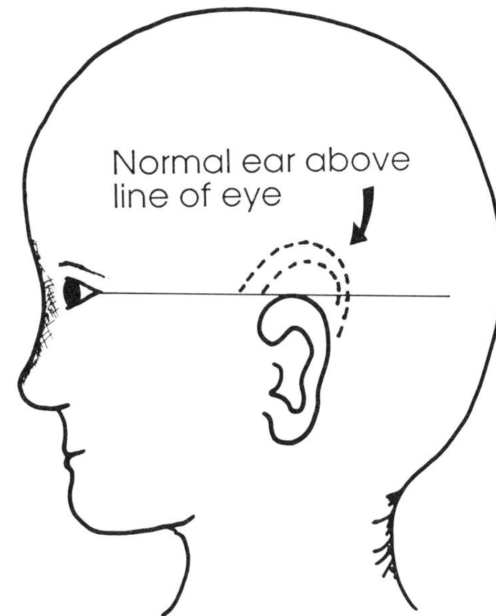

Fig. 10.28: *Low-set ears: this is a common sign in babies with multiple anomalies or inherited syndromes.*

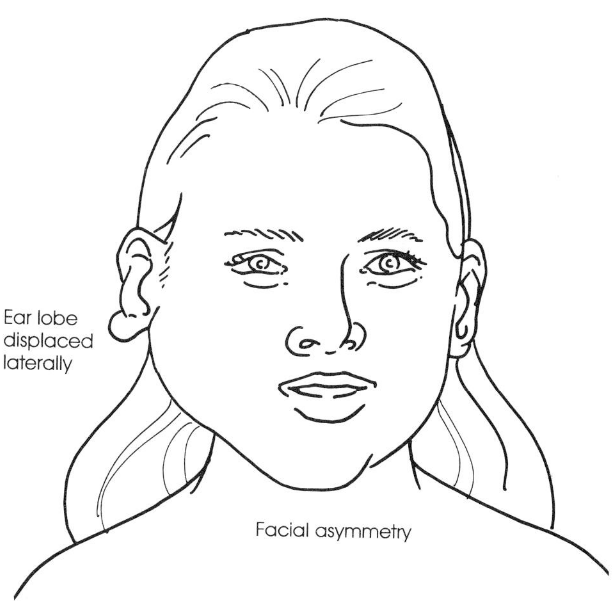

Fig. 10.29: *Anterior view of parotid swelling.*

When the history is of unilateral and recurrent swelling, then the likely diagnosis is sialectasis. Accumulation of saliva within the gland and intermittent bacterial infection occur as a result of an ectatic duct system. Stasis of saliva allows infection to persist. The gland is swollen and painful when saliva production is maximal, such as with the thought of food or during eating. The side of the face becomes swollen (Fig. 10.29), forms a 'J' around the antero-inferior part of the pinna, and covers the angle of the mandible (Fig. 10.30). Inflammatory signs (heat, redness) are not conspicuous because the infection is low-grade and contained by the parotid capsule. Proof of the presence of sialectasis is obtained by examining the opening of the parotid duct inside the mouth (Fig. 10.31). The duct opens in the superior buccal sulcus opposite the second molar. When the gland is massaged, pustular fluid exudes from the opening, which may be slightly inflamed. The ease with which the infected saliva can be squeezed out of the gland is the reason why massage is so helpful in its treatment.

Enlargement of lymph nodes in the substance of the parotid gland must be distinguished from swelling of the gland itself (Fig. 10.32). Lymphatic enlargement produces discrete masses, whereas parotid swelling causes the whole area to enlarge. Lymphatic swellings may be caused by acute (bacterial/viral) infection, or chronic (MAIS) infection. On occasions, neoplasms occur in the parotid lymphatics, and the characteristic signs are described in the section on neck lumps (Chapter 9).

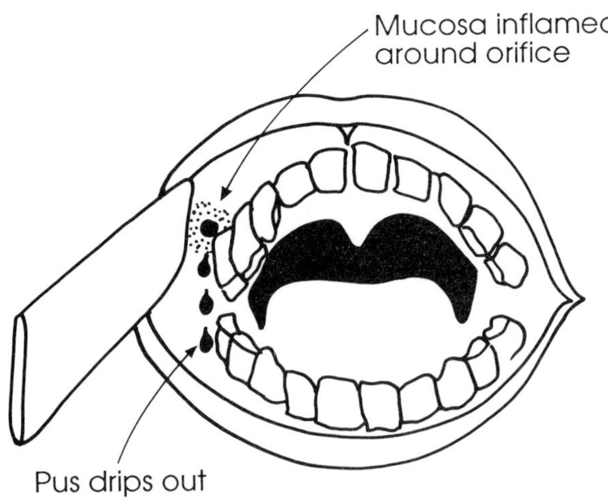

Fig. 10.31: *Examination of the opening of the parotid duct in sialectasis. 1. Pull the cheek laterally with a spatula. 2. The duct opening is opposite the second upper molar. 3. A pustular discharge and periductal inflammation signify sialectasis.*

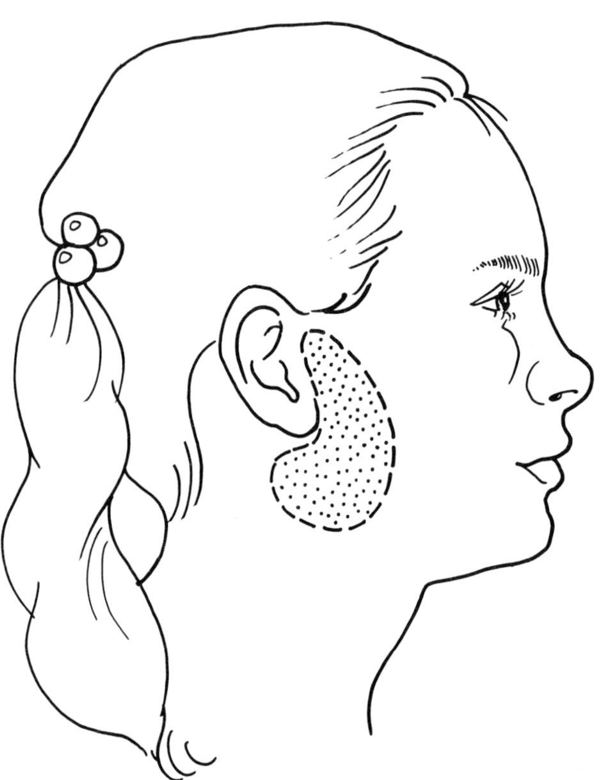

Fig. 10.30: *Lateral view of parotid swelling showing its relationship to the ear and angle of the mandible.*

GOLDEN RULES

Hydrocephalus

(1) Hydrocephalus produces a big head only before closure of the sutures.
(2) Hydrocephalus produces raised intracranial pressure after closure of the sutures.
(3) Headache, vomiting and papilloedema are the cardinal features of raised intracranial pressure: depression of consciousness is a late feature and its absence should not divert the examiner. Low pulse and high blood pressure are very late signs of raised intracranial pressure in childhood.

Face

(1) Beware of infections of the face: speedy diagnosis and aggressive treatment is required to prevent thrombophlebitis spreading to the cavernous sinus.
(2) Beware the fluctuant angular dermoid: it may have an intracranial extension.
(3) Beware 'cysts' over the glabella: they may contain meninges and brain!
(4) Remember to search for a punctum (it may be hidden by hair) when an abscess occurs in front of the helix of the ear.

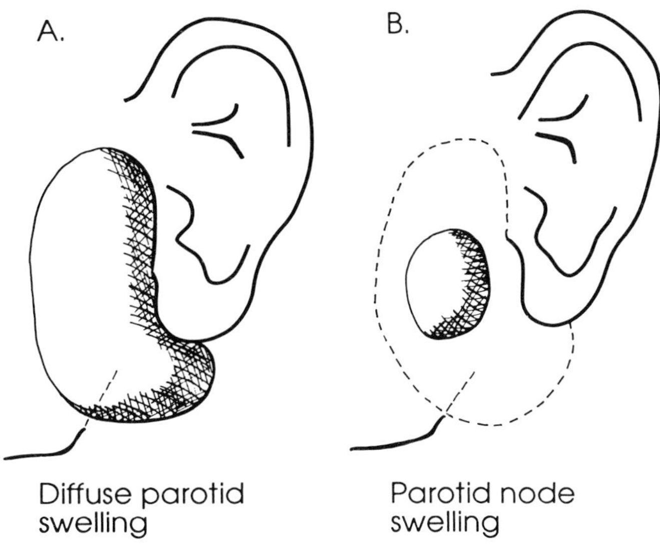

Fig. 10.32: *The difference between a diffuse parotid gland swelling* (A), *and a swollen lymph node in the parotid area* (B). *A localized lump is a lymph node infection or tumour.*

(5) Always test the hearing in microtia: the presence of an inner ear may permit a hearing aid.
(6) Beware low-set ears in the baby: other congenital anomalies may be present.
(7) Unilateral or recurrent parotid swelling is more likely to be sialectasis than atypical mumps.
(8) The mouth must always be examined in patients with parotid lesions: infected saliva can clinch the diagnosis of sialectasis.

11 The mouth

Surgical conditions arising within the mouth form a heterogeneous collection (Table 11.1), and the approach to diagnosis, therefore, depends initially on inspection of the site of origin of the lesion. Specific points in the examination of each lesion are described separately according to their site.

THE TONGUE

Tongue-tie

Tongue-tie is caused by a very short frenulum extending from the tip of the tongue to the floor of the mouth. The frenulum appears as a tight pale band which fetters the tip and, in severe cases, prevents protrusion of the tongue beyond the lower incisor teeth. The tongue may be anchored so closely to the floor of the mouth behind the lower gum that the frenulum is difficult to see. It can cause minor interference with speech, but never affects swallowing as this is a function of the posterior part of the tongue.

The aim of examination is to determine how far the tongue can protrude. Articulation is impaired when the tongue cannot protrude past the teeth (Fig. 11.1), when attempts at poking it out simply result in it rolling up (Fig. 11.2). It is, therefore, its relationship to the incisor teeth which determines the necessity for surgical division of the frenulum.

Macroglossia

Macroglossia describes real or apparent enlargement of the tongue. It is a well-known feature of

Table 11.1 PATHOLOGICAL CONDITIONS IN THE MOUTH

Site of origin	Common conditions	Uncommon conditions
Tongue	Tongue-tie	Macroglossia Lymphangiomatosis Lingual thyroid
Floor of mouth	Ranula Lymphangioma	Dermoid cyst Submandibular calculus
Gums	Alveolar abscess	Dentigerous cyst
Lips	Mucous retention cyst Cleft lip	Papilloma Cavernous haemangioma
Palate	Cleft palate	Submucous cleft palate
Oropharynx	Tonsillitis	Quinsy Retropharyngeal abscess

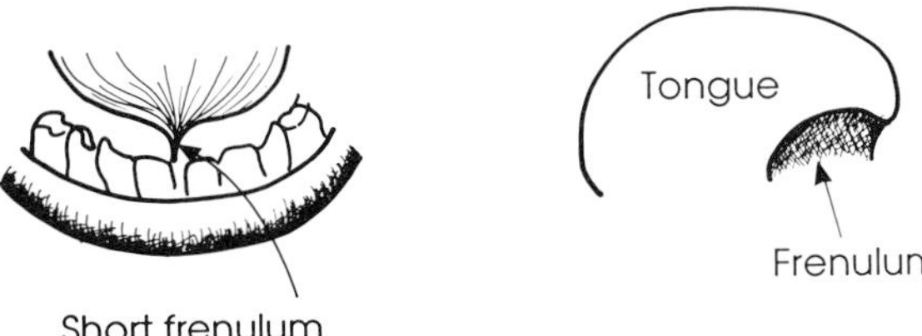

Fig. 11.1: *Tongue-tie, with a short frenulum, anchors the tip of the tongue to the floor of the mouth.*

Down's syndrome. Any space-occupying lesion inside the tongue will produce macroglossia. Alternatively, a normal tongue within a small oral cavity will appear relatively large as in Pierre Robin syndrome (Table 11.2). Macroglossia may occur as part of a generalized syndrome, e.g. hypothyroidism, Beckwith-Wiedemann syndrome, or as a manifestation of local pathology, e.g. lymphangiomatosis.

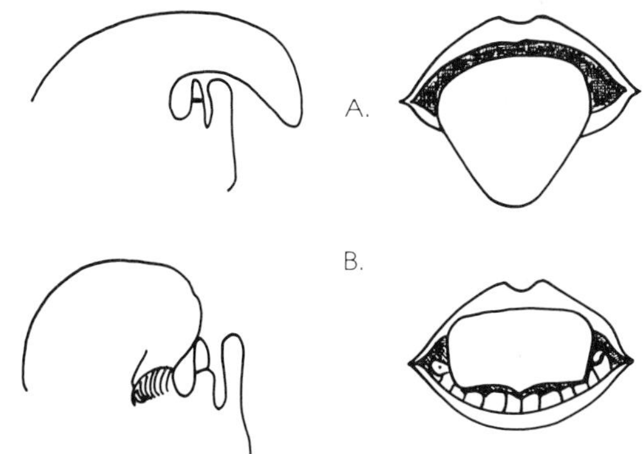

Fig. 11.2: *Protrusion of the tongue as the diagnostic test for tongue-tie requiring treatment. Normally the tongue protrudes well beyond the teeth* (A), *but in severe tongue-tie the tongue cannot be protruded past the teeth and tends to roll up* (B).

Table 11.2 THE CAUSES OF MACROGLOSSIA

Condition	Reason
Lymphangioma	Space-occupying lesion
Lymphangiomatosis	Oedema and inflammation
Haemangioma	Increased blood flow leading to overgrowth
Beckwith-Wiedemann syndrome	Muscle overgrowth from fetal insulin
Pierre Robin syndrome	Normal tongue but small mandible
Neurofibroma	Space-occupying lesion
Cretinism Down's syndrome	Large tongue – mechanism unknown

Inspection and palpation of the tongue should determine whether there is a space-occupying lesion. Where a localized lesion is found, further examination determines whether it is composed of lymphatic fluid (may transilluminate or have multiple 'blebs' on the surface), blood (vascular spaces which empty on compression) or solid tissue (feels hard and may be due to a neurofibroma or rare tumour, e.g. rhabdomyosarcoma). When the tongue is enlarged uniformly, a general examination to identify the cause involves looking for organomegaly (Beckwith-Wiedemann syndrome) or features of Down's syndrome (Fig. 11.3).

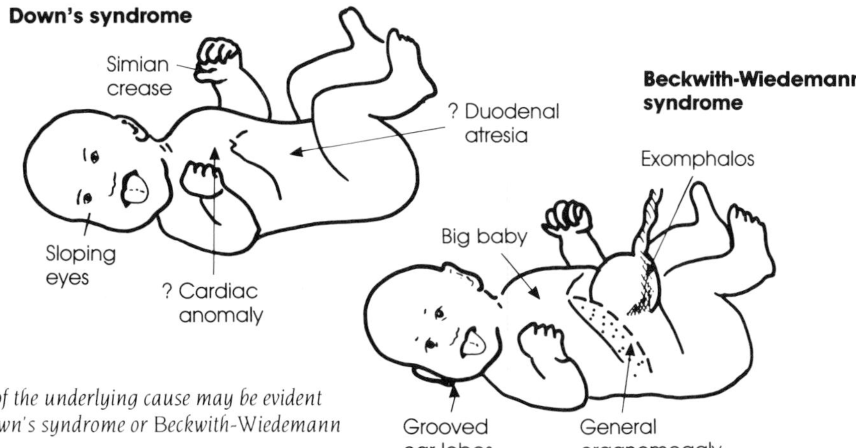

Fig. 11.3: *Macroglossia: diagnosis of the underlying cause may be evident on general examination, such as in Down's syndrome or Beckwith-Wiedemann syndrome.*

Micrognathia and a rectangular defect in the palate confirms the diagnosis of Pierre Robin syndrome (Fig. 11.4).

Lingual thyroid

The lingual thyroid is a rare congenital anomaly of the thyroid gland where it has failed to migrate from the floor of the oropharynx to the neck. It is located on the posterior aspect of the tongue producing a swelling which differs in colour and texture from the surrounding tongue. It is not always apparent until the patient is asked to protrude the tongue. It can be observed more easily if, on tongue protrusion, the anterior half of the tongue is held with a gauze swab (Fig. 11.5). The importance of the lingual thyroid is that it is the only thyroid tissue present and should not be excised. Part of the examination, therefore, involves looking at the lower part of the neck for evidence of normally sited thyroid tissue.

LESIONS IN THE FLOOR OF THE MOUTH

Ranula

Ranula is believed to be caused by mucus retention or obstruction of a sublingual salivary gland. It presents as a painless soft fluctuant swelling, easily visible beneath the tongue. There may be a predominance on one side, but it can extend across the midline beneath the frenulum of the tongue (Fig. 11.6). It has a translucent blue or grey appearance and the submandibular duct may be seen draped across its superficial surface. Larger cysts lift the tongue up towards the roof of the mouth, or extend downwards producing a lump under the chin (the 'plunging' ranula). There may be some disturbance in speech or swallowing. Most ranulas are 2-4 cm in diameter and lie immediately beneath the thin mucosal lining of the floor of the mouth. Ranulas may rupture with exudation of clear mucus and then reaccumulate over several days or weeks.

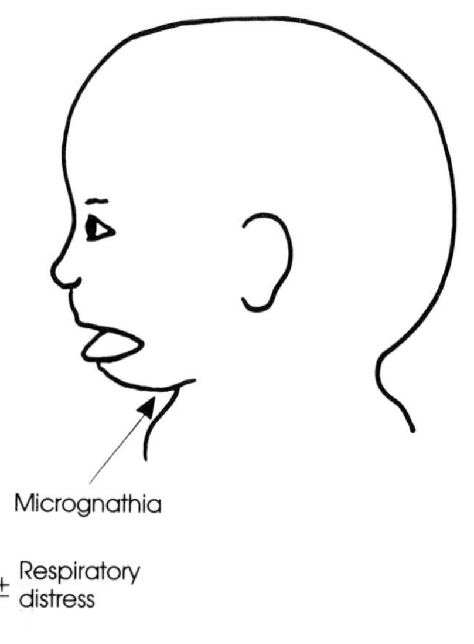

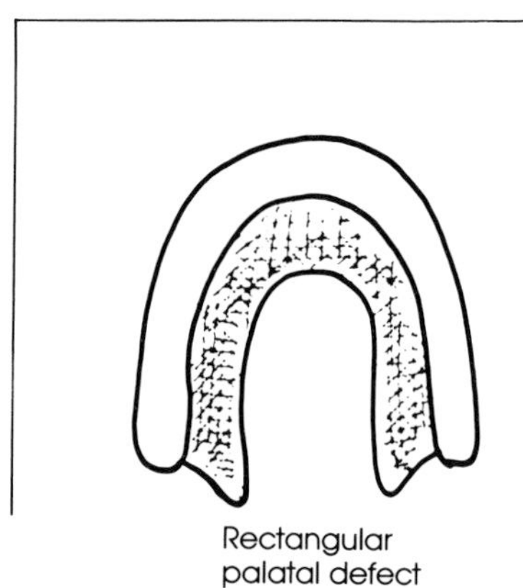

Fig. 11.4: *Micrognathia (Pierre Robin syndrome) as a cause of apparent macroglossia. The tongue is pushed up and interferes with palatal development, leading to the large cleft palate.*

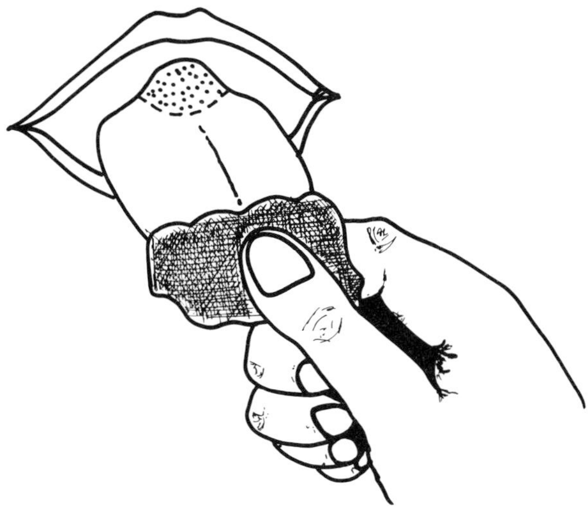

Fig. 11.5: *The technique of examining the tongue for lingual thyroid by holding the tongue forwards with a gauze swab.*

On examination, ranulas should be distinguished from dermoid cysts and lymphangiomata of the tongue. The rare dermoid cyst is firm, deeper within the tissue of the tongue and usually in the midline. There may be a tiny punctum on the surface of the tongue. A lymphangioma is less well defined and lacks the extremely superficial and discrete appearance of the ranula. The ranula is best thought of as being on top of the floor of the mouth, while the lymphangioma is in the floor of the mouth. The cystic hygroma of the floor of the mouth usually has a substantial cervical component.

Salivary duct calculus

Stones of the salivary glands are limited almost entirely to the submandibular duct. The calculus gets stuck at the narrowest part of the duct which is immediately proximal to the orifice in the floor of the mouth, lateral to the frenulum. The calculus is visible through the thin layer overlying it as a white or yellow hard lump about 2-5 mm in diameter (Fig. 11.7).

Where the calculus blocks the flow of saliva, the ipsilateral submandibular gland is enlarged and tender. It is recognized as a submandibular swelling which becomes painful immediately before and during meals. If the duct is massaged with the examining index finger, the stone may move and saliva or pus (if infection has supervened) will be extruded through the orifice. Care must be taken not to allow the stone to be lost proximally within the duct.

The thickened and inflamed submandibular duct proximal to the obstruction, and indeed the submandibular gland itself, can be palpated bimanually as shown in Fig. 11.8.

LESIONS OF THE GUMS

Alveolar abscess

The alveolar abscess results from a deep-seated infection around a permanent tooth, particularly a lower molar. The infection causes severe pain,

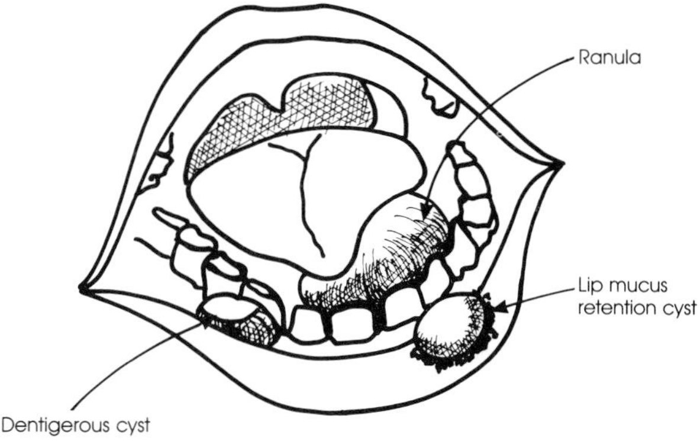

Fig. 11.6: *The three cysts within the mouth: mucus retention cyst of the lip, ranula and dentigerous cyst.*

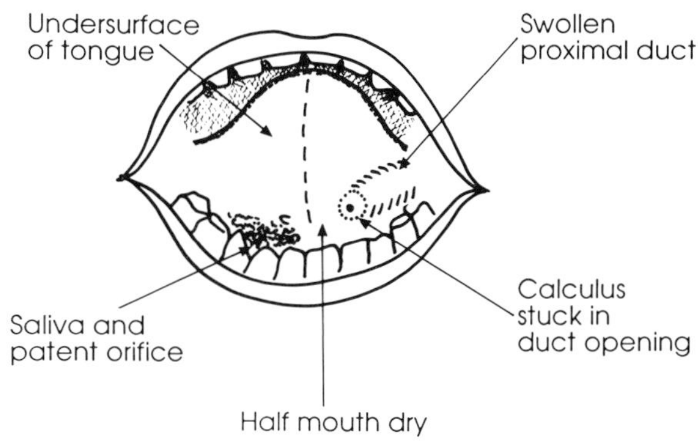

Fig. 11.7: *The signs of a submandibular duct calculus.*

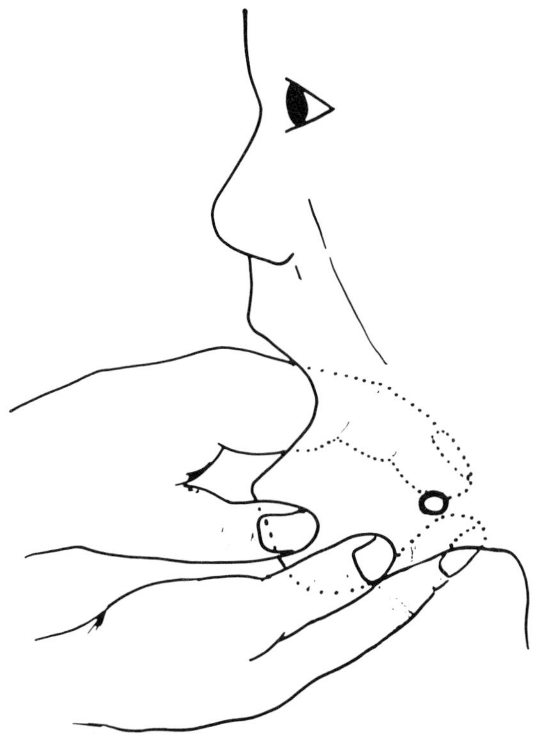

Fig. 11.8: *The technique for bimanual palpation of the floor of the mouth and the submandibular gland.*

local tenderness and fever. Uncontrolled inflammation may spread to produce a brawny cellulitis extending into the surrounding soft tissues of the mouth and jaw.

Dentigerous cyst

This is a cystic swelling surrounding an unerupted permanent tooth and is usually on the external side of the alveolus (Fig. 11.6). It is painless and is seen in children 10–12 years of age. It can be distinguished from an alveolar abscess because it causes no discomfort and shows no evidence of inflammation.

LESIONS OF THE LIPS

Mucous retention cyst

The mucous retention cyst occurs most commonly on the inside of the lower lip, but may occur anywhere on the mucosal lining of the cheek including in the gingivolabial sulcus. It tends to be smaller than the ranula and rarely exceeds 1 cm in diameter (Fig. 11.6). The retention cyst is painless (unless traumatized) and has a discrete margin. It is elevated and sometimes pedunculated (Fig. 11.9).

Two lesions may be confused with a mucous retention cyst: papilloma and cavernous haemangioma. A papilloma is a mucosal tag which results from the repeated trauma of malocclusion. A small cavernous haemangioma may lie beneath the mucosa of the lip and appear similar to a retention cyst except that it empties on pressure ('sign of emptying'), whereas a retention cyst does not. This sign may be difficult to demonstrate in small lesions because of rapid refilling, but can be displayed well if a small blunt instrument, e.g. a ball-point pen or a thermometer, is pressed firmly against the lesion.

Upper Lip Frenulum

A short upper lip frenulum may extend between the two halves of the maxillary arch and may

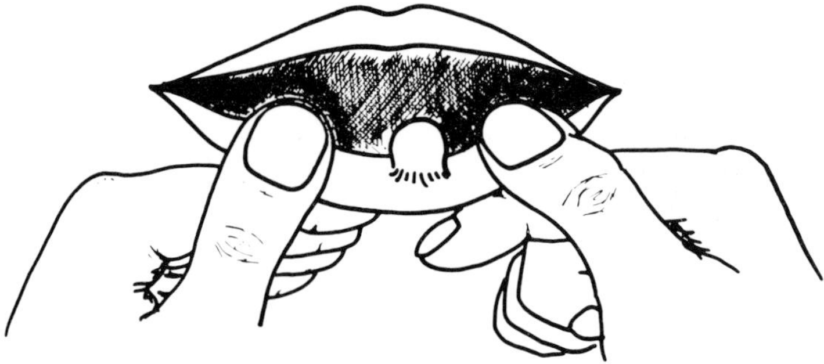

Fig. 11.9: *The technique of lip eversion to identify mucous retention cysts or pigmented spots on its inner surface.*

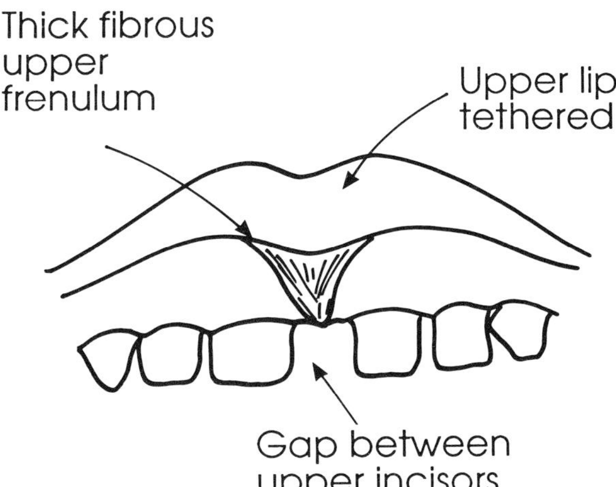

Fig. 11.10: *The short upper lip frenulum: a common but trivial anomaly.*

cause separation of the upper incisor teeth (Fig. 11.10). It tethers the upper lip and may interfere with facial expression, and it is easily traumatized. Despite these features, it is a trivial anomaly often best left alone.

Pigmentation of the lips (Peutz-Jeghers syndrome)

The presence of multiple tiny brown or black spots on the inner surface of the lips, and extending over the vermilion border onto the perioral skin, suggests Peutz-Jeghers syndrome. Pigmentation is seen sometimes on the dorsum of the fingers and on the perianal skin, and these areas should be examined too. The pigmented speckles are the external manifestation of a condition of which the most important abnormality is polyposis of the small intestine, although other parts of the bowel may also be involved. The polyps may cause intermittent colic, intussusception or rectal bleeding.

Isolated cleft lip

The upper lip is formed by the coalescence of the centrally placed globular and frontonasal processes with the laterally placed maxillary processes (Fig. 11.11). Failure of this mesenchymal consolidation results in cleft lip which may be either unilateral or bilateral. It is seen more commonly in boys, particularly when combined with cleft palate.

Isolated cleft lip may involve one or both sides, and presents as a deficiency in the lip which, in the severe case, extends to the nostril. In this situation, the side of the nose is wide and flat and the nasal septum is deviated towards the unaffected side (Fig. 11.12). The vermilion margin is drawn up with the cleft towards the nostril to produce an apparent foreshortening of the upper lip and facial asymmetry. The cleft may extend through the gums into the hard palate immediately behind the incisors, causing rotation forwards of the premaxillary portion of the alveolus. When less severe, there is a notch in the lip with no gum deformity. In bilateral cases, the degree of deformity may be

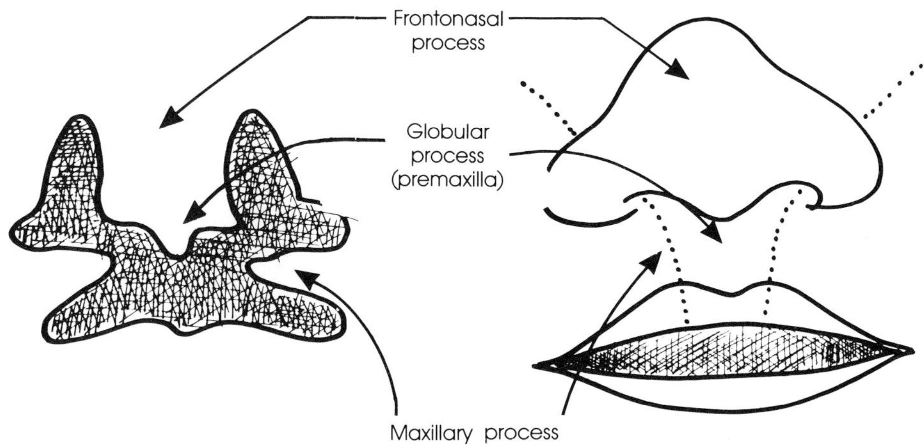

Fig. 11.11: *Development of the nose and upper lip.*

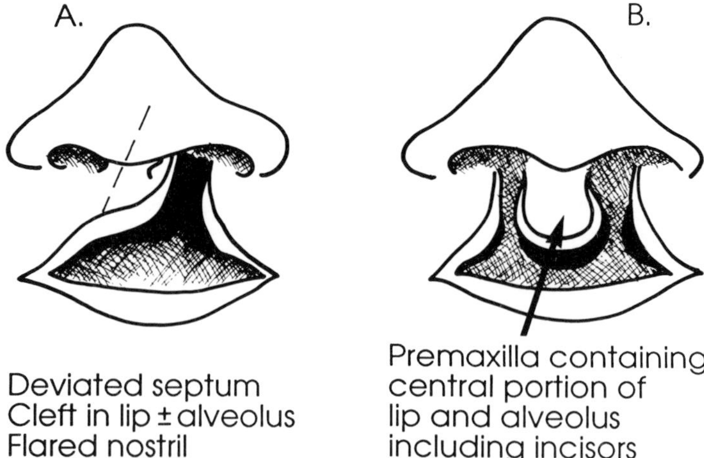

Fig. 11.12: *The features of unilateral (A) and bilateral (B) cleft lip.*

different on each side, resulting in an asymmetrical picture. Cleft lip in association with cleft palate is described in the next section.

LESIONS OF THE PALATE

Isolated cleft palate

In early gestation, the plates of the maxillary bones hang vertically beside the tongue and in the ensuing weeks, as the tongue sinks into the floor of the mouth and moves fowards, the plates acquire a horizontal plane and fuse (Fig. 11.13). Failure of this fusion results in cleft palate. Clefts of the palate can occur as isolated lesions and extend anteriorly only as far as the incisive foramen, or may be associated with anterior defects in the alveolus (gum) and lip.

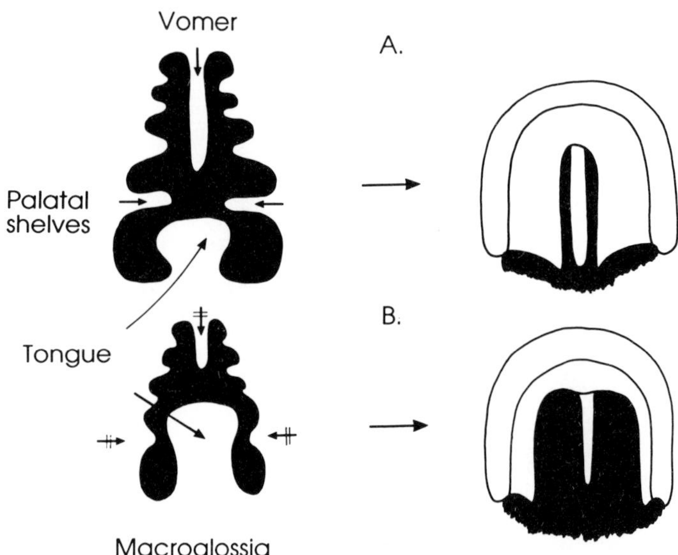

Fig. 11.13: *Development of the hard palate. A. Primary failure of fusion of the palatal shelves and vomer produces the common slit-like cleft, through which the lower edge of the vomer is visible. B. Secondary failure of palatal fusion caused by overgrowth (macroglossia) or upward displacement (micrognathia) of the tongue.*

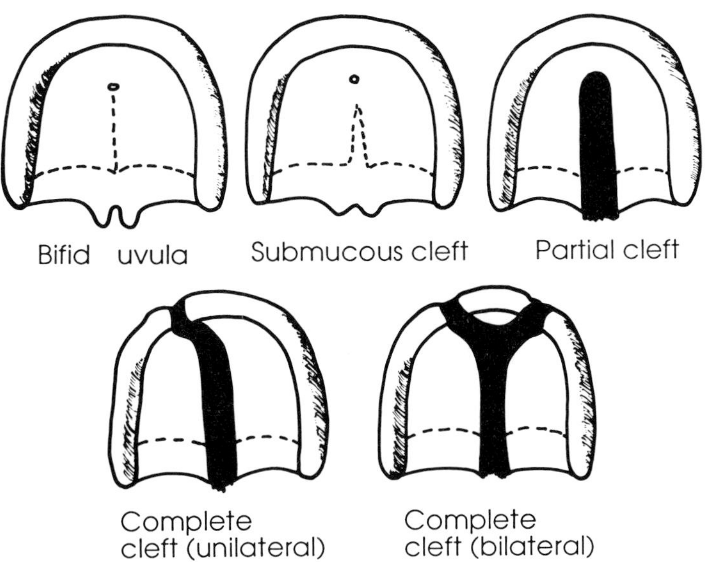

Fig. 11.14: *The clinical variations in cleft palate.*

As with cleft lip, the severity of deformity is variable (Fig. 11.14). The observation of a bifid uvula is suggestive of a submucous cleft. This condition is missed easily because the palate appears intact at first glance but, on closer examination, a notch can be felt in the midline at the posterior edge of the secondary or hard palate, and there is a midline groove in the soft palate where the two edges of the palate are joined only by mucous membrane. In the older child with a previously unrecognized submucous cleft, the palatal speech impediment is obvious.

The more severe and common lesion is the palatal cleft which extends anteriorly as far as the incisive foramen immediately behind the gums. This is obvious when the infant cries.

Isolated cleft palate occurs also as part of the Pierre Robin syndrome. It is due to failure of the tongue to sink into the floor of the mouth which prevents fusion of the two halves of the palate (Fig. 11.13). The other features of the syndrome include micrognathia and a posteriorly positioned tongue with respiratory distress at birth.

Clefts of both lip and palate

Fifty per cent of patients with a cleft lip have an associated cleft palate. The lesions may be unilateral or bilateral, and 'incomplete' or 'complete', according to their extent and severity.

In bilateral cleft lip and palate, the premaxilla – which is derived from the globular process – is suspended from the anterior part of the nose. It tends to protrude even further anteriorly, thereby losing its relationship to the hard palate which is derived from the maxillary processes.

The cleft extends up either side of the nasal septum to produce an open communication between the oral cavity and both nasal cavities.

LESIONS OF THE OROPHARYNX

Tonsillitis

The tonsils are conglomerations of lymphoid tissue and vary in size according to age. They are not apparent at birth, increase in size during childhood and start to decline at puberty. In the absence of infection, their 'normal' size varies considerably from individual to individual, but this increases dramatically with episodes of inflammation and infection.

To view the tonsils, the tongue is depressed with a spatula while the child says 'Ahh'. A good torch for lighting is essential. The view can be improved by using a second spatula to retract the anterior pillar of the fauces laterally. The size and appearance of the tonsils should be noted: a white

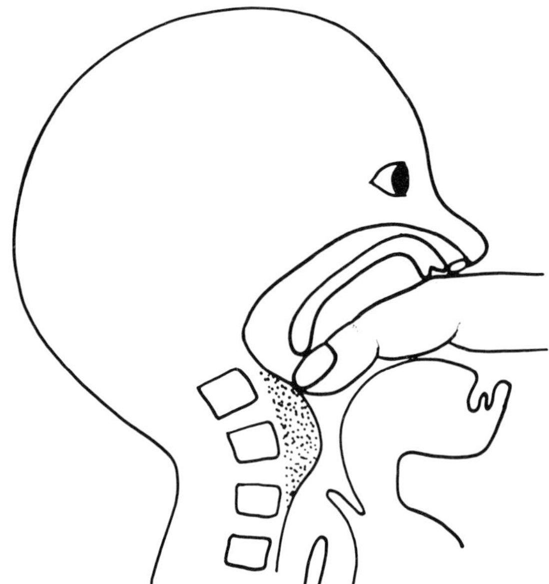

Fig. 11.15: *The technique of palpating a retropharyngeal abscess. Note the hyperextended neck, which is the position adopted by the child to keep the airway open.*

exudate may be a normal finding, whereas pus suggests infection.

In tonsillitis, the patient complains of a sore throat and neck. The tonsils are enlarged and inflamed and covered with a purulent exudate. Pain causes difficulty in swallowing. The child often looks flushed and toxic with systemic features of infection: tachycardia and fever. There is enlargement of the submandibular, tonsillar and jugulodigastric lymph nodes which are tender to palpation.

Quinsy

Quinsy is a peritonsillar abscess above and medial to the upper pole of the tonsil with extension across the soft palate.

The presentation of quinsy is characteristic: there is usually a history of a recent episode of tonsillitis with sore throat and pain on swallowing, which has failed to improve. The child dribbles saliva from a partially open mouth and holds the head forward and extended. Speech is awkward and attempts at swallowing are frequent and painful. The child looks unwell and usually has a fever. Trismus makes examination of the back of the mouth difficult, but perseverence reveals an extremely tender and fluctuant swelling of the ipsilateral soft palate and fauces. The swollen and oedematous palate bulging into the mouth establishes the diagnosis. The draining cervical lymph nodes are enlarged and tender.

Acute retropharyngeal abscess

The retropharyngeal space contains lymph nodes which drain the oropharynx and nasopharynx. They may become infected and suppurate, leading to the development of a retropharyngeal abscess. This usually occurs in the child under two years of age. The abscess extends to the glottis and may cause respiratory obstruction and, if not recognized, death. The infant or small child holds the mouth open and the head in full extension; this posture is an early clue to the diagnosis. He is febrile and toxic. Occasionally, depression of the tongue enables the abscess to be seen as a unilateral swelling in the pharynx: the tight fascial septum which connects the posterior surface of the pharynx to the prevertebral fascia, confines the abscess to one side.

The abscess is palpable if the index finger is inserted into the mouth (Fig. 11.15), a manoeuvre which will reveal a firm spongy mass protruding from the posterior wall of the pharynx.

Chronic retropharyngeal abscesses result from cervical tuberculous infection or tuberculous retropharyngeal lymph nodes.

GOLDEN RULES

(1) Tongue-tie requires no treatment unless the tongue cannot be protruded beyond the teeth.
(2) Beware the lingual thyroid: its odd position invites excision but it should not be removed because there is no normal thyroid.
(3) A ranula is on top of the floor of the mouth, while a lymphangioma (cystic hygroma) is within or below the floor of the mouth.
(4) Lip pigmentation in association with intussusception indicates Peutz-Jehgers syndrome with intestinal polyposis.
(5) Cleft lip/palate are common features of recognizable syndromes.
(6) Beware the dribbling child with neck extension: peritonsillar or retropharyngeal abscess may be present.

12 Trauma

Children are particularly susceptible to injury. Their perception of danger and their ability to recognize a potentially hazardous situation have not developed adequately, and their motor response to that danger may be neither appropriate nor effective. Furthermore, their dependence on adults and lack of physical prowess makes them vulnerable to abuse and maltreatment, which in turn may produce significant physical (as well as mental) injuries. The types of trauma children suffer differ from those of the adult in a number of important respects which are discussed in this chapter.

To perform a goal-oriented examination of an injured child, the clinician needs to know the mechanism of injury. Since the severity and type of pathology produced varies with the type of injury, an exact account of the accident allows certain injuries to be predicted. Moreover, the type of injury provides information about the nature of the trauma, which may be a key step in the diagnosis of child abuse. Pedestrian accidents are an example where certain injuries can be predicted even in the unconscious child (Fig. 12.1). Likewise, motor accidents where the child is wearing a lap seat-belt cause predictable injuries

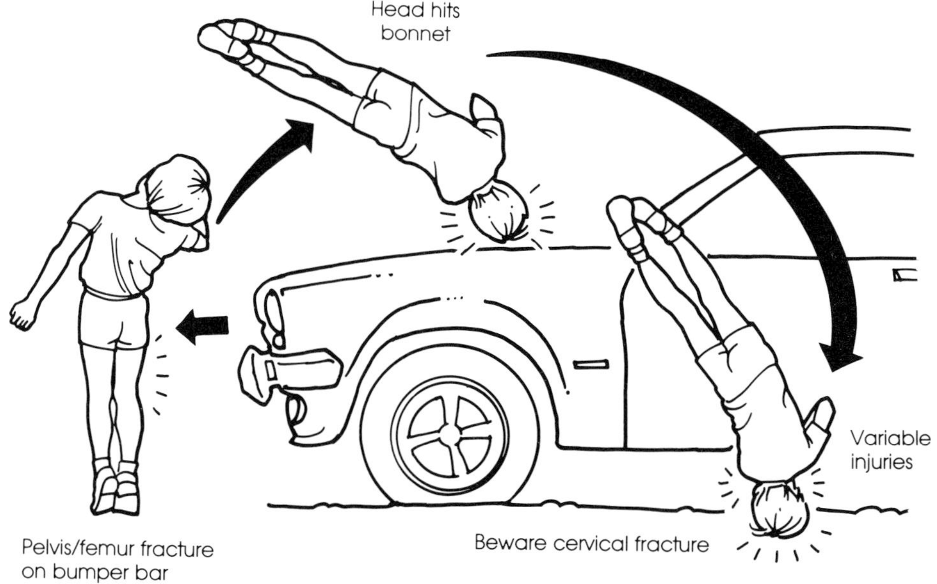

Fig. 12.1: *The mechanism of pedestrian injury in a collision with a fast moving car.*

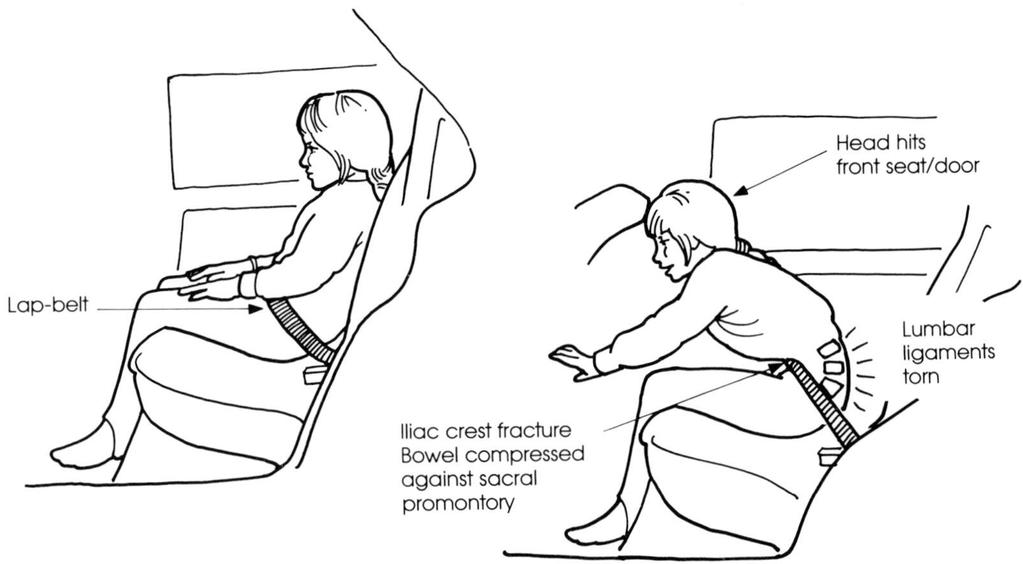

Fig. 12.2: *The mechanism of lap-belt injury. Acute hyperflexion of the spine may tear posterior vertebral ligaments. The bowel may burst from compression against the sacral promontory.*

(Fig. 12.2). A fall off a bicycle may produce a handle-bar injury (Fig. 12.3) with an isolated injury to the spleen or liver. Three general principles should be applied to all cases of trauma:

(1) Look for injuries which match the severity and type of accident.
(2) Suspect child abuse if the history of the 'accident' does not match the severity of the injuries or is inconsistent with the stage of development of that child.
(3) Repeated clinical examination is required to diagnose injuries not apparent initially.

INITIAL ASSESSMENT OF THE SEVERELY INJURED CHILD

The initial approach of the clinician to the severely injured child may be life-saving (Table 12.1). In all situations, the highest priority is the establishment and maintenance of an airway, for without this, anoxia will develop and all other manoeuvres become futile. Once a patent airway is established, ventilation must be adequate to ensure oxygenation. Attention is then turned to the assessment and stabilization of the circulatory state. External bleeding must be arrested, either by pressure or elevation. Subsequently, the whole body is examined for evidence of other injuries, but it must be emphasized that this examination must not delay treatment of the life-threatening injuries.

A. Ensure a patent airway

The first priority is to rule out upper airway obstruction. Severe obstruction causes cyanosis, while lesser degrees are evident as a rapid respiratory rate, restlessness, anxiety and an increase in respiratory effort manifested by indrawing of the ribs, sternal retraction and use of the accessory muscles of respiration. The tongue may fall backwards and obstruct the oropharynx in the supine child. This can be overcome by lifting the chin

Table 12.1 PRIORITIES IN THE ASSESSMENT OF THE SEVERELY INJURED CHILD

A	Airway patency
B	Breathing established
C	Circulation stable
D	General and neurological examination

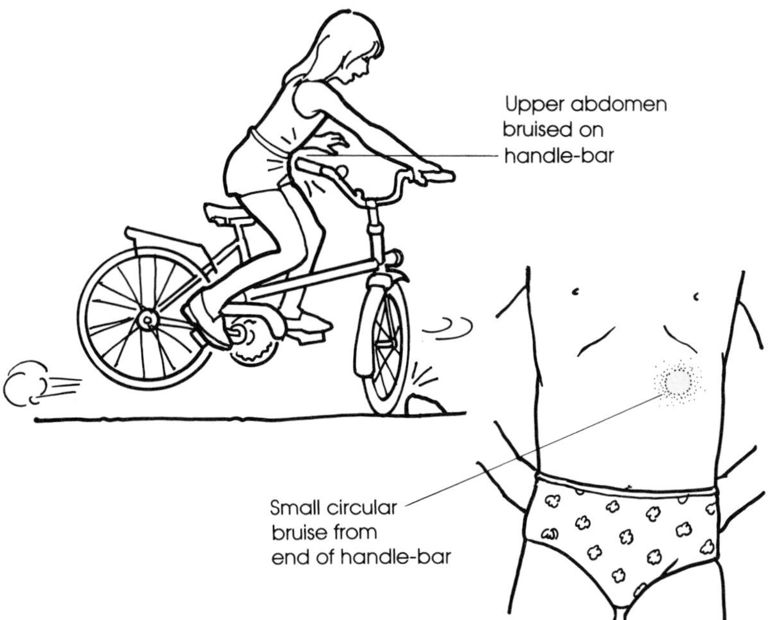

Fig. 12.3: *The handle-bar injury to the abdomen may produce localized spleen, liver or pancreatic damage.*

upwards or by pulling the mandible forwards with the fingers behind the angle of the jaw (Fig. 12.4). Secretions, blood and vomitus also may obstruct the upper airway: the mouth and pharynx should be inspected and suctioned clear if necessary. Insertion of an oropharyngeal tube may be necessary to maintain airway patency or, in the unconscious child who is unable to breathe, endotracheal intubation should be performed.

B. Ensure ventilation is adequate

Effective ventilation can be achieved only once the airway is patent. Ventilation is assessed by observing the movement of the chest wall and abdomen, feeling the moist warm air of expiration, and by checking the colour of the patient for cyanosis. Inadequate breathing may require additional oxygen or assisted ventilation (e.g. 'bagging' by mask, or endotracheal intubation).

C. Stabilize the circulation

External bleeding can be controlled by direct pressure over the wound, digital pressure of the regional artery against a bony prominence (e.g. control of the femoral artery by pressure in the groin, and the branchial artery by pressure against the medial aspect of the mid-humerus) or by elevation of the injured limb. Internal bleeding is suspected from the nature of the injury, superficial bruising and evidence of blood loss (tachycardia, pallor, poor peripheral perfusion, cool periphery and hypotension). Common sites of significant

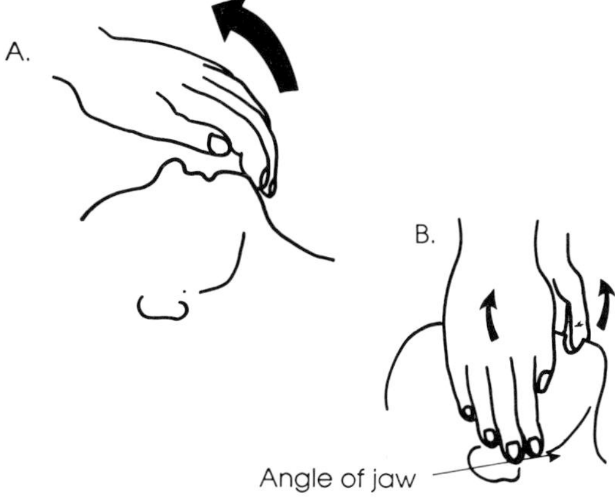

Fig. 12.4: *Maintenance of a clear upper airway by elevation of the chin* (A), *or lifting the angle of the mandible forwards* (B).

internal bleeding are the chest, abdomen, pelvis, thigh and, in the infant, the head.

ABDOMINAL TRAUMA

Abdominal trauma may occur as an isolated injury or as part of a multiple trauma situation where there are injuries to other organs outside the abdomen. Usually, it will be apparent from the history and preliminary examination as to which of these groups the patient belongs. Abdominal trauma most often affects boys, and is blunt and non-penetrating in 99% (except in societies with high gun use, where bullet wounds are common). In 85%, the injury occurs during a motor vehicle accident, during sport or play, or following a fall. If the cause and circumstance of the trauma are not clear, or if the injuries do not match the history provided, then child abuse should be considered.

Examination of a child with abdominal trauma includes examination of the genitals, perineum and back.

How do I know that there is trauma to the abdomen?

Where the injury is isolated, there will be a clear story of direct trauma to the abdomen, e.g. a kick in the belly or fall onto a bicycle handle-bar (Fig. 12.3), and the patient will complain of abdominal pain. Often, the story will be of progressive pain starting at the time of, or shortly after, the accident. The discomfort may be localized to one part of the abdomen.

The abdomen should be inspected closely for external evidence of trauma such as abrasions, bruising and lacerations. Palpation of the abdomen will demonstrate tenderness.

Which organ is involved?

The age of the child, the mode of injury and external signs will suggest which organ is likely to be injured. For example, a kick to the loin with overlying bruising might suggest a renal injury, whereas a fall onto a handle-bar bruising the left hypochondrium would raise the possibility of splenic trauma (Fig. 12.3). Injury to specific organs results in specific effects: the spleen, liver, kidney and great vessels bleed; the bowel leaks its contents; the urinary tract leaks urine; and the pancreas releases exocrine enzymes. Determination of which of these processes has occurred provides further clues as to the affected organ. More specific details are obtained through imaging investigations or laparotomy.

How do I know that bleeding has occurred?

A child can compensate for moderate blood loss without showing clinical evidence of shock, a fact which leads the inexperienced clinician to underestimate the amount of blood loss. There is a rise in the pulse rate which the unwary may attribute entirely to pain. The blood pressure is normal until a relatively late stage, but then it may drop rapidly. The limbs remain surprisingly warm and well perfused despite moderate blood loss. Remember, however, that limb temperature in a child depends partly on the ambient air temperature and the amount of clothing worn, and should be assessed accordingly.

Major blood loss causes pallor, but again other factors contribute to the child's colour – if vomiting has occurred, many children look pale without any blood loss. Sweating and poor peripheral perfusion are seen with greater degrees of blood loss. In short, it is difficult to estimate the amount of blood loss in children from their general signs until a late stage. Yet, it is important to estimate the amount of blood lost so that adequate fluid resuscitation can be implemented before cardiovascular collapse occurs. Careful examination of the abdomen, therefore, is required to assess the presence and extent of bleeding there.

The signs of intraperitoneal bleeding are (1) distension, and (2) tenderness. The distension increases with continued bleeding. Assessment of abdominal distension involves first removing any clothes or blankets which are obscuring the abdomen, and then observing the degree of protuberance whilst the patient is lying relaxed in a supine position. The girth can be measured by placing a tape-measure around the trunk and under the lumbar lordosis. The exact position of the tape during the first recording should be marked on the skin of the flanks and abdomen. Subsequent measurements at regular intervals will identify progressive abdominal distension. The child's smaller abdominal cavity makes serial girth measurements more sensitive than in the adult, but is subject to certain limitations: free blood within the peritoneal cavity causes a temporary paralysis and dilatation of the bowel (ileus), which increases distension. Likewise, air-swallowing increases abdominal distension and makes girth measurements taken in isolation less valuable in the detection of continued intraperitoneal bleeding.

The location of maximal tenderness to palpation should be recorded, and its severity and extension to other parts of the abdomen observed. Blood irritating the undersurface of the diaphragm causes pain which is referred to the shoulder tip, reflecting the cervical innervation of the muscle.

Retroperitoneal haematomata occur as a result of injury to retroperitoneal organs, the commonest of which is the kidney. The degree of anterior abdominal tenderness on examination is less than with intraperitoneal bleeds, but abdominal distension still occurs because of the retroperitoneal haematoma itself and as a result of the secondary ileus that it produces. Further confirmation of intra-abdominal bleeding may be seen on plain x-rays of the abdomen where fluid displaces adjacent loops of bowel, and on observing a fall in the haemoglobin level during the first 12–48 hours.

How do I know that bowel contents are leaking?

When perforation or laceration of the bowel occurs, intestinal contents leak, usually into the peritoneal cavity. These may be gastric juice, bile, small bowel fluid or faeces according to the site of injury, and each produces signs of rapidly progressing peritonitis. The child looks unwell and toxic. Within hours, the abdomen becomes distended and, while tenderness may be localized initially, it rapidly becomes generalized, severe and accompanied by involuntary guarding. It should be apparent that the signs of perforated bowel and haemoperitoneum are not dissimilar except in:

(1) degree – the tenderness with perforation is very marked;
(2) progression – leaking of bowel fluid into the peritoneal cavity persists and causes rapid progression of signs, whereas with rupture of a solid viscus the bleeding usually ceases spontaneously and the physical signs change slowly or are static;
(3) other signs of blood loss – the signs of shock are less evident with peritonitis;
(4) mode of injury – occasionally, knowledge of the mode of injury is helpful.

Nevertheless, it is often very difficult to distinguish the two situations, in which case careful reappraisal of the clinical signs, serial examination at short intervals, and recourse to other investigations may be necessary. An abdominal x-ray showing free gas would confirm gut perforation.

Retroperitoneal duodenal injury may occur after a lap-belt accident and presents as a high bowel obstruction (duodenal haematoma obstructing the lumen) or with progressive but nonspecific signs of sepsis (duodenal laceration and retroperitoneal abscess formation). Pancreatic injuries often present late with a tender epigastric mass, representing a pancreatic pseudocyst.

How do I know that there is urinary tract damage?

Direct trauma to the back and loins is more likely to damage the urinary tract than the gastrointestinal tract. A fracture of the pelvis, particularly if it involves the pubic rami, may injure the bladder or urethra. Unless there has been complete interruption of the urethra, there will be haematuria. Therefore, examination of the urine is mandatory where the possibility of urinary tract trauma exists. Injury to the kidney may result in major retroperitoneal haemorrhage causing abdominal tenderness and distension, and signs of blood loss. Disruption of the pelvicalyceal system or transection of the ureter allows urine to leak into the retroperitoneal space, contributing to the retroperitoneal collection. The urinary tract can be outlined by performing an intravenous pyelogram (IVP) at the time of a plain x-ray of the abdomen. Extravasation of urine is evident as contrast outside the normal urinary tract. In other situations, a computed tomography (CT) scan or nuclear medicine scan may be more appropriate.

When should specific investigations be performed?

The necessity for further investigations depends on:

(1) the suspected lesion as determined on clinical grounds;
(2) the general condition of the patient;
(3) the facilities available.

The organs most commonly injured are the spleen and liver. Where splenic injury is suspected, a nuclear scan has the advantage of being able to outline the liver at the same time. Where clinical examination suggests that splenic injury is likely to be an isolated lesion and the child is stable, surgery is not required immediately and splenography can be performed as a non-urgent procedure. Alternatively, the liver and spleen can be outlined with ultrasound or CT scan.

THORACIC INJURIES

Major thoracic injuries are uncommon in childhood and tend to occur in association with multiple injuries of other organs, e.g. the head and abdomen. The elastic and pliable rib cage of the child results in compression injuries of the intrathoracic structures (Fig. 12.5). Consequently, multiple rib fractures are not seen often, whereas the upper abdominal organs and lungs are damaged frequently (Fig. 12.6).

Thoracic injury should be suspected in any child with multiple system trauma, respiratory difficulties or evidence of blood loss (Fig. 12.7). Again, the first priority is to rule out upper airway obstruction by inspection of the mouth and pharynx for secretions, blood and vomitus, and by confirming that the tongue is not obstructing the oropharynx. There are a number of complications of intrathoracic injury which may be life-threatening, and although not common, must be recognized and treated promptly. (Table 12.2).

Sudden severe respiratory distress

Compression injury of the chest may cause a tear in a major airway with leakage of air into the mediastinum and pleural cavity. Movement of air into the pleural space occurs with each inspiration and remains there during expiration. The volume of air increases with a corresponding rise in pressure (tension). The ipsilateral lung collapses, there is a shift of the mediastinum to the contralateral side, compression of the contralateral lung, and interference of venous return to the heart (Fig. 12.8). If uncorrected, inadequate ventilation of the lungs and decreased cardiac output will cause death. Fractured ribs may also lacerate the lung and cause a tension pneumothorax.

Tension pneumothorax should be considered in any patient with a thoracic injury or fractured ribs who develops sudden increasing respiratory distress. Careful clinical examination will confirm

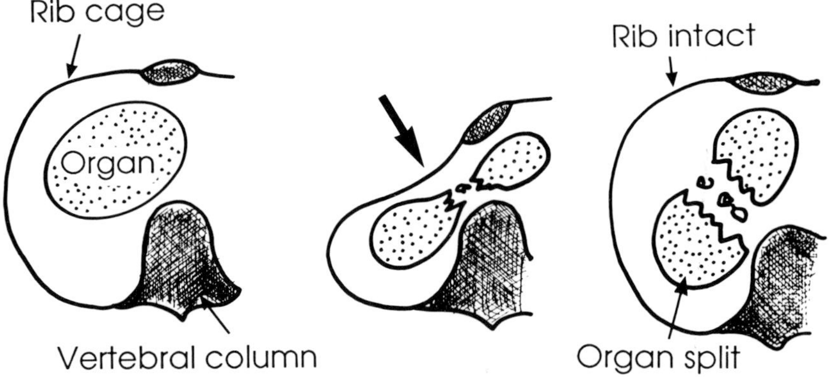

Fig. 12.5: *The mechanism of injury of upper abdominal and thoracic organs without rib fracture. The elasticity of the ribs in childhood allows significant distortion without breaking.*

Table 12.2 CONSEQUENCES OF INTRATHORACIC TRAUMA

EARLY LIFE-THREATENING COMPLICATIONS	1. Tension pneumothorax	
	2. Major haemothorax	(uncommon)
	3. Cardiac tamponade	(uncommon)
	4. Flail chest	(very rare)
	5. Open pneumothorax	(very rare)
UNDERLYING INJURIES	1. Pulmonary contusion	
	2. Pneumothorax	
	3. Haemothorax	
	4. Fractured ribs	
	5. Traumatic asphyxia	
	6. Tracheobronchial tear	
	7. Oesophageal tear	
	8. Diaphragmatic tear	
	9. Aortic tear	
	10. Myocardial contusion	

the diagnosis. The chest wall moves less on the side of the pneumothorax, with a decrease in ipsilateral breath sounds and hyper-resonance on percussion. Mediastinal shift is detected clinically by deviation of the trachea at the level of the suprasternal notch (Fig. 12.9), and in left-sided lesions, the heart sounds become audible more easily in the right chest. Increased intrathoracic pressure impedes venous return as shown by distended neck veins. The diagnosis can be confirmed on chest x-ray, but in an emergency, immediate insertion of a 14 or 16 gauge needle in the fourth intercostal space at the anterior axillary line, and subsequent insertion of a chest tube

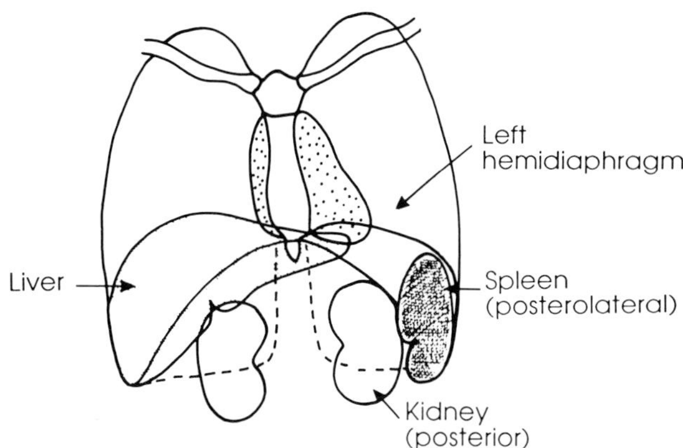

Fig. 12.6: *Surface markings of organs likely to be damaged by rib compression: the organs at greatest risk are actually below the diaphragm.*

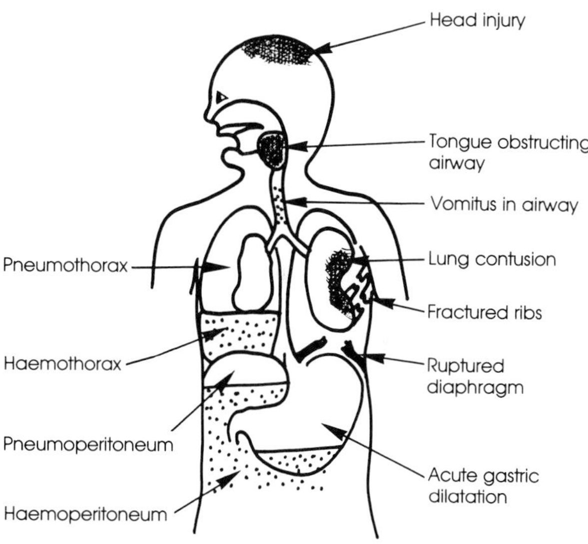

Fig. 12.7: *The causes of respiratory distress in trauma.*

connected to an underwater drain, will alleviate the symptoms. The child should be given high-flow oxygen.

Laceration of an intercostal artery associated with fractured ribs causes major blood loss into the thorax (haemothorax). The signs are similar to those seen in tension pneumothorax except that:

(1) there is evidence of hypovolaemic shock
(2) the neck veins are flat
(3) the ipsilateral chest sounds dull on percussion, rather than hyper-resonant.

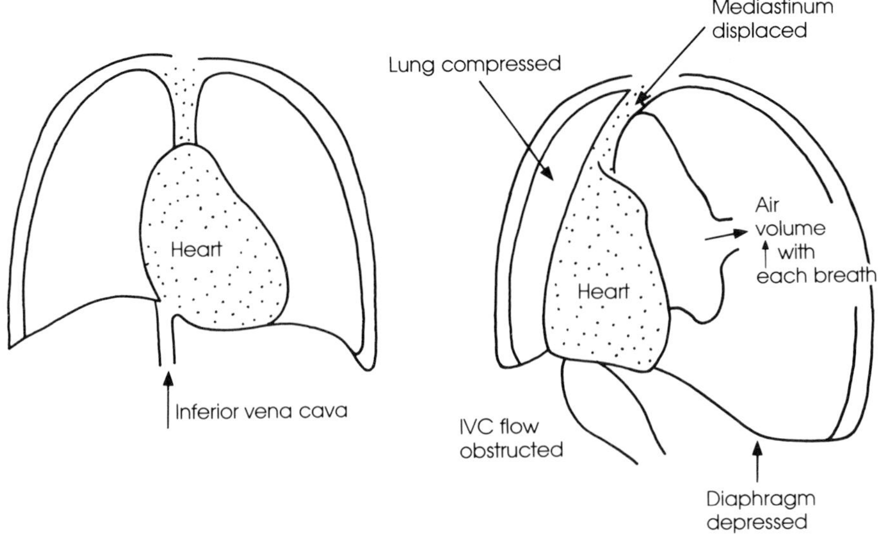

Fig. 12.8: *The effect of tension pneumothorax on ventilation and venous return.*

The diagnosis is confirmed on chest x-ray. Management involves resuscitation followed by a chest drain or thoracotomy if the major intrathoracic bleeding continues.

Respiratory distress, with hypotension and distended neck veins

In some injuries, the heart is compressed between the chest wall and the vertebral column causing myocardial contusion with bleeding into the pericardial sac. Much less commonly in children, penetrating wounds (e.g. stab wounds) also may cause bleeding into the pericardium (cardiac tamponade). The pericardial sac prevents effective contraction and refilling of the chambers of the heart and causes hypotension with poor cardiac output. The pulse pressure is narrow, and the pulse volume decreases with inspiration (pulsus paradoxus). The most striking feature is the grossly distended neck veins in the presence of severe pallor and shock. The heart sounds are muffled and difficult to hear.

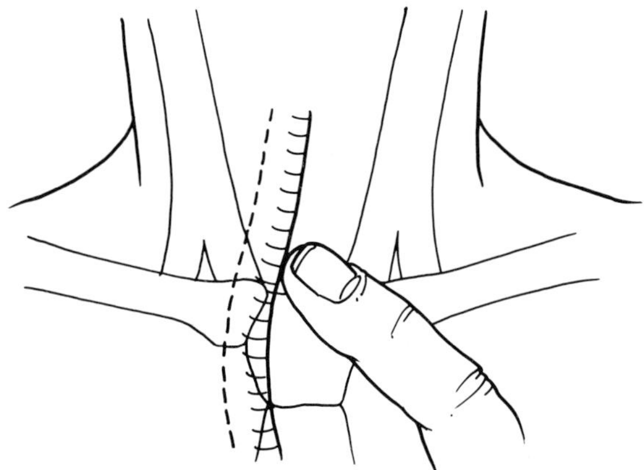

Fig. 12.9: *Mediastinal shift determined by palpation of the position of the trachea in the suprasternal notch. This may be difficult in young children.*

A diagnostic and therapeutic manoeuvre involves the insertion of a needle just below the xiphisternum directed towards the left shoulder at an angle of 45° to the skin. Aspiration of blood from the pericardium causes immediate and dramatic improvement in the child's condition until a thoracotomy is performed.

Flail chest

Flail chest is extremely uncommon and seen only in the older child with multiple rib fractures. There is asymmetric movement of the chest wall and a flail segment which moves paradoxically with respiration. It should be assumed that there is contused lung underlying the ribs. Flail chest may cause a significant haemothorax and mediastinal shift with impairment of venous return to the heart and signs of blood loss.

Open pneumothorax

Open pneumothorax virtually never occurs in children but is readily recognized as a wound which transmits air (bubbles and sucks) during ventilation. The defect should be covered to prevent further air movement and a chest tube inserted.

Traumatic asphyxia

Severe compression of the chest may completely block venous return in the large veins of the thoracic inlet to cause high venous pressures in the head, neck and upper extremities. Small capillaries rupture resulting in petechial skin and subconjunctival haemorrhages. This is relatively common in children and is seen when the child has been run over at low velocity or trapped by a heavy object across the chest. The face, neck and, to a lesser extent, the shoulders and arms are covered with numerous red spots. The cutaneous petechiae resolve after three or four days, whereas the subconjunctival haemorrhages persist for one week or more. There may be no other injuries, apart from a tyre mark.

HEAD INJURIES

Head injury is one of the commonest types of trauma in childhood and is the main cause of morbidity and mortality. Head injuries account for 80% of deaths from trauma, and most children with multiple system injuries have a head injury.

Injury to the brain occurs in two phases: first, there is primary brain damage sustained at the time of the accident; and secondly, there is additional injury which occurs as a consequence of both the local and distant injuries (Table 12.3). Therapeutic measures cannot reverse the damage sustained at the moment of impact but can have a profound effect in reducing the degree of secondary brain injury.

Head injuries in children differ from those in adults in a number of respects:

(1) Head injuries are more common in children than adults because:
   (i) the child's head contributes a greater percentage of body area and weight
   (ii) children are more susceptible to injuries which are likely to cause trauma to the head (e.g. pedestrian accidents, falls and child abuse).

(2) The child's brain is more susceptible to primary injury because:
   (i) the cranial bones are thinner and afford less protection
   (ii) the brain is less myelinated in the infant and small child, making it more easily damaged.

(3) The child's brain is more susceptible to secondary injury because:
   (i) brain injury in children may be associated with a marked degree of hyperaemia and swelling (previously known as 'malignant brain oedema')
   (ii) the high incidence of major associated chest and intra-abdominal injuries may produce hypoxia, hypercarbia and hypovolaemia – all factors which adversely affect cerebral perfusion.

The assessment and treatment of major head injuries in children should be aggressive and aimed at limiting secondary injury to the brain. Secondary brain damage is minimized by ensuring that the surviving cerebral neurons are well supplied

Table 12.3 BRAIN INJURY

PRIMARY (sustained at the time of impact)	
	– laceration of brain parenchyma
	– vascular injury
	– arterial
	– venous
	– axon stretching/shearing
SECONDARY (response to trauma)	
	– cerebral oedema
	– intracranial haemorrhage
	– hyperaemia of the brain
	– temporary cerebral dysfunction
FACTORS CONTRIBUTING TO SECONDARY BRAIN INJURY (adverse effects of distant injuries)	
	– hypoxia
	– hypercarbia
	– hypotension
	– low cardiac output
	– (hypertension)

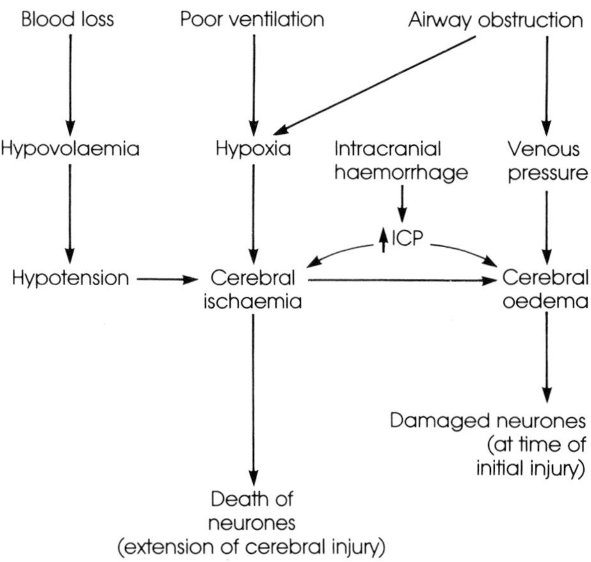

Fig. 12.10: *Mechanisms of secondary brain damage after head injury.*

with oxygen at all times. Several sequelae to trauma may adversely affect oxygenation of the brain (Fig 12.10):

(1) Airway obstruction
(2) Poor ventilation
(3) Hypotension
(4) Brain swelling
(5) Intracranial haemorrhage.

An obstructed airway reduces the supply of oxygen to the brain; hypercarbia increases cerebral blood flow and results in increased cerebral blood volume and raised intracranial pressure; and increased intrathoracic pressure elevates the intracranial venous pressure, further upsetting cerebral blood flow. Poor ventilation exerts similar effects by interfering with normal gaseous exchange, and hypotension from any cause decreases cerebral perfusion. Brain swelling is a normal response to injury, but is exacerbated if hypoxia, hypercarbia, hypotension, hyponatraemia, increased venous pressure or continued ischaemia are allowed to persist. Intracranial haemorrhage reduces further the space available to the brain and causes an increase in intracranial pressure and decrease in cerebral blood flow. Neurones deprived of adequate blood supply become ischaemic and swell further, causing a vicious circle. Because the brain is contained within a confined space (once the sutures have closed), any process which increases the volume of the intracranial contents will ultimately increase the pressure and decrease the blood flow within that cavity.

The early assessment of head injuries, therefore, involves:

(1) estimation of the extent and severity of the primary injury to the brain
(2) observation for events which may compromise adequate oxygenation of the brain and lead to secondary brain injury.

This assessment can be divided into four stages as outlined in Fig. 12.11.

The initial neurological assessment

This is a simple and quick assessment of the neurological status of the child, with a more detailed exmination being deferred until initial resuscitation and stabilization are complete. This initial examination determines the urgency of neurosurgical care and provides baseline information for the assessment of subsequent progress (Table 12.4).

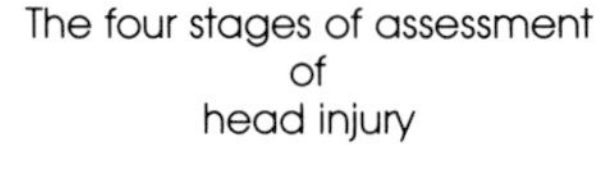

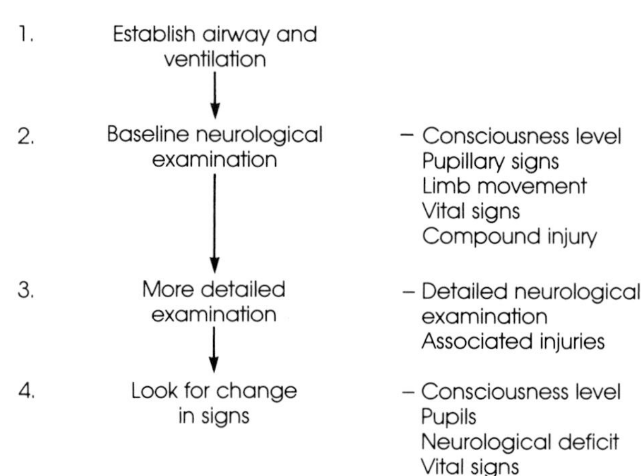

Fig. 12.11: *The four stages of assessment in a child with a head injury.*

Table 12.4 BASIC NEUROLOGICAL ASSESSMENT IN HEAD INJURIES

1. HISTORY	– mechanism of injury – state when first seen – focal signs – deterioration
2. LEVEL OF CONSCIOUSNESS	
3. PUPILS	– size – reactivity to light and accommodation
4. FUNDI	– retinal haemorrhages – (papilloedema)
5. MOVEMENT OF LIMBS	– posture – movement of each limb – flaccidity/spasticity
6. PLANTAR RESPONSE	
7. PULSE RATE	
8. BLOOD PRESSURE	
9. RESPIRATORY RATE	– apnoea – Cheyne-Stokes respirations
10. LEAK OF CEREBROSPINAL FLUID	– otorrhoea – rhinorrhoea

History

The history provides important information about the time and mode of injury, the state of the child immediately after the accident and whether deterioration or improvement in the child's condition has occurred during transport to hospital. Some of this information can be gained from eyewitness accounts, but the most useful source of detail is often the ambulance officer who was first on the scene. It is essential to speak to the ambulance officer before he leaves the emergency department.

Level of consciousness

It is not adequate to describe a child as being 'conscious', 'semi-conscious' or 'unconscious'. The level of consciousness must be described in full (e.g. 'alert and orientated' at one extreme, or 'unresponsive to painful stimuli' at the other extreme). Assessment of consciousness involves observation of the child's motor response to sensory stimuli and evidence of higher cerebral function (verbalization, orientation).

One useful method of documenting consciousness level is to employ the Glasgow coma scale (Table 12.5). This method has gained widespread acceptance throughout the world; it enables the

Table 12.5 THE GLASGOW COMA SCALE

Eye opening	Never	1
	To pain	2
	To speech	3
	Spontaneously	4
Best verbal response	None	1
	Garbled	2
	Inappropriate	3
	Confused	4
	Oriented	5
Best motor response	None	1
	Extension	2
	Abnormal flexion	3
	Withdrawal from painful stimuli	4
	Localizes painful stimuli	5
	Obeys commands	6

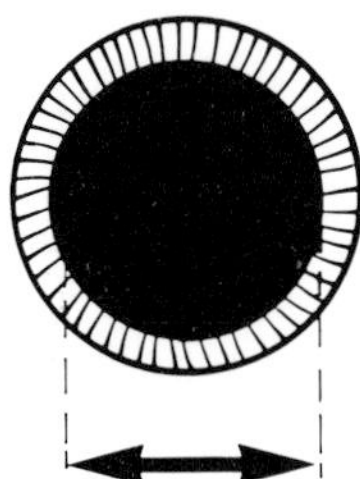
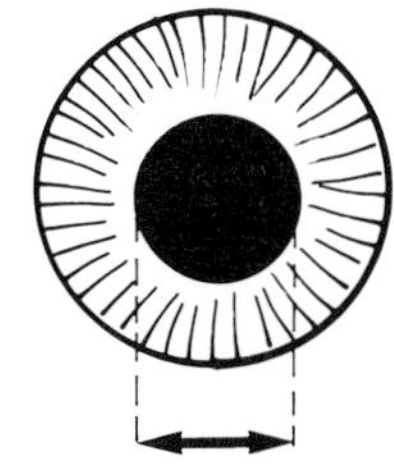
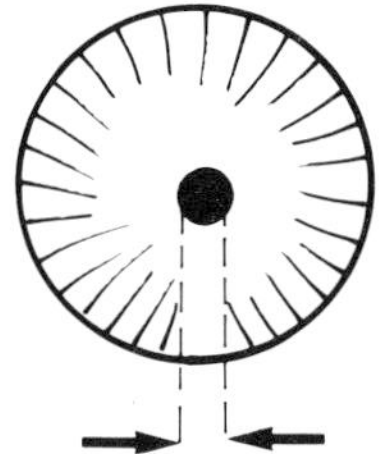

Fig. 12.12: *The size of the pupil is measured in millimetres.*

clinician to assess consciousness level objectively and to monitor its progress with time. It tests neurological function in eye opening, verbalization and motor response. The score of each is recorded along with the time and date at which the observation was made. A cumulative score of 10 or less signifies a serious head injury. In the absence of shock, a decrease in the score of three or more strongly suggests development of a major complication. Although the Glasgow coma scale is widely applicable, determination of the best verbal response of children under three years of age in whom verbal skills are not fully developed, may be difficult. In this situation, it is reasonable to give a verbal score of five if the child cries in response to stimulation.

Pupils

Pupillary size and reactivity afford information on the severity, prognosis and progression of head injury. The size of each pupil is measured separately and its diameter in millimetres recorded (Fig. 12.12). The pupillary reflex is tested by shining a bright light into each eye in turn, and recording the rapidity and degree of pupillary response. If the light is shone into both eyes at once, an intact consensual reflex permits a normal bilateral pupillary response even though one optic nerve may be divided.

There are several causes of fixed dilated pupils (Table 12.6). The fixed, dilated pupils of traumatic iridoplegia and third nerve palsy from direct injury to the eye may be associated with a good neurological prognosis, whereas fixed dilated pupils caused by cerebral ischaemia or increased intracranial pressure signify severe injury to the brain, and have a very poor prognosis. An expanding intracranial space-occupying lesion (e.g. extradural haematoma) may produce initial dilatation of one pupil and may be followed shortly by dilatation of the contralateral pupil. These findings frequently will be accompanied by a decrease in the level of consciousness, bradycardia, increase in blood pressure and change in respiration. The most useful criterion in assessing the pupils is

Table 12.6 CAUSES OF FIXED DILATED PUPILS

TRAUMATIC IRIDOPLEGIA	– damage to the orbit and eye – associated with direct trauma to the face and head – child is otherwise alert and oriented
DIRECT NERVE DAMAGE	– injury to the third nerve – optic nerve injury
CEREBRAL ISCHAEMIA	– profound shock – cerebral anoxia – 'brain death'
INCREASED INTRACRANIAL PRESSURE	– pressure on the third nerve – intracranial bleeding – gross cerebral oedema

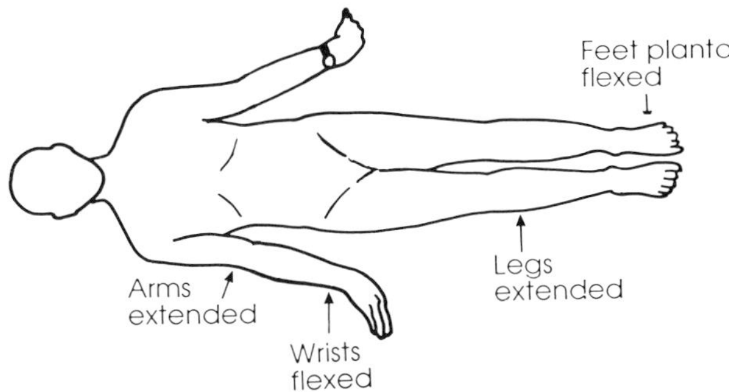

Fig. 12.13: *Decerebrate (extensor) rigidity when the damage is inferior to the basal ganglia.*

progressive deterioration of the reflexes.

Testing of oculocephalic reflexes (doll's eye movements), although valuable in assessing the severity and prognosis of the head injury, should be reserved until after the integrity of the cervical spine has been established.

Fundi

Detailed examination of the optic fundi can be delayed, but the observation of retinal haemorrhages suggests major head injury and may be seen with subarachnoid haemorrhage or an acute subdural haematoma. In a child less than one year of age with an unclear history of trauma, the presence of retinal haemorrhages is strongly suggestive of child abuse.

Acute papilloedema developing within two hours of a head injury signifies grossly elevated intracranial pressure which is usually fatal. Fortunately, papilloedema rarely appears within 12–24 hours.

Movement of limbs

The limbs should be examined for their resting position, spontaneous movement and tone. Complete flaccidity (loss of muscle tone) is seen with severe injury of the brain stem or high spinal cord transection, and no spontaneous movement is observed. Various patterns of rigidity occur, including decerebrate rigidity (Fig. 12.13) and decorticate rigidity (Fig. 12.14). In a high brain stem lesion, rigidity usually is bilateral, whereas in injury to one cerebral hemisphere it may be unilateral with the head turned to the contralateral side (Fig. 12.14). Failure to move one or more limbs should be noted. Absence of spontaneous or induced movement of the limbs is described as monoplegia (one limb only), hemiplegia (the limbs of one side), paraplegia (the lower limbs), or quadriplegia (all four limbs). Lesser degrees of

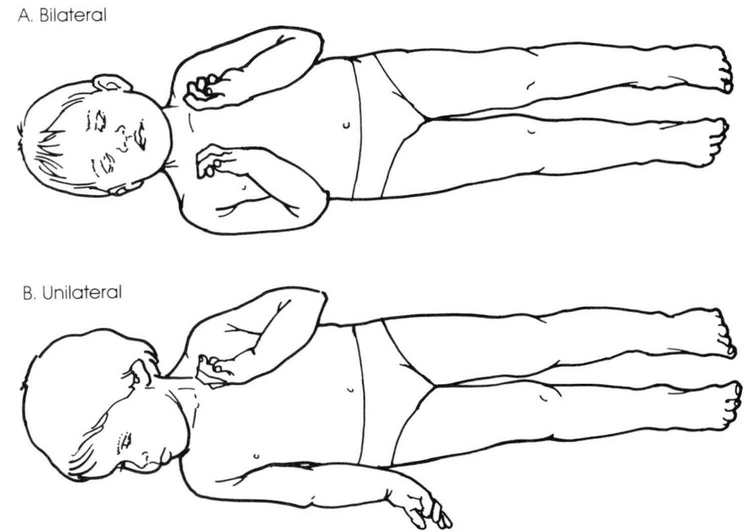

Fig. 12.14: *Decorticate rigidity with injury above the basal ganglia, representing loss of cortical influence.*

impairment of movement also should be noted, and may be caused by spinal cord injury, nerve root injury or limb fractures.

Plantar response

Plantar responses are determined by stroking the lateral aspect of the sole of the foot with a hard, blunt, pointed instrument (Fig. 12.15). The extended thumb, a key or the handle of a reflex hammer are all suitable. The response is recorded as being up-going, down-going or equivocal. In small children, the pressure required to elicit the response is not great and excessive pressure simply causes withdrawal of the limb. A down-going response is considered normal except in infants, and an up-going response in the older child is abnormal. Where the response is equivocal, the examination should be repeated periodically.

Pulse rate

A rapid pulse usually indicates blood loss (which may be concealed). The possibility of haemorrhage into the chest, abdomen and pelvis, or from long bone fractures, should be considered. Scalp bleeding may be profuse and cause shock but can be controlled by direct pressure and the application of pressure dressings. In some open skull fractures, the dural sinuses may be torn; in this situation, an external pressure dressing must be applied before elevating the head to prevent air embolism.

The development of bradycardia in the presence of increasing blood pressure is a late sign of increasing intracranial pressure and often indicates the need for neurosurgical intervention. Other signs of deterioration may have appeared already.

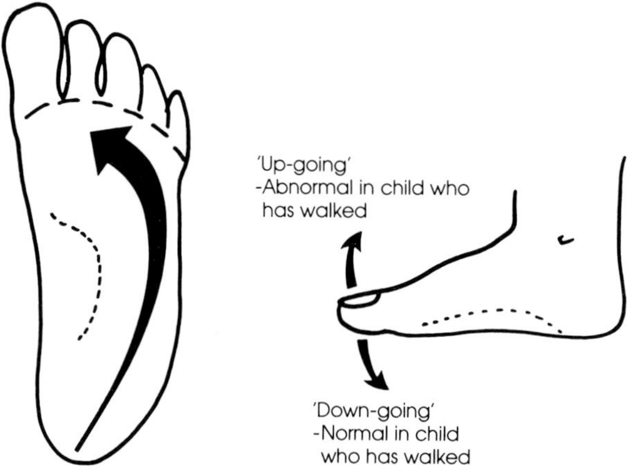

Fig. 12.15: *Testing the plantar response. 1. Use a thumb-nail, key or other blunt object. 2. Stroke the sole firmly but lightly from heel to toes along the lateral aspect. 3. An up-going response is normal in the first year, but thereafter is a sign of an upper motor neuron lesion.*

Blood pressure

Hypotension with a head injury is caused usually by internal haemorrhage elsewhere rather than from intracranial bleeding. The exceptions to this rule are (1) where there is obvious external haemorrhage from the scalp, (2) where a scalp haematoma is present in an infant, or (3) where intracranial haemorrhage occurs in the neonate and infant.

Increasing blood pressure in conjunction with a decline in the pulse rate (Cushing's response) is a late sign of increasing intracranial pressure.

Respiratory rate

Complete absence of respiratory effort after a head injury suggests a major and probably fatal neurological insult or a high cervical spinal injury (phrenic nerve palsy). The coexistence of generalized flaccidity of the limbs and hypoventilation demands careful examination of the cervical spine. Although apnoea is a poor prognostic sign in head injuries, resuscitation should proceed as some of these children recover.

Assessment of the respiratory rate should take into account the age of the patient (Table 12.7). Infants and small children have a much faster rate than older children. At rest, and in the absence of other stimuli, respiratory rate remains relatively

Table 12.7 NORMAL RESPIRATORY RATES IN CHILDREN

Age (years)	Breaths/minute
0–1	25–30
1–5	20
6–12	15
13→	12–15

constant. A pattern of increasing respiration followed by decreasing amplitude with a period of apnoea (Cheyne-Stokes respirations) suggests upper mid-brain or diencephalic derangement and, if it appears following previously normal respiration, is indicative of neurological deterioration.

Leak of cerebrospinal fluid

Otorrhoea and rhinorrhoea should be looked for, and are important because they reflect a dural tear and an increased risk of meningitis. Otorrhoea usually stops spontaneously, but rhinorrhoea may persist and require definitive surgical repair of the dura.

Presentations of head injury

The minor head injury

Head injuries vary in severity and, happily, the commonest presentation is a minor head injury of little long-term significance. The challenge in this group is to detect at an early stage those in whom a complication is likely to occur.

The history is often of a fall from a piece of home furniture, toy or tree, or having been hit by an object during play. The child remains conscious but becomes drowsy and vomits several times. The parents are understandably concerned for the child's welfare and seek medical advice. Examination involves neurological assessment as previously described and a search for other injuries. In the majority of patients, no neurological deficit is identified apart from some drowsiness and perhaps persistent vomiting. The most important aspect of this child's management is careful observation over the next 24-48 hours to exclude serious neurological injury.

When should a skull x-ray be taken? A skull x-ray is not required in every situation but is helpful where there has been documented loss of consciousness or trauma to the temporal area, in an infant less than one year of age, if there are focal neurological signs or signs which suggest a basal skull fracture (blood behind the eardrums, bruising overlying the mastoid process, 'raccoon eyes'), or where there is a possible depressed fracture on palpation, open skull injury, injury from a sharp object, a Glasgow coma scale score of less than 10 or neurological deterioration.

Patients should be admitted for observation if there is (1) deterioration in the level of consciousness, (2) focal neurological signs, (3) a history which does not fit the physical findings, raising the possibility of child abuse, (4) a linear skull fracture, (5) large scalp haematoma in infants, or (6) evidence of leakage of cerebrospinal fluid. Asymptomatic patients with a depressed skull fracture should be admitted for early elevation of the bony fragments.

The severe head injury

A severe head injury is one where the basic neurological examination provides a Glasgow coma scale score of less than 10. Alternatively, there may be focal neurological signs, neurological deterioriation of a mild to moderate head injury in association with major chest or abdominal injuries. Full evaluation involves a comprehensive neurological examination and special investigations (skull x-rays, CT scan) to provide further information on the nature and extent of injury to the brain.

The mild injury which deteriorates

The vast majority of minor head injuries get better without developing complications. The reason these injuries are observed carefully is to detect significant intracranial haemorrhage early and allow prompt neurosurgical intervention before irreversible damage is done to the brain.

An extradural haematoma results from a tear in one of the vessels of the dura and is seen in association with a skull fracture (Fig. 12.16). It should be suspected in a child who has received a blow to the side of the head because this is where the skull is weakest yet intimately related to the middle meningeal artery. Arterial bleeding causes compression of the adjacent cortex, increased intracranial pressure and then herniation of the brain through the tentorium. The patient develops a headache and becomes drowsy. There may be a boggy swelling over the temporal region and some facial weakness. The ipsilateral pupil becomes dilated and fixed, and the level of con-

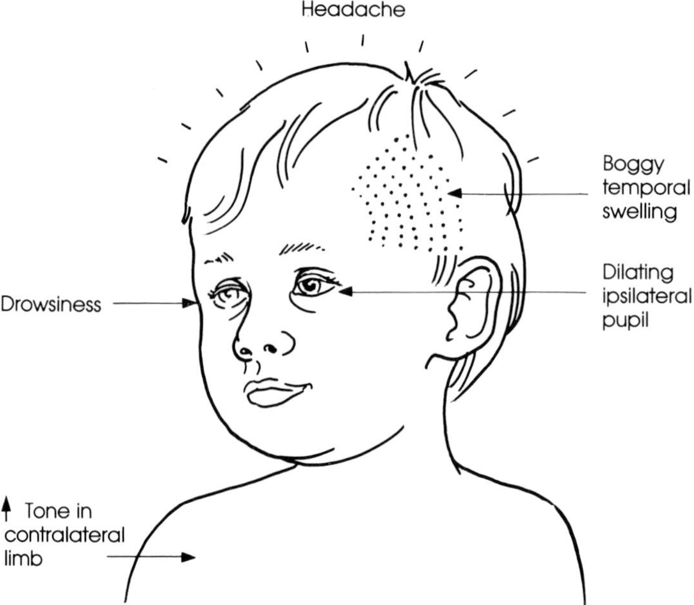

Fig. 12.16: *The signs of an extradural haematoma.*

sciousness decreases. Herniation and compression of the brain causes the contralateral pupil to dilate, and the child may develop decerebrate rigidity (Fig. 12.13). Untreated, death ensues. If the child's condition permits, a CT scan confirms the diagnosis and accurately pin-points the location of the haematoma, which then can be drained surgically and the bleeding point controlled.

Subdural haematomata result from injury to the brain surface, including the bridging veins which run between the cerebral cortex and the dura. They are seen in younger children after high-speed injuries or the violent shaking of child abuse. There is usually a concomitant severe primary brain injury so that deterioration is less obvious. The outcome of a child with a subdural haematoma is not as good as one with an extradural haematoma.

An intracerebral haematoma (a bleed within the parenchyma of the brain itself) presents as slow neurological deterioration one to two days after a severe head injury. It is diagnosed on CT scan, but usually is not amenable to surgical intervention.

Progressive cerebral oedema and hyperaemia over the first two days following a severe head injury also may produce signs of neurological deterioration, particularly if there has been inadequate attention to the prevention of hypoxia, hypercarbia, and fluid and electrolyte imbalance. A CT scan shows profuse oedema with compression of the ventricles and subarachnoid space, with no space-occupying lesions. Treatment involves institution of measures to decrease the intracranial pressure and to increase oxygenation to the brain.

A localized, depressed fracture to the skull may cause local brain damage from the bone ends (Fig. 12.17). This is an important condition, not only because of possible underlying cortical injury, but also because the diagnosis may be overlooked if the depression is assumed to be a scalp haematoma with a soft centre (Fig. 12.18).

Foreign bodies

A foreign body penetrating the skull and lodged in the brain should be left in situ as it is likely to be acting as a tamponade controlling cerebral bleeding. The object is removed by the neurosurgeon in theatre.

LACERATIONS

Lacerations are extremely common in children.

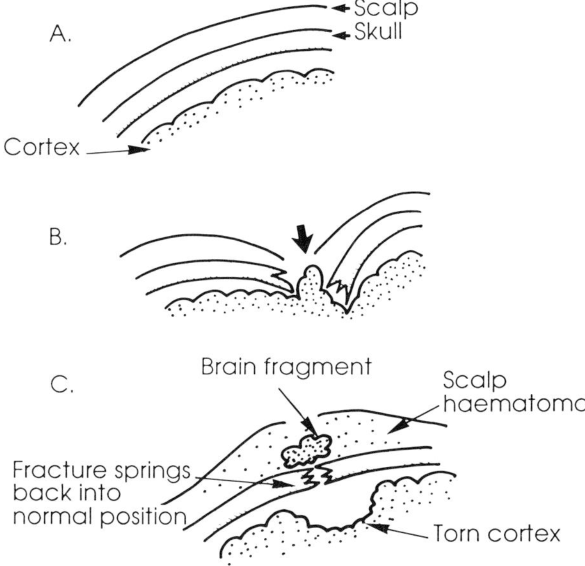

Fig. 12.17: *A localized skull fracture may cause a severe tear in the brain because of the elasticity of the skull bones.*

They are sustained during falls or play, when handling dangerous objects (e.g. scissors, broken glass) or are received during major trauma. The circumstances, site and extent of a laceration may vary considerably but four basic questions must be answered always (Table 12.8).

Lacerations may extend beyond the skin and subcutaneous tissue to damage underlying structures. The most important of these are nerves, vessels and tendons. The anatomical location of the laceration is a clue to the likely structures damaged. For example, a transverse laceration across the anterior surface of the forearm above the wrist is likely to damage the median nerve and flexor tendons. At its medial and lateral extremes, the ulnar and radial arteries respectively also may be involved. Damage to nerves is evident clinically by distal sensory and motor loss. The likely deficit can be predicted from knowledge of the function of the nerve which is damaged. Likewise, it is possible to predict the tendons which may have been severed and specifically to examine the function of each. Even where there appears to be no sensory or functional loss, lacerations should be explored surgically and, where there is evidence of injury to these structures, their exact site and extent must be determined.

Table 12.8 LACERATIONS: THE FOUR BASIC QUESTIONS

1. ?Does it involve – nerves
   – vessels
   – tendons
2. ?Is it associated with a fracture
3. ?Is there foreign material – contamination
   – macroscopic fragments
4. ?Is there dead tissue present

There are two difficulties which may be encountered during the assessment of a small child. First, he may be too small to cooperate or comprehend the manoeuvres in which he is being encouraged to participate. Examination for sensory deficit can be particularly unrewarding, although with patience and perseverance complete sensory loss can be elicited. Assessment is also a problem in the unconscious child or where there are adjacent bony fractures.

Secondly, bruising or stretching of nerves will cause a neuropraxia with temporary loss of function of that nerve, mimicking transection. Likewise, tendons may be incompletely severed but have the appearance of intact function on clinical examination. During exploration of the wound, the true situation is ascertained.

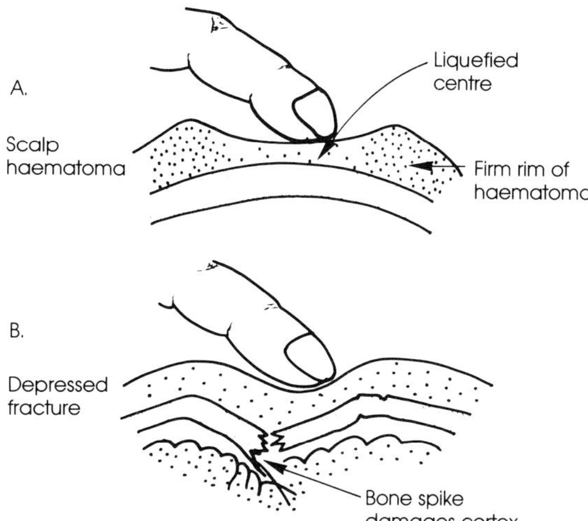

Fig. 12.18: *A scalp haematoma with a liquefied centre (A) may mimic a depressed fracture (B). Diagnosis is made on clinical suspicion and confirmed on oblique x-ray of the skull. The depressed fracture is important because a bony spike may damage the brain and lead to epilepsy.*

In all lacerations, the possibility of an underlying fracture must be considered. In many, the mode of injury will rule this out but in others, particularly head injuries, the possibility must be entertained and appropriate clinical and radiological investigation performed. A laceration in the region of a fracture makes that fracture 'compound', with an increased risk of infection and subsequent osteomyelitis or meningitis: the management of that fracture is altered and antibiotics will be required.

Young children have greater powers of regeneration than adults. This applies especially to finger-tip amputations, where the pulp is able to regenerate provided that the amputation has occurred distal to the midpoint of the distal phalanx (Fig. 12.19). Treatment of finger-tip amputations, therefore, is dictated by age and the exact level of amputation.

Depending on the mechanism of injury, a laceration may be contaminated by foreign material which may be evident on x-ray (e.g. metal, stone or glass fragments). In most cases, however, the presence of foreign material is established during exploration of the wound. It is imperative that foreign material is removed, otherwise infection ensues. Likewise, all devitalized tissue should be removed because it provides a reservoir for infection.

PERINEAL INJURIES

Differences in the anatomy of the perineum and external genitalia between the sexes affect the nature of injuries sustained to the perineum. For this reason, each sex is considered separately (Table 12.9)

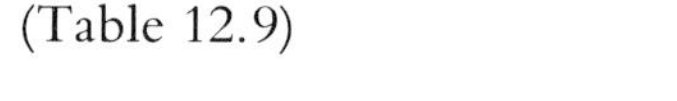

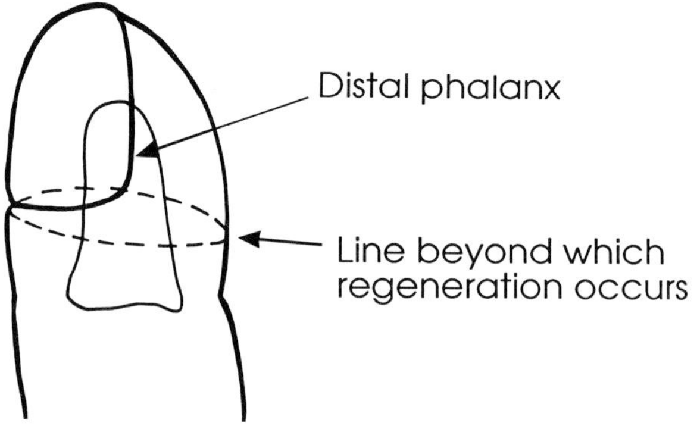

Fig. 12.19: *A finger-tip laceration with distal amputation. In small children, the finger-tip will regenerate completely.*

Male

Straddle injury

A boy who slips while walking along the top of a fence or climbing out of a bath (Fig. 12.20), is likely to sustain a straddle injury. The urethra is at risk as it passes through the urogenital fascia to lie superficially in the perineum. A straddle injury causes bruising in the perineum behind the scrotum, and oedema or bruising of the scrotum. The testes tend to 'ride with the injury' and are infrequently damaged because of their mobility. The important question is: 'Has the urethra been injured?' It may be contused or ruptured. A drop of blood at the meatus strongly suggests major urethral injury and, if it occurs in association with acute urinary retention and an enlarged bladder, complete urethral transection should be considered (Fig. 12.21). Blood-stained urine indicates urethral injury without complete disruption. When the anterior urethra is torn, urine leaks into the space deep to Colles' fascia (the membranous layer of the subcutaneous tissue) to cause swelling

Table 12.9 PERINEAL INJURIES

Type of injury	Male	Female
Straddle	?Urethral injury	?Vaginal tear
Penetrating	?Rectal/urinary injury	?Vaginal/rectal tear
Foreign body		Discharge from the vagina
Sexual abuse	Rare	Common

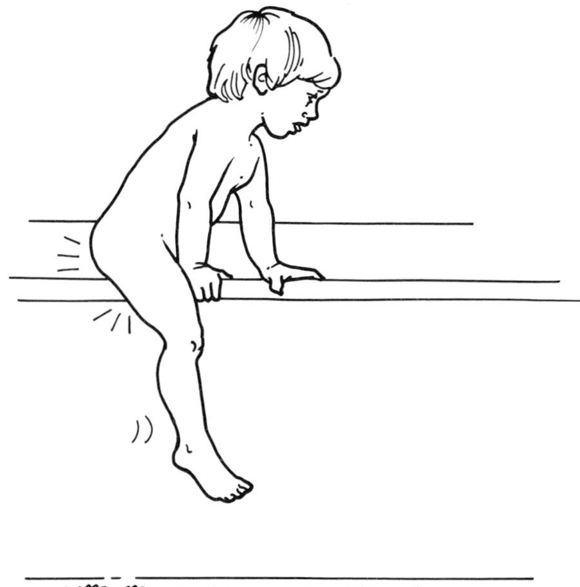

Fig. 12.20: *A common cause of perineal injury – slipping while climbing out of bath.*

of the scrotum and penis with extension to the ventral abdominal wall. The urinary extravasation produces a progressive, diffuse boggy swelling which becomes inflamed (from tissue reaction to urine), bruised (from blood in addition to urine) or frankly infected. Where urethral trauma is suspected, referral to hospital enables a urethrogram to be obtained so that the continuity of the urethra can be established. The surgical management of a urethral injury is dependent on its site, exact nature and associated bony or urinary tract injuries. Where perineal contusion has occurred without urethral injury, adequate analgesia normally permits continued voiding, and no further treatment is required.

Penetrating spike injury

Boys, in particular, may jump from a tree onto an exposed branch, or land on a picket fence while attempting to hurdle it, and sustain a penetrating injury of the perineum. Although any perineal and pelvic structure can be involved, the main danger is penetration of the rectum which may cause severe pelvic peritonitis and death if not recognized. For this reason, all penetrating perineal injuries should be explored carefully, usually under anaesthesia. One finger or a probe is inserted into the wound at the same time as another finger is inserted into the rectum. This allows the examiner to assess the relationship of the two: if the fingers meet at any point, or if the finger in the wound has faeces on it when it is withdrawn, then rectal injury has been proven. Sometimes the spike may enter the anus to perforate the rectum from within. This is evident from perineal or anal bruising and the presence of blood on the glove after rectal examination. This type of injury should raise the possibility of sexual abuse. If the rectum has been perforated above the peritoneal reflection, faecal peritonitis develops with progressive tenderness and guarding of the abdomen and systemic signs of toxicity. In cases of rectal injury, early recognition will allow a defunctioning colostomy and drainage of the wound, and may prevent the onset of serious peritonitis.

Female

Straddle injury

A straddle injury in a girl is more likely to cause

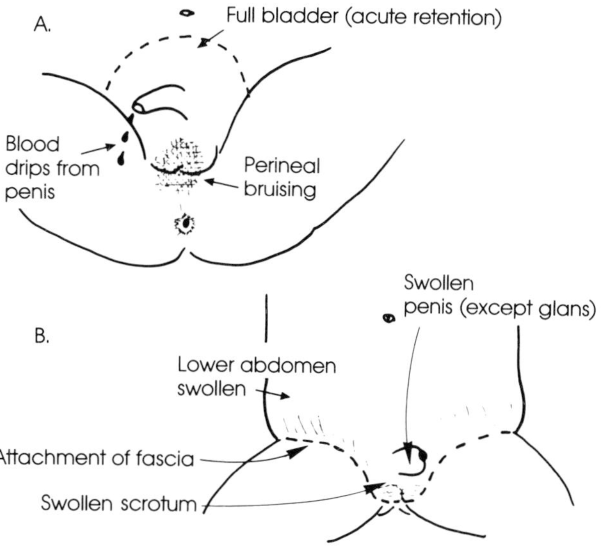

Fig. 12.21: *The straddle injury in the male, showing the early signs of a urethral tear (A), followed by urinary extravasation (B). The attachment of Colles' and Scarpa's fasciae prevent urine spreading posteriorly in the perineum to the anus or down the high.*

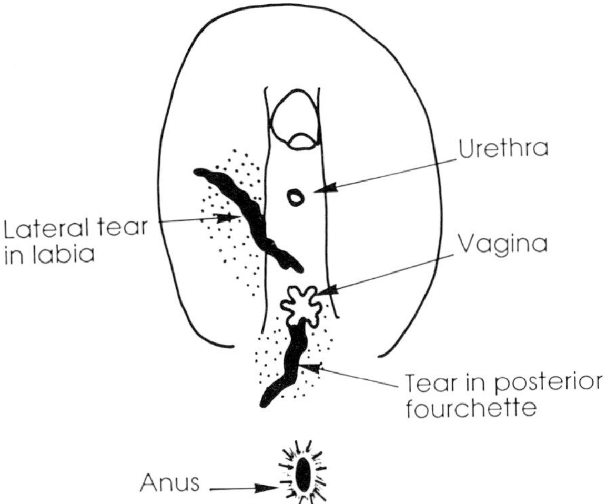

Fig. 12.22: *The two common types of laceration in the female perineum. Adequate examination to ensure the vagina is intact usually requires general anaesthesia.*

bruising or laceration of the introitus than urethral injury (Fig. 12.22). The laceration is either of the labia extending medially to the introitus, or in relation to the perineal body extending anteriorly into the vagina. Fear and pain render the child uncooperative and necessitate general anaesthesia for the examination of all but the most minor injuries. In every case, the possibility of sexual abuse must be entertained. A subcutaneous haematoma will appear as an enlarging dark red swelling, and is treated by local pressure and analgesia. Where a laceration is present, its extent must be established. Laceration of the perineum with extension across the posterior fourchette may indicate a penetrating vaginal injury.

The discharging vagina

Mucopurulent or offensive blood-stained discharge from the vagina is the sign of an unrecognized foreign body. The exploratory and inquisitive nature of the girl may be responsible for the introduction of the foreign material but, as with all female perineal injuries, molestation should be excluded. Treatment involves removal under general anaesthesia. Infections sometimes cause vaginal discharge, but these are rare, and the diagnosis is made from culture swabs after the existence of a foreign object has been excluded.

Sexual abuse

Sexual abuse is an important form of maltreatment which may go unrecognized unless the clinician maintains a high index of suspicion. It includes any sexual activity which a child or adolescent does not fully understand, is unable to give informed consent to, or which violates family and social taboos. Incest is the most common form of abuse, both of adolescents and small children, and is more likely to be concealed at presentation than when abuse emanates from outside the family.

Most children or adolescents who have been abused sexually will not have obvious external injuries and do not present to a surgeon. In a few, the history and nature of injuries lead directly to the diagnosis. However, the more common situation encountered by the surgeon is when a child presents with genital or perianal trauma, or a discharge from the vagina (Table 12.10). The surgeon must then consider the possibility of abuse, and the approach to the clinical assessment of such a child reflects this. The emphasis in the following section relates to the situation just described.

History

Where the presenting symptom is general trauma, a detailed history of the accident should reveal whether or not the story is consistent with the nature and severity of the injury and the child's developmental level. The child should be asked specifically to relate the story, and if abuse is suggested, details of times, dates and places should be sought. Descriptions by the child of sexual activities which are beyond the normal capabilities or experience of a child of that age are likely to be true. A clear history of trauma should exclude straddle injuries to the perineum (see page 145).

The differential diagnosis of perineal injuries or discharge is short (Table 12.11) and a few judicious questions will quickly eliminate urinary infection or a simple accident. A concealed foreign body may masquerade as a venereal infection because of secondary contamination. Self-inflicted injury may be difficult to distinguish from sexual abuse because the child may withhold information through fear or embarrassment.

Table 12.10 PRESENTING COMPLAINT VERSUS LIKELIHOOD OF SEXUAL ABUSE

Symptom/sign	Possibility of sexual abuse
Direct report from child Pregnancy Venereal disease Genital/rectal trauma Precocious sexual interest	Very high
Inappropriate sexual activity Indiscrete masturbation Genital inflammation/discharge	High
Behavioural disturbance Run-away from home	Moderate

Examination

Medicolegal considerations make a detailed examination under controlled conditions essential. Written consent should be obtained first from a parent or guardian, and the examination should be carried out in the presence of a witness of the opposite sex to the examiner. All details, including date, time, place of examination and name of witness, need to be recorded accurately. The impending procedures should be explained to the child as the examination progresses. If forensic specimens, such as vaginal swabs and smears, are likely to be required, the examiner should wear gloves.

The general appearance and emotional state of the child is noted, and obvious injuries should be photographed. Clothing should be removed only in the presence of the clinician and a witness, with the child standing on a sheet of paper, to avoid loss of forensic evidence. The clothing is documented, examined and stored. The face, mouth, throat, head, limbs, thorax, abdomen and buttocks are examined for bruises, abrasions or bite marks. The ear drums require careful inspection to exclude traumatic rupture, which is a common sequel to slapping the side of the face. If the injury suggests recent sexual intercourse, the clothing and skin should be examined under UV light (Woods lamp) since dried semen will fluoresce.

Table 12.11 DIFFERENTIAL DIAGNOSIS OF PERINEAL INJURY AND VAGINAL DISCHARGE

Urinary infection (infected urine pooling in vagina)
Simple accident (straddle injury on fence/bath)
Foreign body (foul-smelling discharge)
Self-inflicted injury (? masturbation)
Sexual abuse (bruising, lacerations, discharge)

The external genitalia and perineum should be examined carefully for semen, blood and mucus as well as for obvious signs of trauma such as bruising or lacerations. The age of bruises should be estimated by their colour. The anus should be examined for signs of rectal trauma. The laxity of anal sphincters is not a reliable sign of anal intercourse in children, since the sphincters are often relaxed normally in sleep.

Where a labial laceration is found in a small girl, examination under anaesthesia is the best way to determine the extent and severity of the injury. In adolescents, a speculum examination of the vagina may be quite satisfactory to identify trauma and obtain swabs.

In cases where sexual abuse appears likely, expert medical and police help should be obtained immediately, so that medical management and forensic and legal proceedings can begin.

FRACTURES

The diagnosis of fractures in older children is

straightforward. However, in small children lack of cooperation and communication may make diagnosis difficult. Soft tissue injuries to the limbs with nerve or tendon damage may be particularly difficult to diagnose because the frightened, distressed infant is not able to cooperate in the physical examination. Even if no deformity is present, it is important to remember that a fracture is more common than a sprain, since the ligaments are much stronger than the bones during childhood. The appearance of the epiphysis and the adjacent cartilaginous growth plate also may lead to confusion during diagnosis, because the cartilaginous parts are not visible on x-ray. Injuries near to or involving the growth plate need referral to someone with significant orthopaedic experience, since inadequate treatment of the fracture may lead to later deformity or limb shortening.

The most important point to remember is that pain along with loss of function in a limb is nearly always caused by a fracture. Minor fractures, such as buckling of the cortex or a greenstick fracture, where the cortex is broken only on one side, are common in childhood and produce little deformity. This type of fracture follows minor accidents around the home or school. More serious fractures through the long bones may occur with a major fall from the roof of a house or a tree, or are sustained in a motor accident. Fractures through the epiphysis are important because they may be 'invisible' on x-ray and the prognosis for growth of the limb following treatment is uncertain. Pathological fractures do occur but are rare in childhood. Benign bony cysts or malignant tumours (osteosarcoma), infection (osteomyelitis) or metabolic diseases (osteogenesis imperfecta) may cause pathological fractures. Children on steroid therapy for malignant disease or chronic inflammatory disease may develop fractures secondary to cortisone-induced osteoporosis.

Fracture of the clavicle is the commonest fracture seen in childhood but does not need to be described at length since its clinical features are identical to those seen in adults. Reduction usually is not needed in children, and the only treatment required is to rest the arm in a sling for two to three weeks.

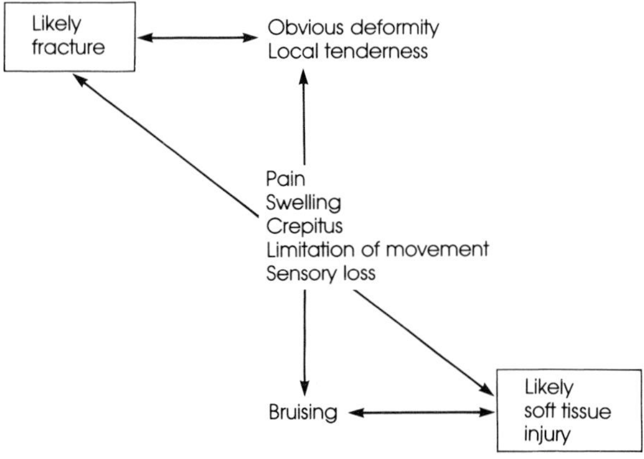

Fig. 12.23: *The signs and symptoms which allow a fracture of the upper limb to be distinguished from a soft tissue injury.*

Upper limb fractures

The superficial location of the bones of the upper limb enables the deformity and bony tenderness of upper limb fractures to be identified readily (Fig. 12.23). Non-specific signs and symptoms include pain, swelling, crepitus, limitation of movement and sensory loss. In fractures, crepitus results from grating of the bone ends on palpation and movement, but may be caused also by a penetrating injury with air under the skin in the absence of a fracture. If bruising alone is present, it is likely that the child has sustained a soft tissue injury rather than a fracture. Bruising secondary to a fracture is rare in the early phases following trauma.

Supracondylar fracture of the humerus

This is a common and important fracture of childhood which follows a fall onto an extended arm. The elbow joint is pushed posteriorly on the humerus and tilted backwards, although the posterior periosteum usually remains intact. The jagged lower end of the shaft of the humerus protrudes forward into the cubital fossa, which is dangerous because of potential damage to the brachial artery or median and radial nerves (Fig.

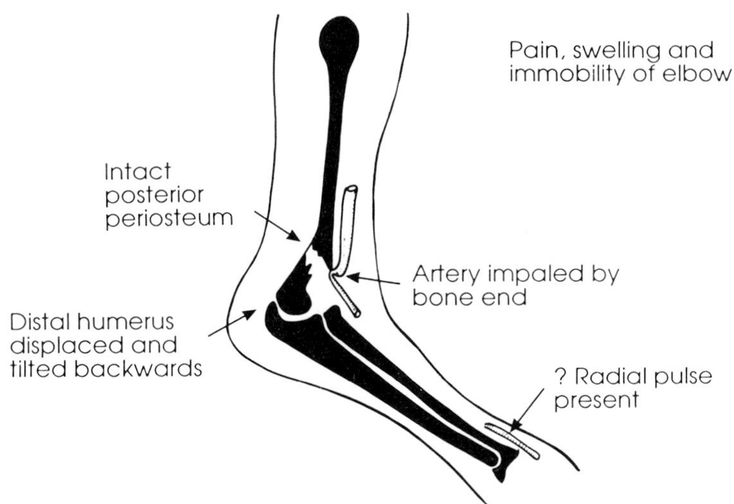

Fig. 12.24: *The signs and symptoms of a supracondylar fracture of the humerus.*

12.24). The child presents with pain, swelling and immobility of the elbow. The most important physical sign to elicit in this or any other fracture around the elbow is the radial pulse. In a supracondylar fracture, the brachial artery may be compressed or damaged by the jagged bone end or may constrict in spasm resulting in a diminished or absent radial pulse.

Loss of blood supply to the forearm causes ischaemic necrosis of the forearm muscles, which are later replaced by scar tissue, producing a clinical syndrome called 'Volkmann's contracture'. Volkmann's contracture is the most important and sinister consequence of inadequate diagnosis and treatment of a supracondylar fracture (Fig. 12.25). Displacement of the humeral shaft leading to arterial occlusion and muscle ischaemia, must be relieved within 6–12 hours to avoid complete infarction of the muscles with subsequent fibrosis and secondary deformity. The physical signs associated with these various stages include deformity, tenderness and swelling by the fracture. Arterial occlusion causes loss of the radial pulse. Ischaemia of the muscle produces severe pain in the forearm, pallor of the fingers, hand and forearm, oedema of the forearm, and paralysis of the hand and forearm muscles. In untreated cases, the fibrosis following muscle infarction leads to a 'claw hand' deformity. The key physical signs are loss of the radial pulse and severe pain in the forearm when the fingers are extended passively; this can be demonstrated between one and 24 hours after the accident. Persistence of the arterial occlusion or spasm can be relieved by splitting or removing the plaster and extending the arm until the pulse returns. Open exploration of the artery is required if this manoeuvre is unsuccessful.

Capitellar fracture of the humerus

The lateral condyle, or capitellum of the humerus, may be fractured following a fall on to the arm (Fig. 12.26). It is misdiagnosed commonly as a sprain because the fracture is through the cartilaginous growth plate, which is not seen on x-ray. The fracture line crosses the epiphysis and enters the joint, but the ossification centre for the capitellum appears intact. The only abnormality on the x-ray may be a small flake of bone from the distal end of the metaphysis. Although the x-rays give a false impression that this is a minor fracture, involvement of the joint means that it must be corrected exactly to maintain normal elbow function. Consequently, this is one of the few fractures in childhood requiring open reduction and internal fixation to realign the displaced joint surfaces. If the capitellum is not displaced, a collar and cuff sling is adequate treatment.

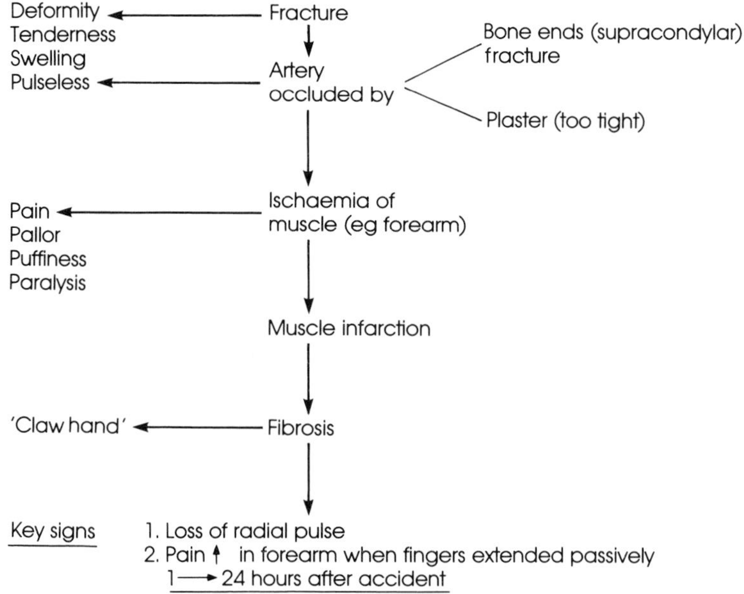

Fig. 12.25: *The mechanism and signs of forearm muscle ischaemia which, if untreated, leads to Volkmann's contracture.*

Subluxation of the head of the radius

Subluxation of the radial head, or 'pulled elbow' occurs when an infant's arm has been pulled hard by an adult in play, during a tantrum or to prevent an accident. The head of the radius is dislocated partially out of the annular ligament, which is caught between the joint surfaces of the radius and the humerus (Fig. 12.27). The appearance of the infant is quite characteristic with the normal arm supporting the injured limb which is held immobile in pronation. There is localized tenderness over the head of the radius. Passive flexion and extension of the elbow may be limited but not totally lost. In contrast, passive supination of the forearm is resisted completely because this induces severe pain in the joint. The head of the radius can be replaced in the joint by twisting the forearm alternately in pronation and supination while pushing the forearm towards the elbow. This manoeuvre simulates handling a screwdriver.

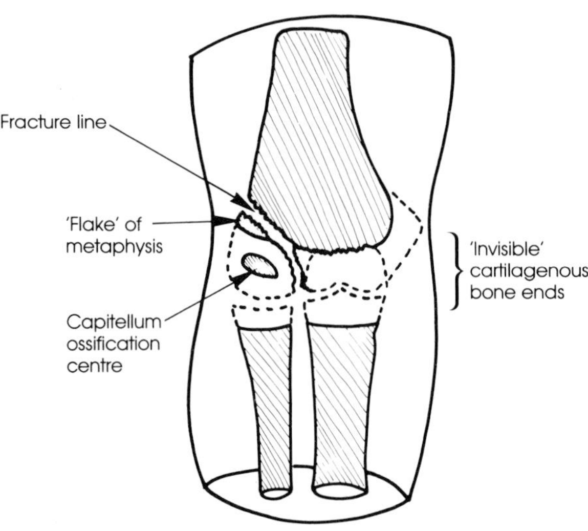

Fig. 12.26: *Capitellar (lateral condyle) fracture of the humerus. This is misdiagnosed easily as a sprain, unless the significance of the flake of metaphysis is appreciated.*

Forearm fractures

The radius and ulna are broken with falls onto the hand or the arm (Fig. 12.28). Fractures of the shafts of these bones are more common than in adults. The commonest type is a greenstick fracture of the lower end of the radius and ulna (Colles' fracture). Where deformity is present it is characteristically the shape of a dinner fork. In a fall onto a pronated forearm or a direct blow to the back of the forearm, the ulna may fracture alone

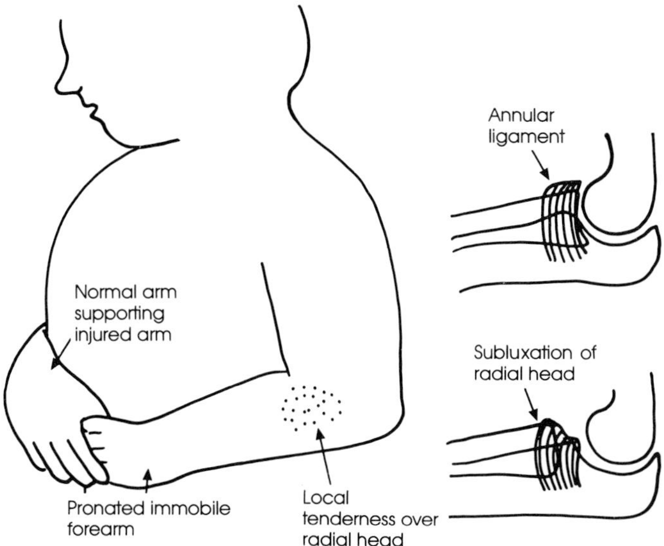

Fig. 12.27: *Subluxation of the head of the radius in an infant.*

and the radial head dislocate, producing a Monteggia's fracture. This is an important injury because the dislocated radial head may be overlooked on clinical or radiological investigations. Biplanar x-rays always should include the joints above and below the injury, and in forearm fractures, this procedure will prevent the dislocated radial head being missed. Forearm fractures are treated by manipulation under general anaesthesia if there is displacement, followed by an above-elbow cast.

Lower limb fractures

Lower limb fractures may be difficult to diagnose because the greater bulk of the lower limb compared with the upper limb precludes direct palpation of the bones. Deformity in association with painful movement provides strong clinical evidence of a fracture (Fig. 12.29). Physical signs which may be present with both bone and soft tissue injuries include pain in the leg on standing, local tenderness, limitation of movement and crepitus. If bruising alone is present, it is likely that the bone is intact.

Fractured femur

Femoral fractures occur with major falls from the roof or a tree, or in a motor accident (Fig. 12.30). Commonly, the femur is fractured in child pedestrians, since the thigh is level with the bumper bar of a car. A strong bone such as the femur requires major force to break it, and therefore it is usually associated with multiple injuries to the head, chest or abdomen. A horizontal blow from a car produces a transverse midshaft fracture, leading to a swollen and painful thigh which cannot weight-bear. The force of the injury is associated with lacerations either from the bone ends or from other penetrating wounds.

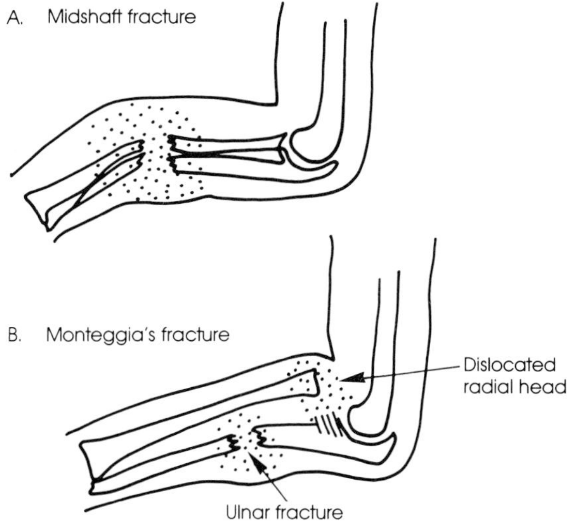

Fig. 12.28: *Fractures of the forearm.*

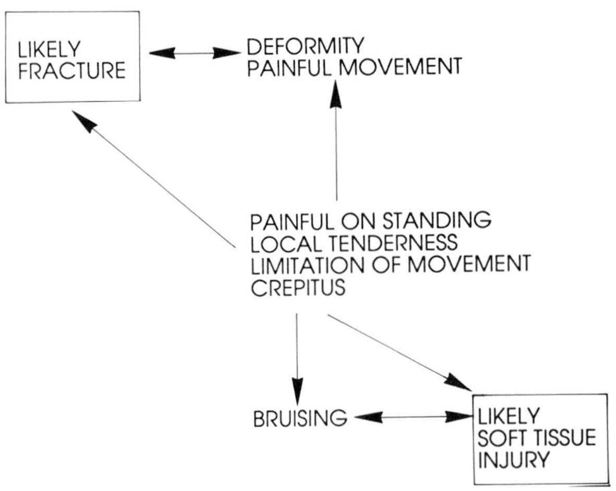

Fig. 12.29: *The signs and symptoms of lower limb fractures and soft tissue injuries.*

BURNS

Three parameters are important in the assessment of the severity of any burn:

(1) The circumstances and type of burn
(2) The area of burn
(3) The depth of burn.

Type of burn

Knowledge of the causative agent is useful in anticipating the likely type and severity of burn. Scalds account for 85% of burns in children less than 10 years of age, and the injury they cause is related to:

(1) The temperature of the liquid at the time of the accident. Had the water just boiled? For how long had the cup of coffee been poured?
(2) The length of time the skin was exposed to the hot liquid. Was clothing removed immediately? How long was it before the burnt area was dowsed in cold water?
(3) The type of liquid involved. Fats are hotter and retain their heat longer than water.

The worst flame burns involve flammable clothing and are proportional to the temperature of the flame and duration of exposure. Synthetic materials often melt, producing molten blobs which become adherent to the skin and cause further damage. In children, chemical burns are received through contact with household or gardening agents, particularly strong alkalis and acids. The severity of burn is dependent on their concentration and the time elapsed before being washed off.

Electrical burns damage all the tissues between the entry and exit points of the current. At low voltage, the skin – being a poor conductor – is less affected than muscle, nerves and blood vessels, belying the gravity of the injury to the deeper structures.

Area of burn

The infant has a proportionally larger head and smaller lower limbs than the older child or adult (Fig. 12.31). When estimating the area of a burn, therefore, a figure chart should be used and the age of the child taken into account. There is a tend-

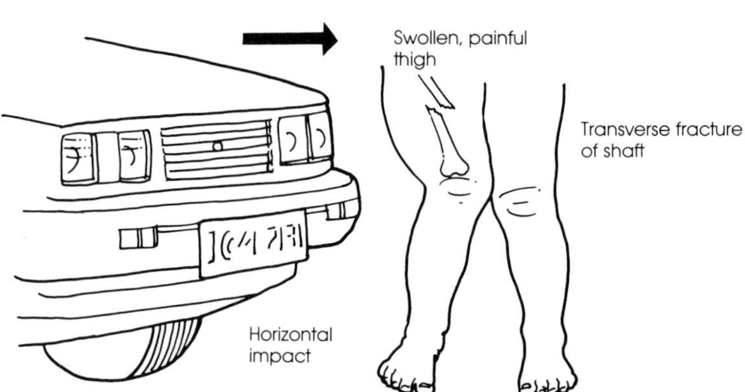

Fig. 12.30: *Fractured femur: transverse shaft fracture is the common injury in childhood.*

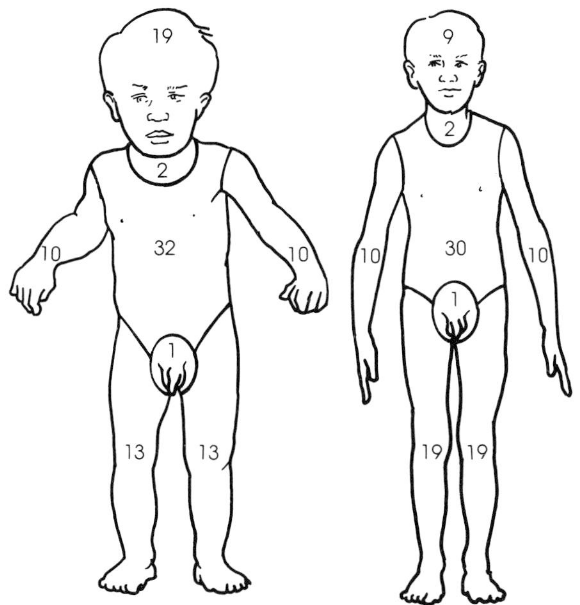

Fig. 12.31: *Estimation of burn area in children of different ages.*

ency to over-estimate the area burned, which is another reason for mapping out the area on a figure chart. This chart should become part of the medical record.

Depth of burn

It is important to know the depth of the burn (Fig. 12.32) because:

(1) the metabolic upset is greater with deeper burns;
(2) healing occurs more slowly with increasing depth of burn;
(3) deep burns (unless small) require skin grafting;
(4) circumferential deep burns, involving limbs, digits or the chest wall, may cause vascular impairment or restrict ventilation, and necessitate urgent decompression with escharotomy.

When assessing the depth of burns in children, it is useful to appreciate that:

(1) small children have thinner skin, and therefore a certain insult will cause greater damage;
(2) skin thickness varies from area to area (e.g. the skin of the back is thicker than that of the forearm, and plantar or palmar skin is thicker than the skin of the eyelids);
(3) parts of the body with good blood supply (e.g. the face) conduct the heat of the burn away more quickly, and heal more rapidly after a burn;
(4) some areas of the skin may be more deeply burned than others.

Burns involving the epidermis alone (first degree/superficial) are painful and appear as a bright erythematous area which has a tendency to blister and is sensitive to pin-prick. Full thickness burns (third degree/subdermal) imply death of all layers of the skin and exposure of the subcutaneous layers. The sensitive nerve endings in the dermis have been destroyed, producing a rela-

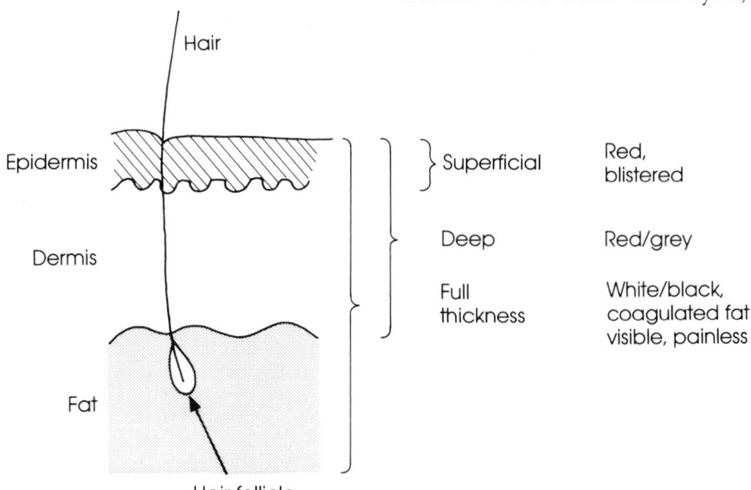

Fig. 12.32: *Assessment of the depth of the burn.*

tively painless lesion which is insensitive to pinprick. When the injury is caused by a scald, the surface appears pale or white with a transitional zone of more superficially burned skin between it and unaffected skin. In flame burns, the surface is black or brown. As the skin lifts or is burnt off, subcutaneous fat becomes visible. Coagulative necrosis and thrombosis of underlying vessels is seen as dark red puncta, and there may be islets of surviving skin. Deep partial thickness burns vary in colour and may be difficult to distinguish both from more superficial and from deeper burns. Blisters are common, but the skin is often grey or a darker red than the erythema of epidermal burns. Where doubt persists, re-examination after about one week clarifies matters.

Table 12.12 CAUSES OF RESPIRATORY INSUFFICIENCY IN BURNS

Site of pathology	Cause
Upper airway obstruction	– coma or shock – posture – associated injuries – laryngeal burns
Lower airway obstruction	– bronchospasm – soot/smoke – mucus plugging
Parenchymal damage	– hot gas – toxic chemical
Impairment of ventilation	– chest wall burns
Pneumonia	– secondary infection

General signs in burns

Restlessness

Superficial burns are extremely painful and may cause restlessness, which must be distinguished from hypoxia or restlessness caused by psychological factors following the accident. In major burns, hypoxia must be suspected and blood gases obtained.

Shock

Thirst, nausea and lethargy are symptoms of hypovolaemic shock which can be assessed clinically by observing general pallor and by measurement of the pulse, blood pressure, quality of peripheral perfusion (warmth of the extremities and rapidity of capillary return), degree of dehydration (moistness of mucous membranes, tissue turgor, sunken eyes, collapsed fontanelle) and urine output. An extensive area of burn (greater than 10–15% surface area), deep burns and young age are factors predisposing to hypovolaemic shock. Hypovolaemia should be anticipated and prevented by the administration of intravenous fluids and blood.

Associated injuries

The possibility of other injuries sustained with the burn must be entertained from knowledge of the circumstances of the accident, and ruled out by clinical examination.

An inhalational injury is caused by hot gas or poisonous smoke damaging the airways and lung parenchyma. Inhalation trauma can be anticipated from the history of the injury, by examination of the nose and mouth for evidence of burns, and by observation for the development of stridor and respiratory distress. Early onset of respiratory symptoms suggests severe injury to the respiratory passages.

A history of smoke inhalation, of being trapped in an enclosed space, or of the combustion of synthetic materials or toxic industrial chemicals, makes inhalation injury likely. Flame burns to the face and mouth suggest that the inspired gases were of high temperature. Look at the nostrils for burns to the nasal hairs, and at the mucous membrane of the mouth and pharynx for oedema, erythema or soot (Fig. 12.33). A hoarse voice indicates an inhalational injury with vocal cord oedema.

Hot gases and toxic agents damage the respiratory passages, causing oedema and bronchial irritation (Table 12.12). The irritated and swollen mucosa of the bronchi produce excessive mucus and bronchospasm. Obstruction of the airways may occur from bronchospasm, soot and mucus plugging, and be exacerbated by poor posture, coma or aspiration of vomit.

The chest should be examined for evidence of hyperexpansion and increased respiratory rate or effort. The use of accessory muscles of respiration and the amount of indrawing that occurs during inspiration should be noted. There may be an audible wheeze and auscultation may reveal few breath sounds, crepitations and rhonchi. A localized area of poor air entry may be caused by mucus plugging and, if unrelieved, becomes an area of atelectasis with crepitations and dullness on percussion.

In major burns, the presence of hypoxia should be detected biochemically before it becomes manifest clinically. The signs of hypoxia are late and imply severe lack of oxygen. The child appears restless, confused and disoriented, or shows a change in behaviour. However, the circumstances of major injury in a child experiencing pain in an unfamiliar and frightening environment, limit the specificity of these parameters. Increasing respiratory effort also may reflect hypoxia or anxiety, pain or another respiratory complication, but cyanosis indicates that severe hypoxia has occurred already.

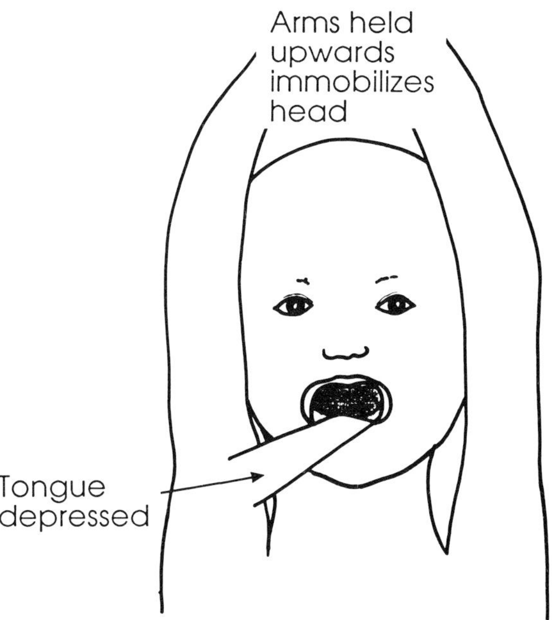

Fig. 12.33: *Examination of the mouth and oropharynx in a small child.*

FOREIGN BODIES

There is a tendency for children under three years of age to put things into their mouths and, as a consequence, to swallow or inhale them.

The child who has swallowed a foreign body

Most swallowed foreign bodies are inert and pass through the gastro-intestinal tract uneventfully. The child is likely to present if (1) ingestion was witnessed, or (2) it has caused symptoms. The symptoms of an ingested foreign body vary according to where its passage becomes arrested. In the mouth and pharynx, it may cause choking and gagging, with dysphagia and excessive salivation. Fish bones often become stuck in the tonsillar region. Foreign bodies in the oesophagus (e.g. coins) cause retrosternal discomfort, excessive salivation and difficulty in swallowing. The child can drink, but attempts at swallowing solid material result in regurgitation and choking. Once a foreign body reaches the stomach, it should pass through the gut unless it is too long to negotiate the duodenojejunal flexure (e.g. bobby-pins or other rigid objects more than 6 or 7 cm long). Rarely, foreign bodies such as large chicken bones and toothpicks may cause perforation of the terminal ileum and produce symptoms similar to those of appendicitis with localized peritonitis. Ingestion of button or disc batteries is considered hazardous because they may leak strong alkali and cause local necrosis and perforation of the bowel.

In the asymptomatic child, where the type of foreign body ingested is known and unlikely to cause complications, no further investigation is required. Where the child has symptoms referable to the mouth, pharynx or oesophagus, the location of the foreign body should be established. The mouth should be examined, including inspection of the fauces and tonsillar region (Fig. 12.33). In the smaller child, examination requires two people – one to hold the child still with the head extended, the other to focus the torch on the back of the mouth with one hand and to manipulate the tongue depressor with the other. Deliberately allowing the spatula to touch the fauces causes the child to gag and may improve visualization of the oropharynx and tonsillar region. This manoeuvre

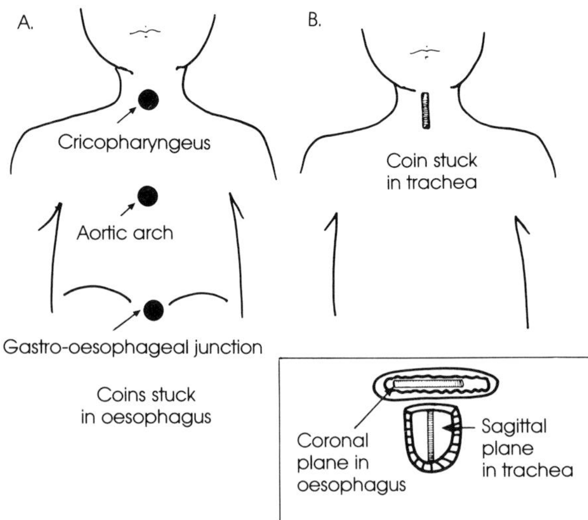

Fig. 12.34: *Coins stuck in the oesophagus* (A) *or trachea* (B).

is only of benefit if the child is restrained.

Where the foreign body is radio-opaque, x-rays are valuable. Where the location of a swallowed foreign body is uncertain, x-rays should include the head and neck, thorax and abdomen, as the foreign body could be located anywhere from the nasopharynx to the anus. Coins, which are amongst the commonest radio-opaque items swallowed, usually become arrested in the upper oesophagus (see Fig. 12.34), and can be shown to be in the oesophagus rather than the trachea by observing the orientation of the coin or by obtaining a lateral x-ray (Fig. 12.34). Coins in the oesophagus are common and lie in a coronal plane, whereas coins in the trachea are extremely rare and have a sagittal orientation. If the coin is below the diaphragm, no further action is required. Foreign bodies lodged in the oesophagus require oesophagoscopy and removal under general anaesthesia. Those which reach the stomach, including open safety-pins, can be allowed to pass spontaneously unless they are very long (Fig. 12.35) or likely to cause secondary complications (e.g. button batteries). In these situations, consideration must be given to their endoscopic removal.

In the rare event that a foreign body causes perforation of the bowel, there is often no history of foreign body ingestion and the diagnosis is made at operation for peritonitis. Retrosternal discomfort and prolonged or progressive dysphagia may be caused by impaction of a foreign body in the oesophagus without complete obstruction. Perforation of the oesophagus produces signs of mediastinitis, which include malaise, fever, pain, and swelling and subcutaneous em-

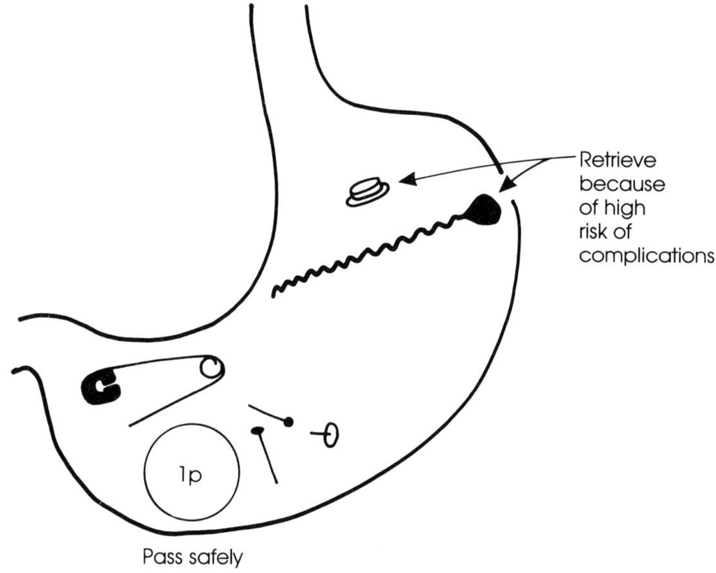

Fig. 12.35: *The approach to foreign bodies in the stomach.*

physema in the neck. Subcutaneous emphysema, caused by air spreading along tissue planes, is diagnosed by feeling crepitus and 'bubbling' in the soft tissues.

Has a foreign body been inhaled?

Most children who have inhaled a foreign body present early, either because of sudden onset of coughing, spluttering and an audible wheeze, or because the object was observed to have been inhaled. In less than one third, the episode of inhalation is not recognized at the time, and the child presents weeks or months later with a wheeze, bronchitis or chronic chest infection.

The usual foreign body inhaled is a peanut, and most children are aged three years or under. Cyanosis is rare, and reflects almost complete obstruction of the trachea or the presence of multiple inhaled particles. The usual symptoms are coughing and a wheeze, although the child may appear to gag and vomit. If there is diagnostic delay, the child may develop pyrexia and chest infections (Fig. 12.36).

An inhaled foreign body may produce a 'ball-valve' effect, whereby dilatation of the bronchus during inspiration allows air in, but no air escapes during expiration. This will cause the lung distal to the obstruction to become hyperinflated while remaining poorly ventilated. Clinically, this can be detected by observing the movement of the chest wall with respiration and looking for asymmetry. There may be an inspiratory stridor and increased use of the accessory muscles of respiration. The child will tend to sit leaning forward, breathing through the mouth, with retraction of the supraclavicular and intercostal areas during inspiration. The increased respiratory effort increases the negative intrathoracic pressure to suck more air past the obstruction into the distal segments of lung. The chest is hyper-resonant on percussion, and auscultation may reveal reduced air entry to one side and a wheeze. Inspiratory and expiratory films, or screening x-rays, confirm the diagnosis. When a peanut is inhaled, it becomes impacted in the bronchus and causes the surrounding mucosa to swell. This leads to collapse of the distal lung and subsequent infection, with signs of consolidation and pneumonia on examination.

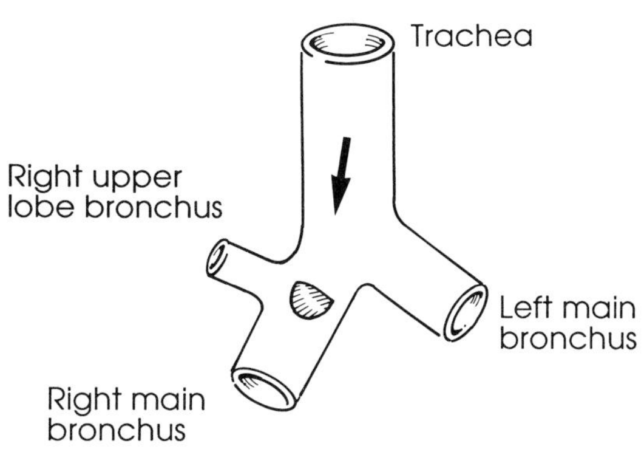

Fig. 12.36: *Inhaled foreign bodies in the trachea. A peanut is the common foreign material, and the right main bronchus is obstructed because it runs almost vertically downwards.*

Has a corrosive been swallowed?

Children between nine months and three years of age are particularly liable to swallow corrosive substances accidentally. In most instances, the toddler is unsupervised during exploration of the kitchen cupboards when he ingests some washing powder or house detergent. The mother's attention is drawn to the accident when the child starts crying and is observed to be drooling excessively, suffers pain on swallowing and refuses to eat, or has blisters on the tongue, lips and around the mouth, and burns to the fingers.

The importance of early recognition of corrosive ingestion relates to the susceptibility of the oesophagus to major damage from strong alkalis. Burns in and around the mouth are suggestive of concomitant oesophageal injury and are an indication for oesophagoscopy to delineate the extent and severity of injury. Therefore, when there is a possibility of corrosive ingestion, the tongue, buccal mucosa, palate and lips must be examined carefully. Failure to recognize and treat major oesophageal burns early is likely to result in oesophageal stenosis from stricture formation that is resistant to dilatation.

GOLDEN RULES

General and resuscitation

(1) The supreme aim of the initial assessment

and resuscitation after any trauma is to ensure that oxygenation of the brain is occurring. A patent airway (A = airway), and adequate ventilation (B = breathing) and perfusion (C = circulation) must be provided.

(2) Beware the battered child: where the history and physical signs do not correlate, consider child abuse.

(3) Beware major blood loss in the child: the small child compensates well for blood loss and there is a tendency to underestimate the amount lost. A child with clinical evidence of shock has suffered major haemorrhage.

(4) Children suffering major trauma should be assumed to have multiple organ system injury, until proved otherwise.

(5) Beware the missed injury: carefully reassess the child after resuscitation is complete to look for skeletal and other injuries not evident at the first presentation.

(6) In multiple system trauma, the most important early investigation is the chest x-ray.

(7) Repeated serial examination of the cardiovascular system, the neurological state and the abdomen, is essential to determine progression of signs.

(8) The clinical demonstration of blood in the peritoneal cavity is not in itself an indication for surgery.

(9) Beware retroperitoneal and renal injury: look for blood in the urine in all cases of abdominal trauma.

(10) Absence of haematuria rules out major urinary tract injury (except in the rare case of transection of the ureter or urethra).

Head and neck injuries

(1) Beware airway obstruction: hypoxia in the small child with concussion may cause coma.

(2) Beware hypoxia, hypercapnioa and hypotension in the head injury: these factors have a devastating effect on the injured brain and may extend the neurological damage.

(3) Beware severe hypotension in association with a head injury: look for bleeding into the chest, abdomen or long bones.

(4) Beware complete absence of respiratory effort: the child may have a high cervical spinal injury. Look for flaccidity of all limbs and hypotension.

(5) Assessment of head injuries involves repeated examinations at intervals and accurate recording of information: only in this way will deterioration be detected early.

(6) Beware the unilateral fixed dilated pupil: it may represent local damage to the orbit and the nerves of the pupillary reflex arc and be of little neurological significance, or it may be the first indicator of an expanding intracranial lesion and increased pressure.

(7) Beware the scalp laceration: the child may have a compound fracture of the skull.

(8) Beware the child who becomes drowsy and vomits after an apparently minor head injury: he may have intracranial haemorrhage.

Perineal injuries

(1) Beware the female perineal injury: has sexual abuse occurred?

(2) Beware the straddle injury in a boy: the urethra may have been damaged.

(3) Beware a boggy swelling of the perineum, scrotum and penis after perineal trauma: urine extravasation from penile injury has occurred.

(4) Penetrating perineal injuries should be explored to rule out rectal or lower urinary tract injury.

(5) Beware the laceration extending across the posterior fourchette: deeper vaginal or intraperitoneal injury may have occurred.

Limb injuries

(1) Beware femoral fractures in infants: child abuse is likely.

(2) Acute loss of function and pain in a limb indicates a fracture until proven otherwise.

(3) Beware pallor/anaemia in femoral fractures: internal haemorrhage is present.

(4) Beware the supracondylar fracture: look for evidence of distal ischaemia and neurological loss.

(5) Beware loss of finger movement in elbow injuries: the medial, ulnar or radial nerves may be damaged.

(6) Beware persisting pain after reduction of a fracture: muscle ischaemia is present.

(7) Beware loss of capillary circulation: muscle ischaemia is present.

(8) All potential fractures should be x-rayed, including the joints above and below the

injury, and in two planes.

(9) Beware the 'sprain': this is usually a fracture without displacement, since bones are weaker than ligaments during childhood.

(10) Beware the 'dislocation': these occur only at the elbow in childhood.

(11) All lacerations should be explored for evidence of tendon, nerve or vascular injury.

Burns

(1) Severity of burn depends on the temperature and duration of exposure to the causative agent, the area involved and the depth of the burn.

(2) Knowledge of the circumstances of a burn provides useful information for determining the severity of injury and predicting likely complications and sequelae.

(3) Beware burns to the head in the infant: the head accounts for one fifth of the surface area.

Foreign bodies

(1) Virtually all ingested foreign bodies pass spontaneously.

(2) Radiography for a swallowed object should include the head and neck, thorax and abdomen.

(3) Beware the long rigid foreign body: it may get stuck at the duodenojejunal flexure.

(4) Beware the mercury oxide micro-battery which has been swallowed: disintegration releases corrosive substances which damage the bowel wall.

(5) Oesophagoscopy is indicated for all foreign bodies impacted in the oesophagus.

13 The limbs

Abnormalities in the limbs affect the legs more frequently than the arms, except for fractures (see Chapter 12). There are many problems which are minor aberrations of shape during growth, both before birth (e.g. compression deformities) and during childhood (e.g. 'bow legs' and 'knock knees'). This chapter discusses the common anomalies (1) as they present at birth, and (2) in early childhood, as well as the important pathological conditions (e.g. osteomyelitis) which may occur at any time throughout life.

THE LIMBS AT BIRTH

Abnormalities of the hip joints or the shape of the feet at birth are common. The attention of the physician often will be directed to misshapen feet, but the more important abnormality to detect is congenital dislocation of the hip. This is one area in paediatric surgery where a 'screening' examination is very helpful because the hip treated at birth (by splinting) will grow normally, whereas diagnosis of a dislocation after the child has learnt to walk (with a limp) may be too late to preserve function.

The hip joint

The Ortolani test is used to diagnose dislocation of the hips (Fig. 13.1). The baby should be relaxed with the pelvis held still between the thumb and fingers of one hand while the other hand holds the thigh with the thumb in the groin (anteriorly) and the middle finger on the greater trochanter (posteriorly). The hip is flexed to 90° and then abducted to 45°. In this position, forward pressure with the middle finger will tend to push the femoral head into the joint, while backward pressure of the thumb will tend to dislocate the head posteriorly. When the femoral head relocates, there is an audible and palpable 'clunk'. The baby should be referred for an orthopaedic opinion and application of a harness (e.g. Pavlik) to hold the femoral head within the joint until dislocation can no longer occur.

Foot deformity

Most abnormalities are caused by extrinsic compression of the feet within the uterus and resolve spontaneously after birth (Fig. 13.2). These postural deformities can be recognized on examination by a normal range of passive movement. The deformity may be caused by abnormalities of fetal position or of the uterus (e.g. septum or fibroids), and will be predisposed to by oligohydramnios, a small amniotic cavity (especially with chromosomal abnormalities), or paralysis/stiffness of the legs (e.g. spina bifida, arthrogryposis). Weak legs cannot kick hard enough to allow the feet to maintain their normal posture *in utero*. Consequently, all babies with deformed feet must be examined carefully for (1) major chromosomal defects, (2) multiple joint abnormalities (arthrogryposis), and (3) myelomeningocele.

Particular postural deformities, such as calcaneovalgus, are of themselves trivial but may signal associated dislocation of the hip, since the position of the dislocated leg *in utero* predisposes

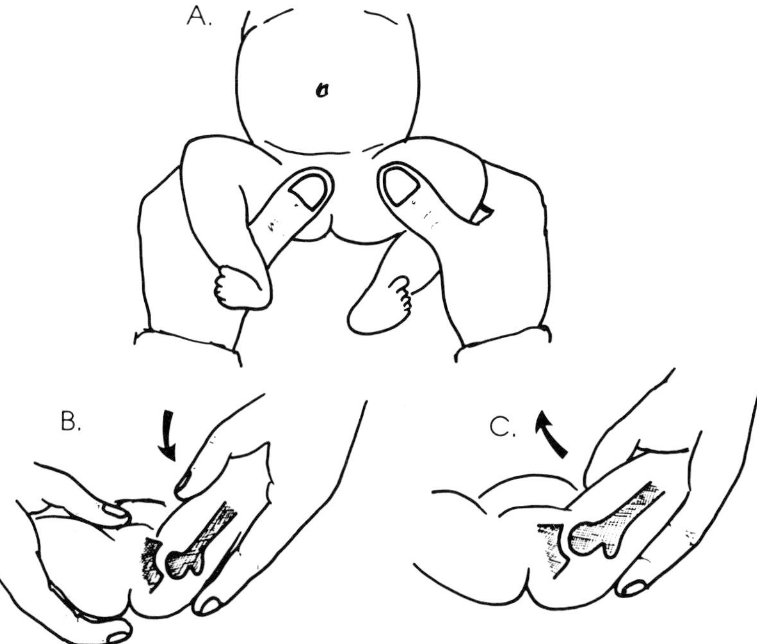

Fig. 13.1: *The Ortolani test for diagnosis of congenital dislocation of the hip(s). A. How to hold the pelvis and legs. B. The thumb on the groin pushes the femur posteriorly. C. The middle finger on the greater trochanter pushes the femur forwards and may cause a 'clunk' as the head re-enters the joint.*

to this deformity. Metatarsus adductus (metatarsus varus) is a relatively minor angulation deformity of the foot caused by compression of the foot around the contralateral leg. If the foot has full passive movement, casts or splints should not be needed.

Talipes equinovarus, or 'club foot' (Fig. 13.3), needs to be assessed carefully, since any limitation of passive movement indicates that immediate treatment is required. This is because the lax joints in the first week of life allow rapid correction with serial plaster casts or splints. If the foot cannot be

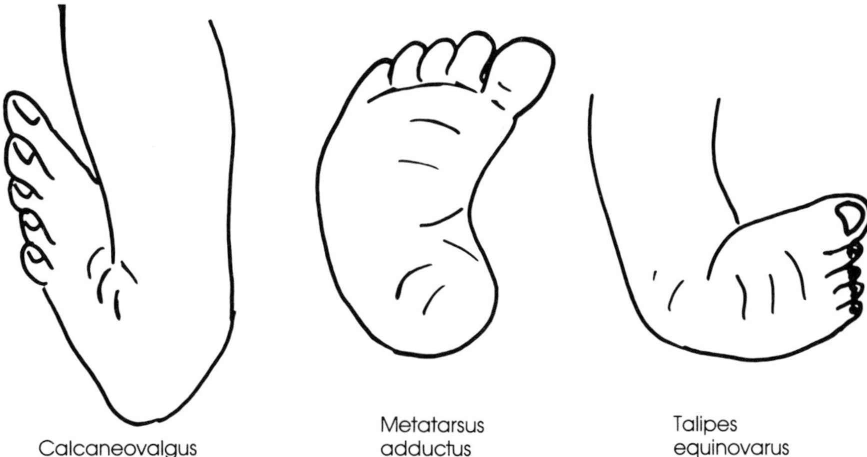

Fig. 13.2: *The three main types of foot deformity at birth.*

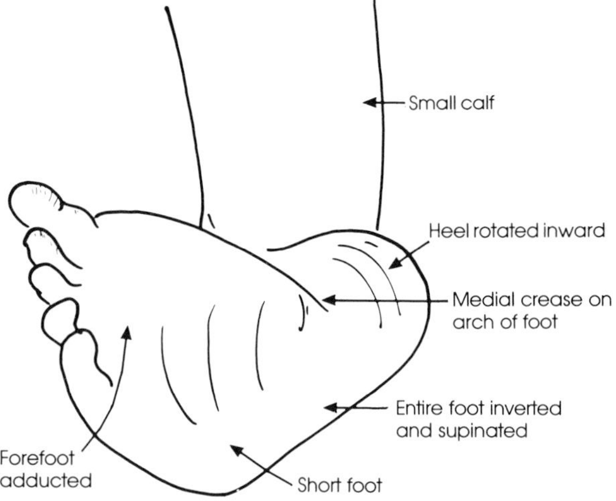

Fig. 13.3: *Abnormalities in talipes equinovarus.*

pushed into the calcaneovalgus position easily, an orthopaedic surgeon should be consulted.

The digits

A common concern both of parents and of medical attendants at birth is whether the fingers and toes are normal. The likely problems are (1) incomplete separation of the fingers or toes (syndactyly), (2) duplication of the digital rays to produce an extra digit (polydactyly), (3) curly toes, and (4) trigger thumb (described later).

Where syndactyly is present, the examination should include all limbs as well as enquiry about other family members, because of the likelihood of familial inheritance. In addition, syndactyly is a common feature of recognized syndromes, and therefore other abnormalities should be sought during the general examination (see Chapter 2).

With polydactyly, the examination should determine whether the extra digits have a bony connection with the rest of the hand or foot. Where the base is narrow and contains no bone, ligation of the base at birth is satisfactory. Extra digits containing bone, or with a wide base, need referral for excision at a convenient time after the neonatal period.

THE LEGS IN EARLY CHILDHOOD

Most children learn to walk between 10 and 18 months of age. The legs grow rapidly during this time and minor aberrations of this process account for much parental anxiety.

The common problems are (1) in-toeing ('pigeon-toes'), (2) bow legs, (3) knock knees, and (4) flat feet.

In-toeing

This may be caused by (1) metatarsus adductus (medial angulation of the forefoot), (2) tibial torsion (spiral twist of the tibia), or (3) femoral torsion (spiral twist of the femur) (Fig. 13.4). Metatarsus adductus usually reflects deformity *in utero*, and is recognized easily by inspection of the shape of the foot. It may first be noticed at the time of walking. The tibia of an infant normally grows with a slight outward curvature and a degree of internal twist or torsion. Internal tibial torsion may be exacerbated by the baby sleeping face down with the feet tucked inwards underneath, or by the infant sitting on the in-turned feet. Elimination of these postures should allow the tibia to straighten normally with growth. Internal femoral torsion ('in-set hips') is in part an inherited condition common in girls, made worse by sitting with the legs rotated outwards for long periods of play or kindergarten activities. It resolves spontaneously with maturation of the pelvis and femur.

The history should include questions about (1) a family history of leg deformity, (2) any functional impairment of normal activities (there should be no impairment unless there is an underlying cause, e.g. occult spina bifida, muscular dystrophy), and (3) the common sleeping and sitting positions (are these making it worse?).

Clinical examination of a child with in-turned toes is structured to answer four questions: (1) '*How severe is it?*' The gait angle should be assessed by observation of the feet during walking and is best done by watching from directly in front (Fig. 13.5). The normal angle between the feet during walking is 10° of external rotation. (2) '*Is it the tibia or the foot?*' The infant is placed prone on the couch with the knees bent. The feet are observed from above. Metatarsus adductus is revealed by the shape of the sole (Fig. 13.5). Internal tibial torsion is determined by the angle between the thigh and

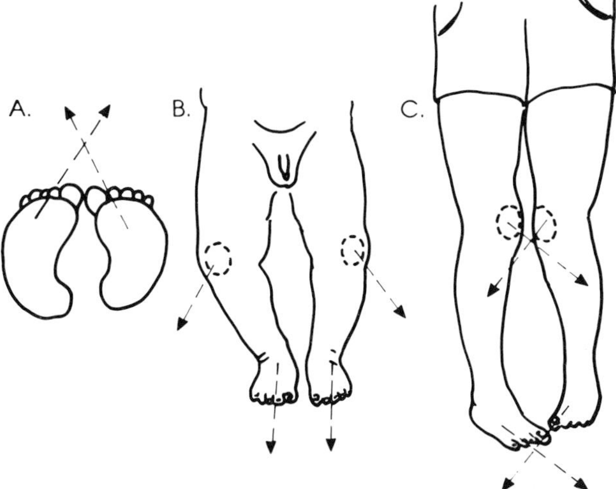

Fig. 13.4: *The three causes of in-toeing ('pigeon toes'). A. Metatarsus adductus (varus). B. Internal tibial torsion (associated with bow leg). C. Internal femoral torsion ('in-set hips'). The direction of the toes should be compared with the direction of the heel or patella.*

the foot, which is normally 0-30° of external rotation. (3) '*Is it the femur?*' With the knees still bent, the clinician crouches down and examines the degree of hip rotation, using the lower leg as the marker (Fig. 13.6). The normal range is 45° of internal rotation (the tibia appears *externally* rotated because the child is prone rather than supine) to 30° external rotation (looks like *internal* rotation). Where internal femoral torsion is present, the legs may lie easily on the couch (i.e. 90° internal rotation) and external rotation will be limited. (4) '*Are there other abnormalities?*' Hip abduction should be tested to exclude an unrecognized dislocation of the hip as the cause of in-toeing. Weak muscles causing or exacerbating the deformity should be excluded by instructing the child to sit on the floor, and then to stand up (Fig. 13.7). Use of the hands in levering himself up

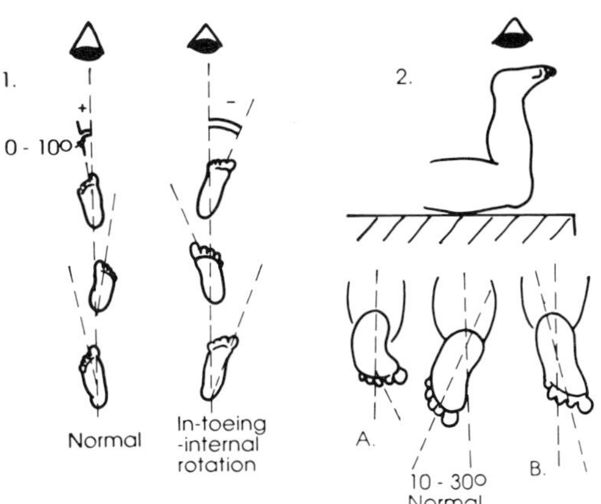

Fig. 13.5: *Examination of pigeon toes. (1) Observe the gait angle from in front to assess the severity. (2) Place the child prone with the knee bent and observe the foot from above. Metatarsus adductus (A), or internal tibial torsion (B), can be diagnosed by the shape or angle of the foot with the thigh.*

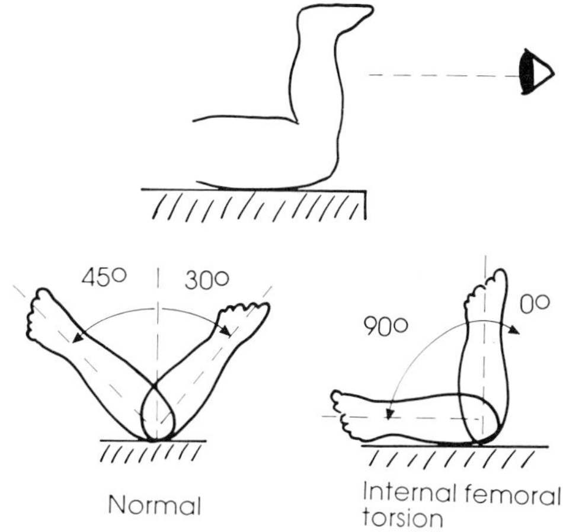

Fig. 13.6: *Observe the leg flexed from behind to diagnose 'in-set hips' (internal femoral torsion).*

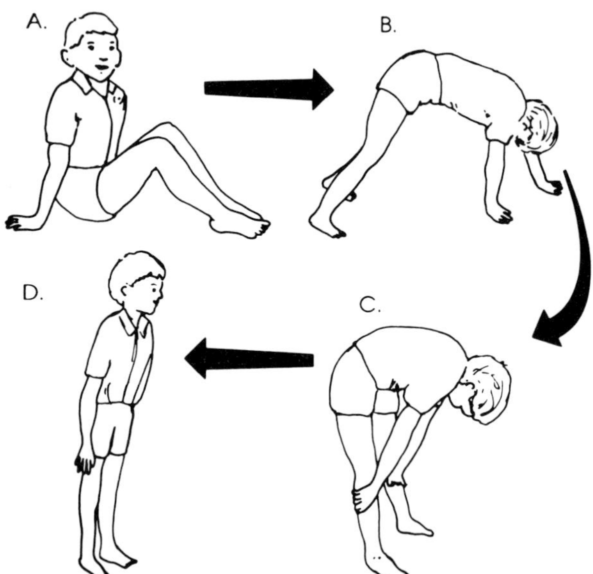

Fig. 13.7: *Gowers' test. The child sits on the floor and is asked to stand up (A). A positive test is seen when the child has to lever the trunk up using the hands on the floor (B) and on the legs (C), to reach the standing position (D). A positive Gowers' sign indicates weak leg muscles (as in muscular dystrophy).*

(positive Gowers' sign) indicates general or specific muscle weakness (e.g. muscular dystrophy). Finally, the lumbosacral spine should be examined for external stigmata of occult spina bifida (see Chapter 18).

Bow legs [genu varum]

Bowing of the tibia is extremely common before two years of age, and resolves spontaneously in most children as the growth of the bones responds to weight-bearing. Usually, it is associated with internal torsion of the tibia (Fig. 13.4B). Rickets (vitamin D deficiency) may cause bow legs because of bone softening, but this is now rare where milk is supplemented with vitamin D. Enlargement of the growth plates at the wrists or the costochondral junctions ('rachitic rosary') would confirm this rare cause.

The degree of severity of bowing of the tibia can be assessed by placing the infant supine after removal of all clothes from the waist down. The legs are held with the knees extended, the knee caps pointing towards the ceiling and the medial malleoli touching each other. The distance between the knees is determined with a tape-measure.

Knock knees [genu valgum]

This is nearly always a normal variant during growth of the femoral condyles between two and seven years, and only rarely is knock knee caused by rickets. The deformity produces no symptoms, and clumsiness is more likely to be related to neuromuscular development. The deformity reaches a peak at three and a half years, after which relative growth of the lateral condyle increases and the level of the knee joint becomes horizontal causing the legs to straighten.

The severity of the deformity is measured with the child standing and the knees touching (Fig. 13.8). The normal distance between the medial malleoli may be up to 10 cm. The feet appear to be flat because the knock knees shift the weight-bearing onto the medial side of each foot.

Flat feet

In fat toddlers, the feet often appear flat because of

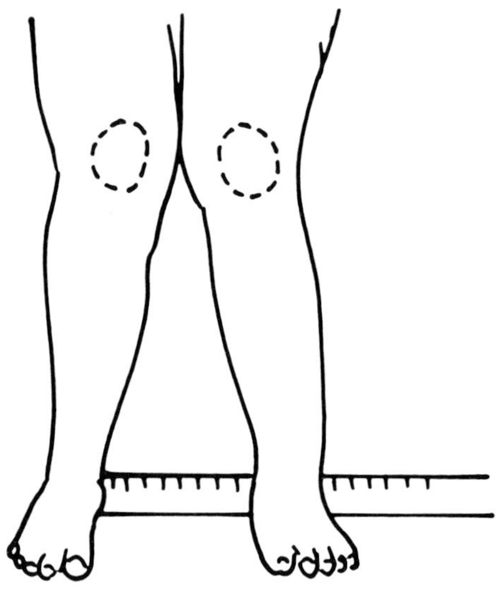

Fig. 13.8: *Knock knees. The distance between the medial malleoli should be less than 10 cm, otherwise specialist opinion should be sought.*

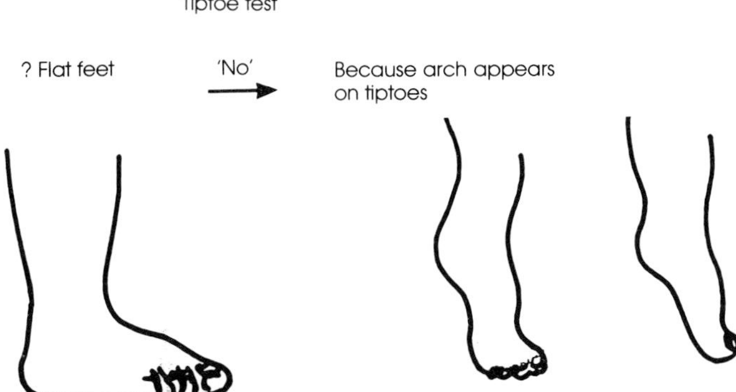

Fig. 13.9: *The tiptoe test for flat feet. The foot is normal if the arch appears on tiptoes.*

a thick fat pad on the sole. The deformity is common early in childhood when the ligaments are loose. Once walking (and weight-bearing) is established, the strength of the arch ligaments increases, making the foot appear normal by five to seven years.

Many 'flat' feet become normal when weight-bearing is maximal, such as when standing on tiptoes. These children have flexible joints with loose ligaments, but muscle strength and bony structures are normal. Pathological causes include muscle weakness or imbalance (cerebral palsy, muscular dystrophy) or rare intrinsic bony abnormalities (e.g. 'rocker-bottom' feet where the talus is abnormally vertical). The latter deformity may be associated with major chromosomal defects.

The feet are observed while first walking normally and then on tiptoe, when the arch will appear in normal feet with flexible joints (Fig. 13.9). Neuromuscular defects are excluded by general examination and Gowers' test. Incoordination abnormalities (which may be blamed on 'flat feet') are excluded by the child being able to hop on one leg.

THE ACUTE LIMB

The acutely painful arm or leg is a common problem in paediatrics, and usually indicates infection (Table 13.1). Cellulitis of the superficial tissues (e.g. infected abrasion) produces obvious signs of inflammation with little difficulty in diagnosis. However, osteomyelitis and septic arthritis, which are the two common skeletal infections, may be difficult to diagnose because the signs of inflammation are hidden. The acutely painful limb also may be caused by an unrecognized fracture, particularly in toddlers where a spiral hair-line fracture of the tibial shaft presents as an acute limp or painful leg, but with no signs

Table 13.1 THE DIFFERENTIAL DIAGNOSIS OF THE ACUTE LIMB

Pathology	Frequency	Clue
Cellulitis	Common	Obvious inflammation
Osteomyelitis	Common	} ± inflammatory signs
Septic arthritis	Common	
Spiral tibial fracture	Occasional	Local tenderness, callus
Generalized arthritis	Uncommon	Multiple joints
Tumours	Rare	Lump/pathological fracture

of systemic infection. On examination, there is tenderness over the shaft of the tibia, and an x-ray will confirm the spiral fracture.

Generalized causes of arthritis include (1) juvenile rheumatoid arthritis, (2) viral arthritis, (3) Henoch-Schönlein purpura, (4) rheumatic fever, and (5) scurvy. They are distinguished by their associated features, and the fact that multiple joints are usually involved. Malignant bony tumours also may produce an acutely painful limb, especially osteosarcoma, leukaemic infiltration, neuroblastoma and Ewing's tumour.

OSTEOMYELITIS

The metaphysis of a long bone is a common site for spread of infection, either from the blood stream or a local abrasion. *Staphylococcus* is the usual causative organism, and the lower femur and the upper tibia are the two most common areas involved. The natural history of osteomyelitis is shown in Figure 13.10.

The initial infection in the metaphysis causes local oedema with elevation of the adjacent periosteum. There is generalized fever and malaise, and the child holds the limb still. The elevated periosteum produces exquisite local tenderness. As the disease progresses, pus begins to collect under the periosteum to form a subperiosteal abscess. The inflammatory swelling within the bone compresses the blood supply to the bone and may cause local ischaemia. The physical signs of a subperiosteal abscess include swelling, local heat, redness, fluctuance and very severe pain. If the disease remains untreated or misdiagnosed, particularly in older children, a chronic form of osteomyelitis may develop. The subperiosteal abscess eventually ruptures through the periosteum and drains through a sinus on the skin. The area of ischaemic bone becomes necrotic, forming a sequestrum. New bone (the 'involucrum') begins to form around the cavity and under the elevated periosteum, resulting in obvious bony deformity.

Clinical picture

The clinical presentation of osteomyelitis depends on the duration of infection (Table 13.2). In the early phases, the child has pain, a high fever, an immobile limb and refuses to weight-bear. On

Table 13.2 THE SIGNS AND SYMPTOMS OF OSTEOMYELITIS

	Symptoms	Signs
Early:	Pain	Local tenderness
	Fever	No spontaneous movement
	Limb held still	Normal passive movement
	Refusal to weight-bear	Bone scan positive
Late:	Severe toxicity	Swelling
	Fever	Tenderness
	Immobile limb	Fluctuance
		Overlying erythema
		Nearby joint effusion
		X-rays positive

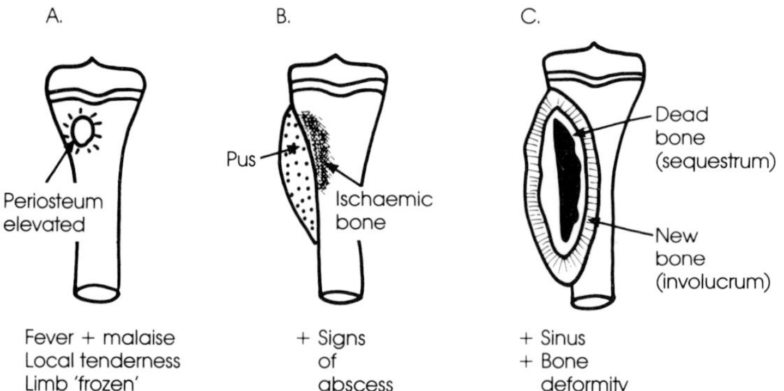

Fig. 13.10: *The natural history of osteomyelitis, from initial metaphyseal infection (A), to a subperiosteal abscess (B). If untreated, this may progress to a chronic discharging sinus (C).*

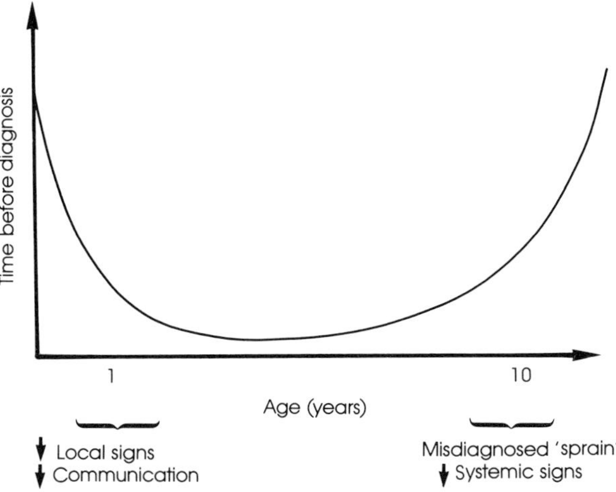

Fig. 13.11: *The relationship between delay in the diagnosis of osteomyelitis or septic arthritis and the age of the child. Both infants and adolescents may present difficulties which hamper early diagnosis.*

examination, there is reduced spontaneous movement with exquisite tenderness and swelling usually over a metaphysis. Examination of the adjacent joints shows a normal range of passive movement. If x-rays are taken at this stage, they usually show no abnormality since the pathological changes that are seen on x-ray take at least 10 days to develop. (By contrast, the bone scan is positive at an early stage). In the later phases of infection, the degree of toxicity and fever may be increased and the limb is completely immobilized. The physical findings usually demonstrate the presence of a subperiosteal abscess, with marked swelling and tenderness over the affected bone and a fluctuant, hot, red mass. The adjacent joint has an effusion. Once a subperiosteal abscess has formed, x-ray changes usually are evident.

Although osteomyelitis and septic arthritis may occur at any age during childhood, the diagnosis is often delayed in infants (Fig. 13.11). In addition, the pain in adolescents is often misdiagnosed as a sprain or other minor injury. Systemic signs may be less obvious than in younger children because the infection is localized more effectively. In neonates and infants, the natural history of the disease is somewhat different (Table 13.3). Local signs are less obvious because the periosteum is less tightly fixed to the bone and is more easily elevated by oedema or pus. When pus is not under high pressure, it causes less pain. The inflammatory response spreads rapidly through the leg to produce diffuse redness and oedema. These inflammatory signs are easily recognized, but commonly are misdiagnosed as cellulitis. Temperature control in small infants is less stable, such that systemic infections may reduce rather than elevate the temperature. Radiological signs appear at an earlier stage because bony changes occur more rapidly than in older children.

Clinical examination

When osteomyelitis is suspected, the clinical routine which should be followed is shown in Figure 13.12. If the child can walk, the gait should be observed for a limp. The common situation, however, is refusal to weight-bear or walk, and the parents will carry the child. If the child is old enough, the examiner should ask him to point to the tender area. In more than 50% of cases, this will be localized to the femur or tibia. Next, the area should be examined for evidence of inflammation (swelling, redness, heat) or an entry site for organisms, such as superficial abrasions. The presence of increased local heat caused by the inflammatory response is assessed by feeling the

Table 13.3 THE PROBLEMS IN DIAGNOSIS OF OSTEOMYELITIS IN NEONATES OR INFANTS COMPARED WITH OLDER CHILDREN

Problem	Explanation
1. Fever variable	Temperature more unstable in neonates
2. Local signs less evident	Loose periosteum easily elevated by oedema causing less pain
3. Oedema greater and more diffuse	Periosteum does not restrict the spread of inflammation
4. X-ray signs 'earlier'	? Faster bone destruction ? Missed diagnosis

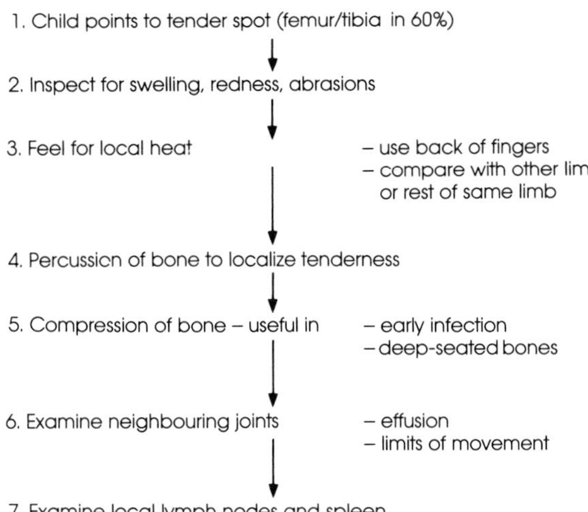

Fig. 13.12: *Examination of a child with possible osteomyelitis. A preliminary step is to observe the gait for a limp, but commonly the child refuses to walk and has to be carried by a parent.*

limb with the back of the fingers and comparing the two limbs to detect even minor elevations in local temperature. In addition, the fingers should be run up and down the limb past the affected area to demonstrate that the whole limb is not equally affected. Palpation of the full length of both limbs will enable any local swelling to be recognized. Local tenderness often is diagnosed best by percussion, particularly in areas where the bone is superficial. If bony percussion fails to elicit local tenderness, the bone can be squeezed directly by manual compression. This may be useful if the infection is early, or if the bone is deep within the limb. Once the area of local tenderness has been identified precisely, the neighbouring joints should be examined for the presence of an effusion and for limitation of movement. This is important because the joint may be affected by direct spread from the metaphysis, particularly the hip and shoulder joints. Alternatively, the diagnosis of osteomyelitis may be incorrect and the origin of the infection is the joint itself.

Finally, the lymph nodes draining the area involved should be examined for local enlargement and tenderness as a guide to the rate and extent of spread of the infection. Splenomegaly should be sought since this may accompany a severe systemic infection such as osteomyelitis. Splenomegaly also may be present with systemic disorders, such as rheumatoid arthritis or leukaemia.

SEPTIC ARTHRITIS

Suppurative infection of the joint may occur from blood-borne spread, a skin wound, or from adjacent osteomyelitis (Table 13.4). The three common organisms, *Staphylococcus, Haemophilus* and *Streptococcus*, produce a clinical picture of generalized illness with fever, malaise, rigors and collapse, with local signs of synovitis. This causes pain and local tenderness over the distended joint capsule, restriction of all joint movements and signs of inflammation, including redness and heat in the overlying skin.

The cardinal signs of septic arthritis are refusal to move the joint and extreme tenderness along the line of the joint surfaces. In most joints in the body, this is determined easily, although the hip may provide some difficulties (Fig. 13.13). Septic arthritis of the hip is common in neonates following an episode of bacteraemia or septicaemia. The inflammation spreads rapidly beyond the synovium and joint capsule in a way analagous to that seen in neonatal osteomyelitis, which almost always is present as well, and can cause the hip to sublux or dislocate. Marked inflammation in the adjacent soft tissues produces a swollen thigh, and the distension of the joint capsule pushes the femur into a position of flexion, abduction and external rotation. This is the so-called 'frog'

Table 13.4 SEPTIC ARTHRITIS

Aetiology	Symptoms	Signs
Blood-borne	Malaise, fever	All movement restricted
Skin wound	Rigors	Tender, swollen joint
Osteomyelitis	Limb held still	Overlying heat, redness
– hip	Will not walk	+ pain
– shoulder		
– elbow		

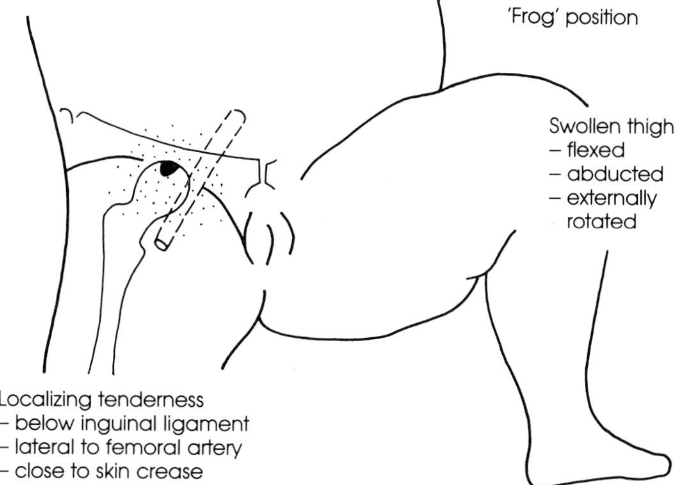

Fig. 13.13: *Septic arthritis of the hip in infancy. The swollen joint capsule pushes the leg into the frog position. Exquisite tenderness is localized to the femoral head, with the diagnosis confirmed on joint aspiration and culture.*

position, and is quite characteristic. The diagnosis of septic arthritis can be confirmed by pain with movement (and decreased mobility because of pain), and the demonstration of tenderness over the anterior surface of the femoral head. This is identified below the inguinal ligament, lateral to the femoral arterial pulse and adjacent to the femoral skin crease which, in the infant, corresponds to the level of attachment of Scarpa's fascia. As in other forms of arthritis, the diagnosis is proven by aspiration and culture of the joint fluid.

LIMP

Osteomyelitis, septic arthritis and trauma occur throughout childhood, but there are some diseases which have a predilection for specific age groups (Fig. 13.14). The two common conditions affecting the head of the femur, i.e. Perthes' disease and slipped upper femoral epiphysis, affect boys more commonly than girls (four to one), with Perthes' disease being the common abnormality in boys aged less than 10 years, while slipped epiphysis

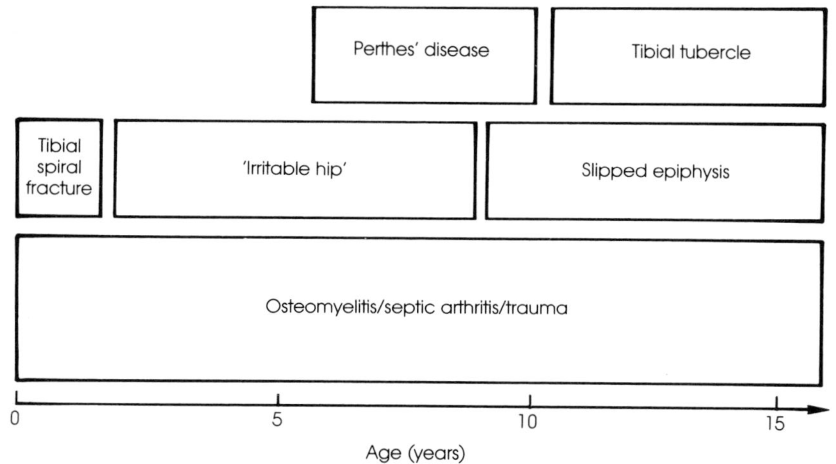

Fig. 13.14: *The effect of age on the frequency of the common orthopaedic conditions.*

affects boys older than 10 years.

A chronic limp may be caused by a congenital abnormality of the leg or by diseases with an insidious onset (Table 13.5). Important causes of a limp from the commencement of walking include congenital dislocation of the hip or a short leg. If undiagnosed before the onset of walking, a dislocated hip produces an unstable hip with a positive Trendelenburg's sign (see below). Neuromuscular diseases such as cerebral palsy, muscular dystrophy or various forms of spastic hemiparesis also will produce a limp, but the aetiology should be determined readily by neurological examination. The two causes of a chronic intermittent limp arising later in childhood are Perthes' disease and slipped epiphysis of the femoral head.

Table 13.5 CAUSES OF A CHRONIC LIMP

Congenital dislocated hip
Spastic hemiparesis
Congenital short leg
Perthes' disease
Slipped epiphysis of the femoral head
Transient synovitis (irritable hip)

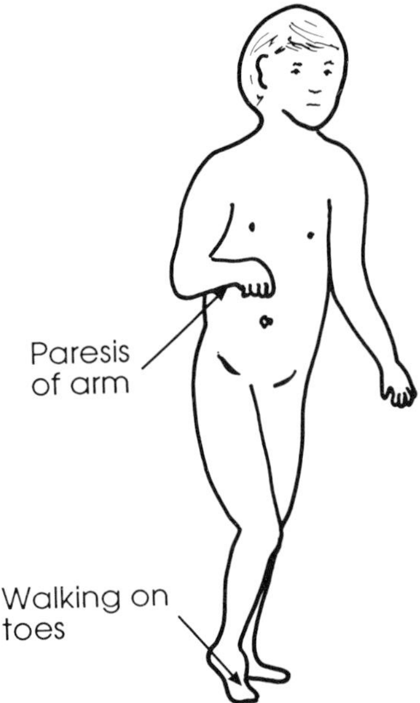

Fig. 13.15: *Spastic hemiparesis as a cause of chronic limp.*

There are five different forms of limp (spastic, antalgic, Trendelenburg, short leg and ataxic), which can be distinguished by observation of the gait (Table 13.6). The gait of a child with spastic hemiparesis or cerebral palsy is characterized by imbalance of the calf muscles with excessive contraction of the achilles tendon, causing the child to walk on his toes. The arm is held flexed at the elbow in a characteristic manner (Fig. 13.15). Where an underlying abnormality causes increased pain on weight-bearing, the child walks with an antalgic or painful hopping gait, transferring the weight rapidly on to the normal leg with each step. The uneven rhythm of this form of walking is easy to recognize. If the hip is unstable, the child walks with a waddling gait, and the pelvis tilts down to the normal side when weight is taken on the abnormal leg. This is called a positive Trendelenburg gait. In contrast, where the leg is shorter on one side, the pelvis tilts down to the affected side on standing still, and on walking the knee of the longer leg will remain slightly bent to keep the pelvis horizontal. Children with neurological diseases, such as posterior fossa tumours, may present with an ataxic gait, poor balance and incoordination. The degree of ataxia can be appreciated readily if the child is asked to make several quick turns, as this will usually produce a fall.

Table 13.6 TYPES OF LIMP

1. Spastic hemiparesis (cerebral palsy) – arm held flexed at the elbow
   – walks on toes
2. Painful weight-bearing – weight transferred more quickly to the normal leg → hopping
3. Unstable hip – pelvis tilts down when weight is on the abnormal leg (positive Trendelenburg's sign)
4. Short leg – pelvis tilted down when standing still
   – opposite knee kept bent during walking
5. Ataxia –poor balance and coordination
   – worse during turning

'Irritable hip'

This is a non-specific synovitis of the hip joint, which is the commonest hip problem in childhood. The aetiology may be viral or traumatic, but this remains unproven. It causes acute onset of a painless limp, usually in a pre-school child. Often, there is a history of a mild ache the night before, and the child wakes up with pain in the groin or front of the thigh and stiffness of the hip joint. There are no obvious signs of inflammation, either clinically or on laboratory testing. The hip is held fixed and the extremes of all movements are limited by pain. The adjacent muscles may be felt to be in protective spasm. The aim of diagnosis is to exclude more serious pathology since an irritable hip improves quickly after a few days' rest.

Perthes' disease

This disease is one of the common forms of osteochondritis juvenilis affecting the epiphyses of growing bones (Fig. 13.16). The blood supply of part or the whole of the epiphysis becomes defective, and slow aseptic necrosis occurs, usually without primary destruction of the articular cartilage. The head of the femur gradually collapses and acquires a mushroom shape, with the epiphysis appearing smaller and irregularly dense on x-ray. Most children affected are boys between three and 10 years of age.

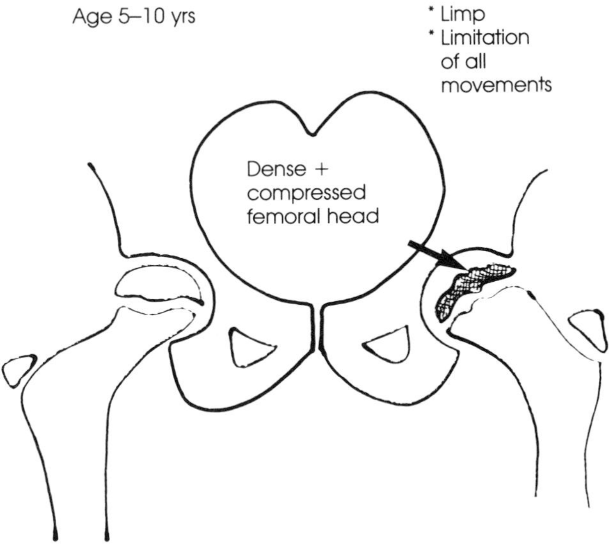

Fig. 13.16: *The features of Perthes' disease.*

The presenting features of Perthes' disease include an intermittent limp, which may be painless or sometimes painful, without evidence of systemic toxicity. If the disease is longstanding, the gluteal muscles on the affected side are wasted slightly and produce a flat buttock. In addition, there may be a positive Trendelenburg test caused by the effective shortening of the neck of the femur from collapse of the femoral head. The greater trochanter may be more prominent than on the normal side. There is limitation of the hip joint movements, particularly abduction of the flexed leg and medial rotation.

In younger children, where only part of the femoral head is involved, the prognosis is good and the disease is self-limiting after one to two years. However, in older children and those in whom the whole femoral head is involved, permanent deformity of the hip joint may ensue.

Slipped upper femoral epiphysis

This is a fairly common cause of pain and limp in the hip joint during adolescence (Fig. 13.17). Most children affected are boys of above average height and weight, with relatively small external genitalia. The epiphysis usually slips off the femoral neck downwards and posteriorly, and causes the leg to be pushed into external rotation. The mechanical disturbance of the hip joint produces a secondary synovitis. In most cases, the onset is insidious with gradual progression of pain and limp involving one or both hip joints, although there is a history of injury in many. In some, the epiphysis slips suddenly and produces more dramatic symptomatology and clinical signs which suggest a sprain or fractured neck of the femur. The cardinal physical sign is the demonstration of some degree of fixed external rotation with definite, painful limitation of internal rotation (Fig. 13.18). Radiological signs may be subtle, with the earliest abnormality being irregularity and widening of the epiphyseal plate. Biplanar x-rays are essential since the abnormalities are often shown clearly only in the lateral view.

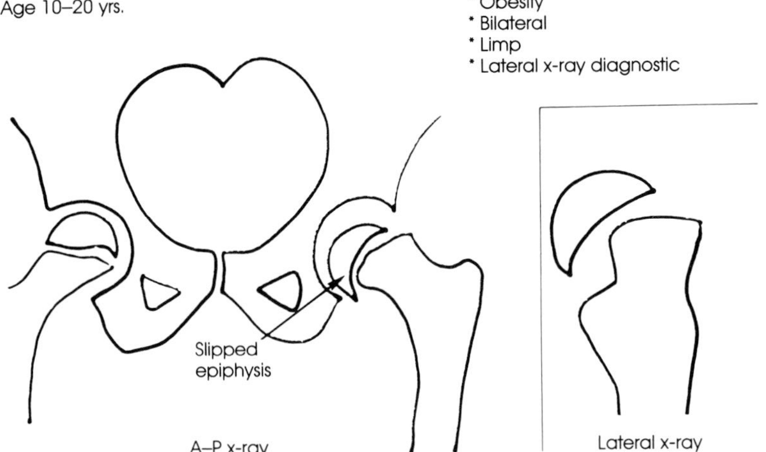

Fig. 13.17: *The features of slipped upper femoral epiphysis.*

Osgood-Schlatter disease

This is another form of osteochronditis juvenilis and affects the tibial tuberosity of boys and girls aged eight to 14 years (Fig. 13.19). The child presents with a tender lump on the tibial tuberosity, usually following vigorous activity. It hurts most on kneeling and on active extension against resistance. The tibial tuberosity appears fragmented on x-rays, but no other physical signs are present.

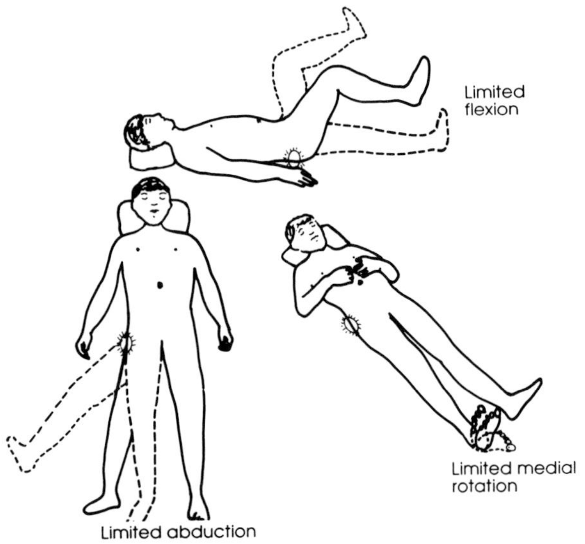

Fig. 13.18: *Testing for limitation of movement of the hip joint in a suspected case of slipped epiphysis.*

Clinical examination of limp

The procedure to be followed in the physical examination of a child with a limp is shown in Table 13.7. The examination may be difficult because of the young child's inability to localize pain causing the limp. It should commence with the child walking to observe the type of limp, as this will often allow the diagnosis to be made immediately. Next, the child should be asked to hop on one leg because trivial causes of a limp will not interfere with hopping. This is a simple test of leg strength and coordination which can be performed in children older than three or four years. Thirdly, the level of the pelvis should be examined to determine the position of the iliac crests, either from the anterior or from the posterior aspect, to exclude a short leg (Fig. 13.20). Pelvic tilt can be corrected by insertion of blocks of different thickness under the foot of the short leg. This provides an accurate measure of the degree of shortening.

An unstable hip can be identified by performing the Trendelenburg test (Fig. 13.21). The examiner stands behind the child to determine the tilt of the pelvis. When the child stands on the abnormal leg, the pelvis tilts downwards under the body weight because the hip abductor muscles are ineffective. The Trendelenburg test is positive in abnormalities which cause paralysis or weakness of the gluteus medius or minimus, but is observed most frequently in patients with a dislocated hip or Perthes' disease. After performing the Trendelenburg test, the buttocks are examined in the

Table 13.7 PHYSICAL EXAMINATION OF A CHILD WITH A LIMP

Standing
1. Observe walking to determine the type of limp
2. Observe hopping on one leg to exclude trivial lesions
3. Examine the level of the pelvis to exclude a short leg
4. Carry out the Trendelenburg test to identify an unstable hip
5. Examine the buttocks and thighs for wasting (hip diseases)

Lying on the couch

6. Examine the area of abnormality/pain
7. Measure leg lengths (short leg, dislocated hip)
8. Carry out Thomas' test (hip disease)
9. Check joints for – range of movement
   – tenderness
   – masses
10. Check bones for tenderness/masses
11. Examine soles of the feet for foreign bodies, plantar warts
12. Examine shoes for – type/degree of wear
    – protruding nails

standing position for signs of muscle wasting, which may indicate a subacute or chronic hip disorder.

Examination is continued with the child lying on the couch. The area of abnormality or pain is examined for signs of inflammation as described previously. The skin creases of the thigh need to be examined for asymmetry caused by dislocation of the hip (Fig. 13.22). The length of the legs should be measured to document the short leg or possible dislocated hip (Fig. 13.23), if this has not been determined already with blocks under the feet while standing. The measurement is taken from the lowest point of the anterior superior iliac spine to the lowest tip of the medial malleolus on each side. The tape-measure should lie evenly along the inner side of the leg so that it is not buckled by the patella.

Fixed flexion deformities of the hip can be identified by Thomas' test (Fig. 13.24). When the child is lying on the couch, the thigh usually will appear to be horizontal, often because the lumbar spine has an increased lordosis. To overcome the compensatory curvature of the spine, the normal leg is flexed passively right up onto the abdominal wall. This corrects the lumbar lordosis, and if a fixed deformity in the hip joint is present, the abnormal leg will lift passively off the couch. The angle of the fixed flexion deformity is defined by the angle between the femur and the couch. The other joints of the limb are checked for their range of movement, joint-line tenderness and swelling which may indicate synovitis. The common joint movements limited by disorders of the hip are abduction (dislocated hip or Perthes' disease) and internal rotation (slipped epiphysis). The long bones are palpated for local tenderness.

Examination is not complete until the soles of the feet have been studied for evidence of foreign bodies or plantar warts. The shoes also should be examined to determine the type and degree of wear, and whether there are any protruding nails or studs on the insides of the shoes which might have caused the limp. Neurological assessment and examination of the back will exclude discitis and disc prolapse.

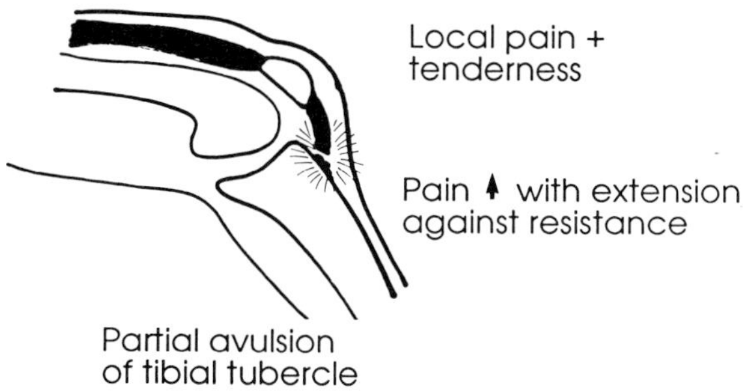

Fig. 13.19: *The features of Osgood-Schlatter disease.*

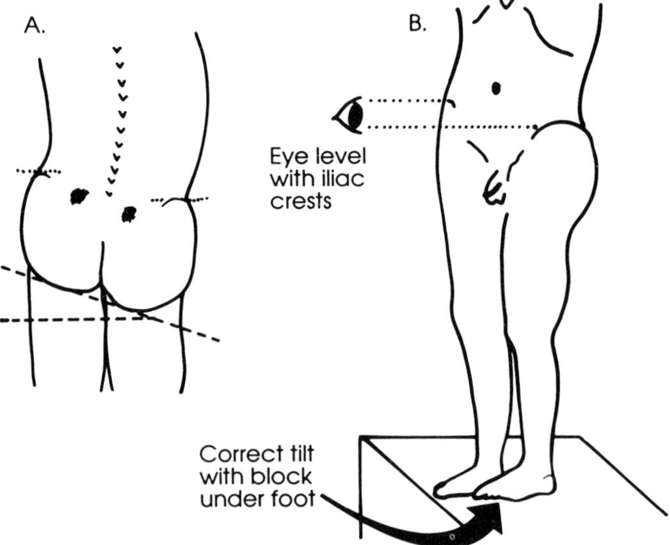

Fig. 13.20: *Examination for a short leg as a cause of limp. Blocks placed under the shorter leg until the iliac crests are level with each other is a simple and accurate way to measure the degree of shortening.*

MISCELLANEOUS PROBLEMS

Semimembranosus bursa

Enlargement of the semimembranosus bursa, which lies between the semimembranosus muscle and gastrocnemius muscle, produces a cystic swelling on the medial side of the popliteal fossa (Fig. 13.25). The swelling is painless, but very obvious if viewed from behind when the child stands. When the presentation is of a lump behind the knee, the position of the lump should be observed with the child standing, after which the child should be lain on the couch with the knee

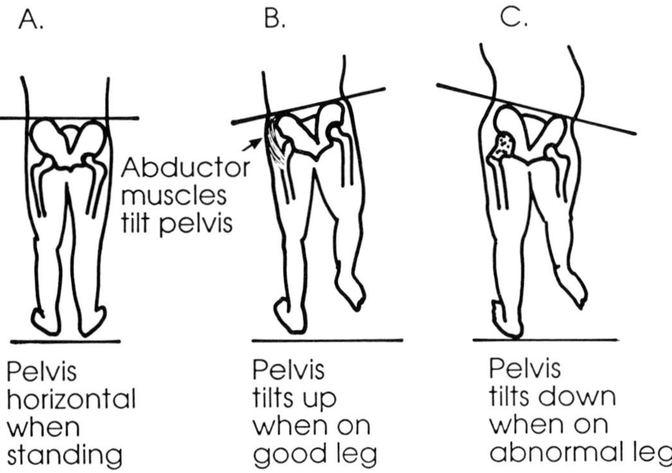

Fig. 13.21: *Trendelenburg test. Stand behind the child and determine the pelvic position, then ask the child to stand first on the good leg, followed by the abnormal leg. A positive result is obtained if the pelvis tilts down instead of up. It is seen where there is weakness of the gluteus medius and minimus, or an unstable fulcrum caused by a dislocated hip or fractured neck of the femur.*

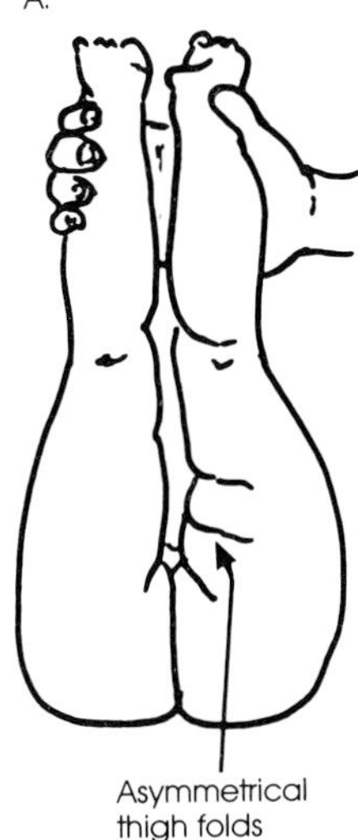

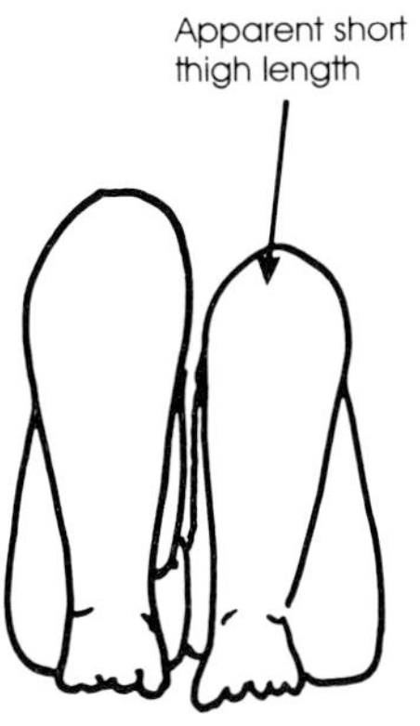

Fig. 13.22: *Late signs in congenital dislocation of the hip. A. Asymmetrical skin creases. B. Apparent shortening of the thigh.*

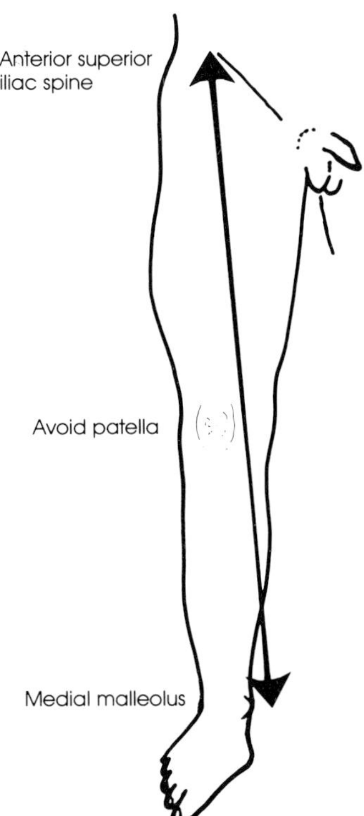

Fig. 13.23: *Measuring the legs. Position the child on the couch to get the pelvis horizontal to the legs. Measure with a tape-measure from the anterior superior iliac spine to the medial malleolus, avoiding the patella by passing the tape medial to it.*

flexed. The cyst is not visible in this position, but once the skin is lax it can be felt easily on the medial side of the knee posteriorly. Transillumination of the cyst confirms that it contains clear fluid, and direct compression of the cyst demonstrates that it does not empty, since it has no communication with the joint space. Almost all resolve spontaneously and do not require removal. Cystic swellings in the popliteal fossa arising from the synovium of the knee joint are rare in childhood.

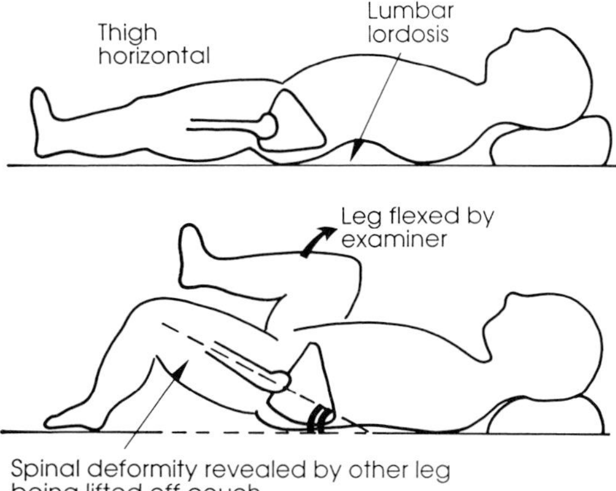

Fig. 13.24: *Thomas' test for a fixed flexion deformity of the hip joint. Compensatory lumbar lordosis may mask the deformity until this is corrected by passive flexion of the normal thigh.*

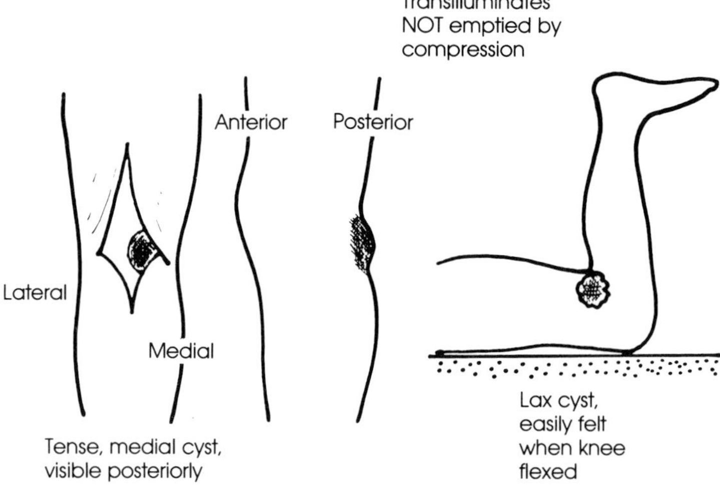

Fig. 13.25: *The features of an enlarged semimembranosus bursa.*

'Trigger thumb'

This is a common abnormality in infants less than two years of age and may be bilateral (Fig. 13.26). A narrowing of the tendon sheath produces a fusiform swelling of the tendon of flexor pollicis longus as it crosses the head of the first metacarpal. The mother may notice the thumb fixed in the flexed position, and when it is passively extended it produces an audible or palpable 'snap'. The hard nodule is sometimes wrongly diagnosed as a dislocation.

GOLDEN RULES

(1) All babies should be examined at birth for congenital dislocation of the hip.
(2) Beware hip dislocation at birth: diagnosis should not wait until symptoms appear at the time of walking.
(3) Beware newborn foot deformity: it may signal a chromosomal defect, multiple joint deformities (arthrogryposis) or paralysis (myelomeningocele).
(4) Beware calcaneovalgus deformity: it may be

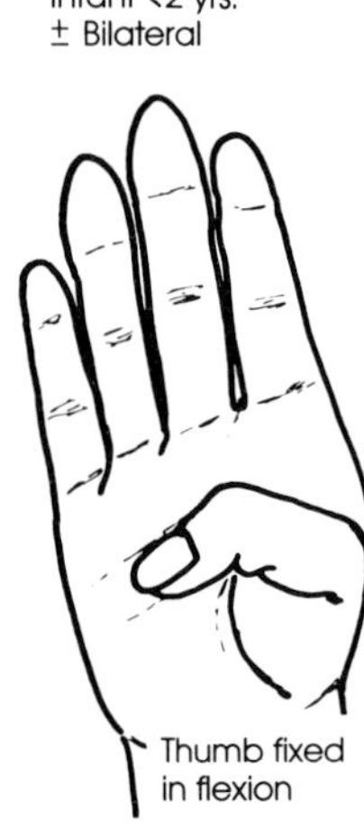

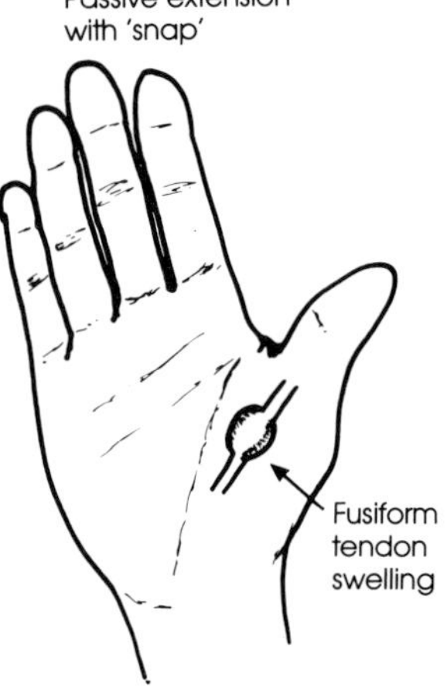

Fig. 13.26: *The features of trigger thumb.*

associated with congenital dislocation of the hip(s).

(5) Deformed feet should be assessed by a specialist unless a full range of passive movement is present.

(6) Beware syndactyly (and polydactyly): a multiple malformation syndrome may be present.

(7) Beware the swollen limb in a neonate: there may be osteomyelitis and/or septic arthritis.

(8) Osteomyelitis should be suspected in any child who refuses to walk.

(9) Increased temperature or tenderness of bone indicates osteomyelitis until proven otherwise.

FURTHER READING

Apley A.G. (1973). A System of Orthopaedics and Fractures, *4th edn. London: Butterworths.*

The Easter Seal Guide to Children's Orthopaedics (1982). Ontario: The Easter Seal Society

14 Urinary tract symptoms

There is marked variation in the presentation and clinical features of infection of the urinary tract. The symptoms in the neonate and infant usually are general in nature and not specific to the urinary tract, whereas in the older child, although general features may be present, there are clinical features suggestive of a urinary tract problem (Table 14.1). This means that urinary tract infection can present in a number of guises, the most common of which are described below.

THE VOMITING NEONATE

Vomiting is extremely common in the neonate and may be of little significance (e.g. minor feeding problems, mild gastro-oesophageal reflux) or serious (e.g. meningitis). Urinary tract infection is one serious cause of sepsis in the infant, and thus it shares with other infections the general features of fever, lethargy or irritability, refusal to feed, malaise and vomiting. These are general signs of sepsis and they suggest that, as in any search for infection, the urinary tract should be excluded by looking for white cells or bacteria in the urine. This can be achieved by obtaining a bag specimen or suprapubic aspirate of urine.

DYSURIA AND FREQUENCY

Dysuria denotes pain in the urethra on voiding and should be distinguished from intra-abdominal pain on voiding, which is discussed below. In the female, the discomfort is perineal and in the male, it is felt as a sharp burning sensation in the penis or glans. The pain persists for a short period after completion of micturition. The severity of pain may cause involuntary interruption of micturition, allowing only the passage of small volumes of urine at one time. The small child may scream at the commencement of voiding and then be seen to 'hold back'. In this situation, severe pain may produce urinary retention with overflow incontinence, and the bladder will be palpable in the lower abdomen.

Table 14.1 PRESENTATION OF URINARY TRACT INFECTION

1. GENERAL FEATURES
   - Vomiting
   - Lethargy or irritability
   - Refusal to feed
   - Failure to thrive
   - Fever
   - Toxicity
2. SPECIFIC FEATURES
   - Dysuria and frequency
   - Loin pain
   - Abdominal pain
   - Wetting
   - Haematuria

Frequent passage of small volumes of urine is known as 'frequency'. It may be caused by overflow incontinence but is more commonly the result of the sensation of imminent voiding or 'urgency', which occurs in urinary tract infection when the bladder becomes inflamed: a small increase in urine volume triggers reflex bladder emptying. The child finds these impulses difficult to suppress and has 'accidents'.

Micturition may cause pain in the lower abdomen if there is inflammation of the pelvic peritoneum in the absence of urinary tract infection (e.g. pelvic appendicitis). It is mandatory, therefore, to identify the site and nature of the pain since dysuria, which refers to urethral pain alone, should not be confused with abdominal pain during micturition.

Where a history of dysuria and frequency has been established, further questioning is directed at ascertaining the presence of haematuria or of cloudy or offensive urine. Cloudy precipitates can be present in normal urine at the end of voiding and are of no consequence, and there is no doubt that normal urine has a characteristic odour. However, opaque urine throughout the stream

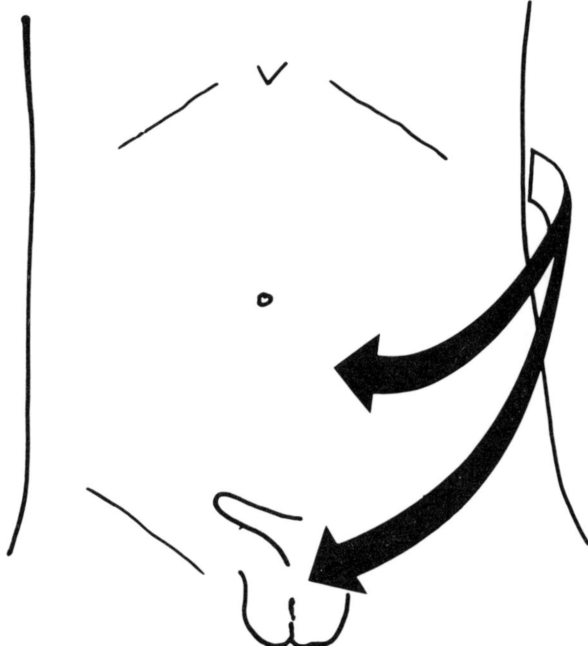

Fig. 14.1: *Radiation of loin pain to the abdomen and scrotum.*

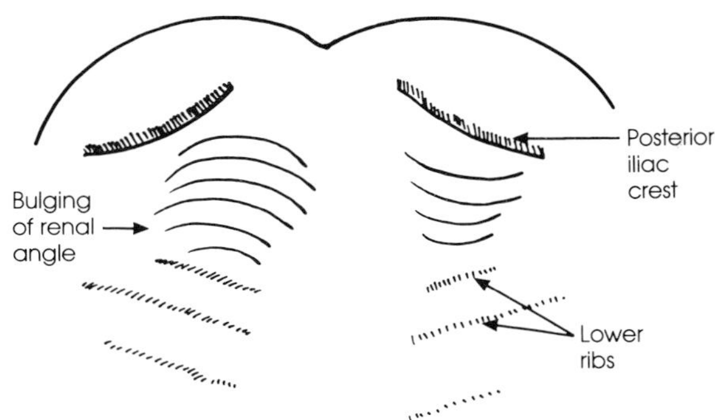

Fig. 14.2: *Assessment of fullness of the renal angle: view from above looking down the patient's back.*

(due to white blood cells and bacteria) and a strong unpleasant odour can be valuable signs of infection even in the absence of dysuria or frequency. Indeed, children with recurrent infections often are able to recognize the infection in this way before other symptoms develop.

LOIN PAIN

The kidneys lie in the retroperitoneum protected by the posterior abdominal wall muscles and lower ribs. Inflammation of the kidney and renal pelvis produces pain in the loin which may radiate around the flank to the ipsilateral iliac fossa or testis (Fig. 14.1). If the bladder is inflamed as well, there may be suprapubic pain. In pyelonephritis, the collecting system and renal parenchyma become inflamed causing severe loin pain and systemic signs of sepsis and toxicity. The patient is febrile, anorexic, tachycardic and appears flushed and unwell. There is loss of the normal concavity of the renal angle (Fig. 14.2), and scoliosis to the affected side (Fig. 14.3). Gentle percussion of the renal angle is extremely painful (Fig. 14.4) and will cause the patient to jerk the spine in extension. Tenderness anteriorly is less marked but does make palpation of the kidney difficult.

Examination and culture of the urine confirms the presence of infection. Plain x-ray of the abdomen will show whether a stone is present, and ultrasound of the kidney may show dilatation of the renal pelvis or swelling of the kidney. In rare instances, where there is infection of the

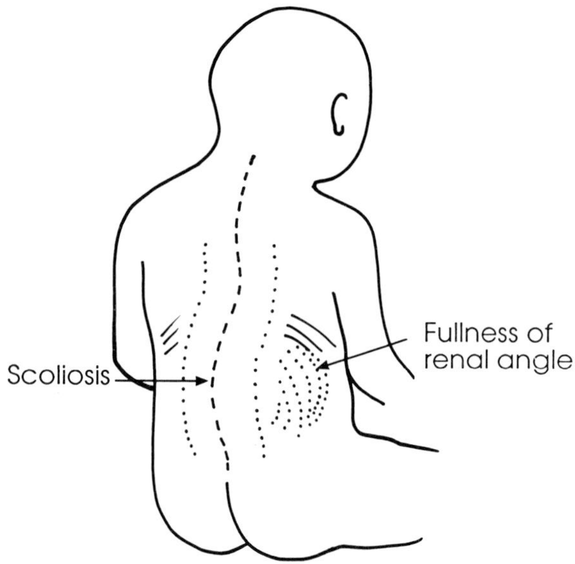

Fig. 14.3: *The signs of pyelonephritis. Sit the patient symmetrically with slight flexion of the back. Look for 1. scoliosis to the affected side, and 2. fullness of the renal angle* (*Fig.* 14.2). *Percuss the renal angle for tenderness* (*Fig.* 14.4).

urinary tract proximal to complete obstruction of the ureter or pelviureteric junction, microscopy of the urine may show little evidence of white cells or bacteria and can be misleading.

COLLECTING A SPECIMEN OF URINE

A midstream specimen of urine is difficult to obtain in a young child and is unreliable unless supervised. Obtaining a catheter specimen of urine is uncomfortable, time-consuming and runs the risk of introducing infection into the bladder and of damaging the urethra. Furthermore, it is not as reliable as a suprapubic aspiration and, for this reason, is used infrequently. A bag collection of urine is the least reliable technique because of contamination from the perineum, and is only significant if the specimen produces no growth. Where culture of a urine specimen produces a pure growth of $>10^5$ organisms/ml, infection is considered to be present. Where a mixed growth of organisms is obtained, the significance becomes less certain and collection of a second specimen is indicated.

Suprapubic needle aspiration

Suprapubic needle aspiration is the most reliable method of obtaining urine in an infant. It relies on the intra-abdominal position of the infant bladder attached to the umbilicus and on the small size and capacity of the pelvis (Fig. 14.5). The technique is simple but attention to detail is important (Fig. 14.6). The bladder can be percussed in the lower abdomen or readily palpated in the relaxed infant, and may extend as far as the umbilicus. The lower abdomen and external genitalia are thoroughly swabbed with antiseptic solution. A 23-gauge needle attached to a 2 ml syringe is introduced perpendicular to the skin in the midline just above the pubis. It is often helpful to place the index and middle fingers of the left hand on either side of the point of puncture to make the skin taut. The needle is introduced with a quick controlled movement enabling the resistence as it pierces the skin and then the bladder to be felt. Once the bladder has been entered, 1–2 ml of urine is aspirated. The needle is then withdrawn quickly from the skin and the syringe sent directly to the laboratory, or the urine transferred to a sterile urine container for immediate transfer to the laboratory. Delay between collection of the specimen and inspection by the microbiologist should be avoided to prevent overgrowth of contaminating organisms.

Bag specimen of urine

The sterile collection bag is attached to the perineum by an adherent watertight rim after the

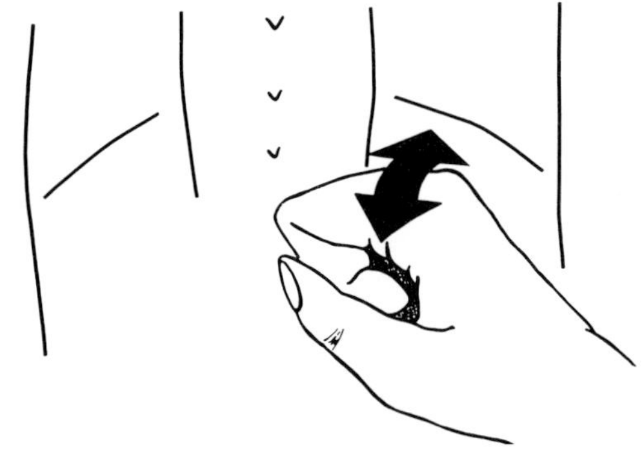

Fig. 14.4: *Percussion of the renal angle with the back of a clenched fist to test for tenderness.*

skin has been cleaned with a mild antiseptic. As soon as the infant or child has passed urine, the bag is removed and the contents immediately placed in the refrigerator or sent to the laboratory for culture. Contamination of the urine by perineal organisms may make interpretation difficult unless culture shows no bacterial growth or a mixed growth of less than 10^3 organisms/ml. This indicates no urinary tract infection. A colony count between 10^3 and 10^5 organisms/ml may indicate urinary infecton or merely represent contamination. Hence, a bag specimen of urine is best used to exclude an infection and should not be used where infection is suspected strongly.

Midstream urine

This technique can be used in children of four years or greater and is appropriate for the routine collection of urine. A midstream urine specimen is obtained because the few bacteria which colonize the urethra are washed out at the commencement of micturition. This method of collection is best in the circumcised male. To minimize contamination in the uncircumcised male, the prepuce should be retracted to expose the glans, and in the female, the labia should be parted (Fig. 14.7). Midstream urine collection is not applicable to younger children because they are unable to initiate and control voiding effectively, and it may be difficult for them to pass an adequate volume on demand.

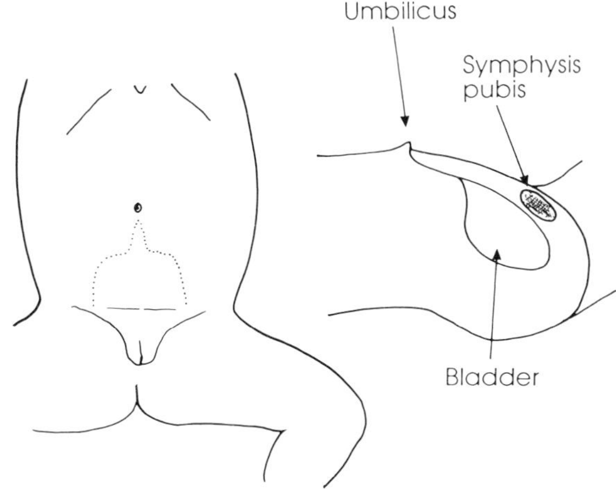

Fig. 14.5: *The full bladder in an infant is an intra-abdominal organ.*

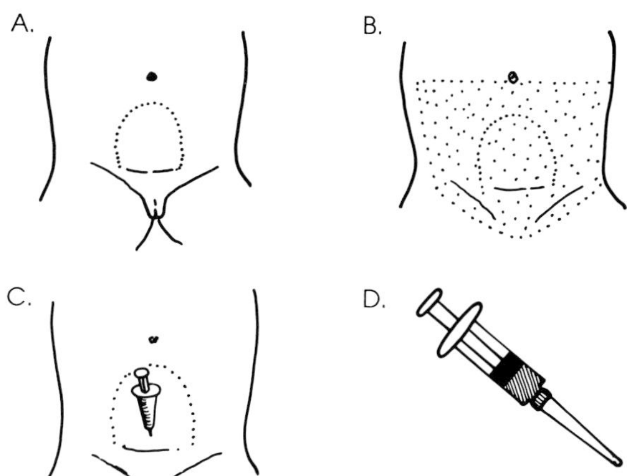

Fig. 14.6: *The technique of suprapubic needle aspiration of urine. A. Percuss the bladder in the lower abdomen. B. Swab the suprapubic region with antiseptic solution. C. Introduce the syringe perpendicular to the skin just above the pubic tubercle, and aspirate urine. D. Replace the cap over the needle, label the syringe with the patient's identification, and immediately send it to the laboratory.*

Catheter specimen

A catheter specimen of urine is more reliable than a midstream or bag specimen because it eliminates preputial and perineal contamination. It suffers from being an invasive technique, however, with the potential to damage the urethra or introduce organisms into the bladder. In the normal child, it is an uncomfortable and distressing procedure. Its place is largely limited to spina bifida children and to children who have a catheter inserted for another reason.

WHAT IS THE SIGNIFICANCE OF PROVEN INFECTION?

In boys, urinary tract infection should be taken as an indicator of a possible underlying congenital abnormality, e.g. pelviureteric junction obstruction, vesico-ureteric reflux, posterior urethral valves, ureterocele or diverticulum. Girls have a much shorter urethra than boys and are more prone to urinary infection in the absence of an underlying lesion. Despite this, many congenital anomalies of the urinary system present with an infection and should be sought by the appropriate radiological investigations.

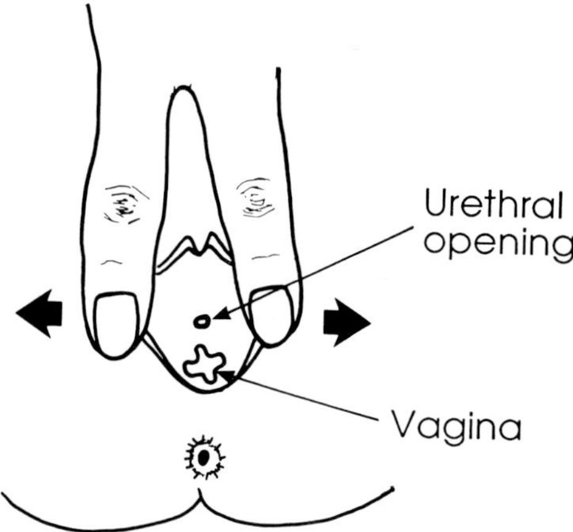

Fig. 14.7: *The technique of labial separation to avoid perineal contamination during midstream urine collection in a girl.*

The significance of urinary infection not only relates to its association with anomalies of the urinary tract, but also to the damage it may cause to the kidneys, with loss of function of renal parenchyma. Therefore, management is directed towards: (1) treatment of proven infection with antibiotics to which the causative organisms are sensitive; (2) investigation of the urinary system for congenital anomalies; and (3) treatment of the underlying abnormality to avoid recurrent infections.

HYPERTENSION

Measurement of blood pressure

The blood pressure should be measured in all children with a urinary tract infection or suspected renal abnormality. A sphygmomanometer is used with a cuff appropriate to the size of the child. The cuff should be wide enough to fit the upper arm comfortably from the deltoid insertion to above the cubital fossa, to enable auscultation of the brachial artery (Fig. 14.8). An excessively large cuff will be difficult to apply, will obscure the cubital fossa and give a fallaciously low recording. Likewise, a narrow cuff tends to produce a falsely high recording. The correct cuff width is two thirds the length of the upper arm. The position of the arm in relation to the heart is important, and the pressure should be taken with the arm at the same level as the heart, i.e. with the child lying in a supine position.

The pressure is interpreted in relation to the normal range for that age (Fig. 14.9), since this varies considerably and in all children is less than in adults.

Sometimes, a child presents with hypertension detected in the absence of known renal disease during routine examination, or where there are symptoms of hypertension, e.g. headaches and epistaxis. When this occurs, other causes of hypertension have to be considered (Table 14.2).

'WETTING'

Wetting is a term used to describe a perceived inadequate level of urinary continence. A child with wetting is a frequent concern to parents, often resulting in resort to medical opinion, but is rarely of pathological significance.

At birth, infants do not have voluntary control over voiding but do micturate at intervals and are dry between voids. Neurological development is

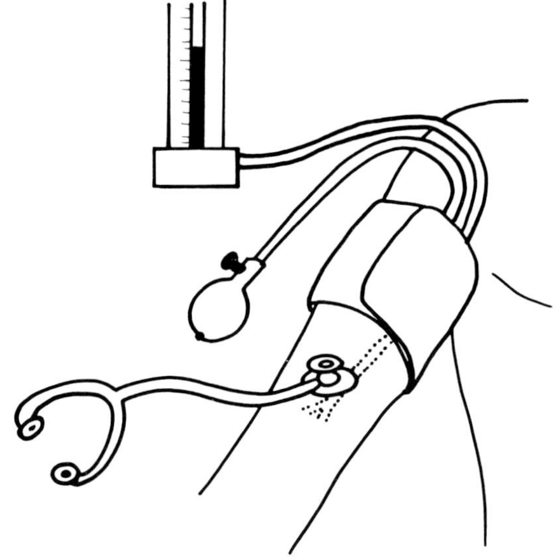

Fig. 14.8: *The measurement of blood pressure in a child. 1. Choose a cuff size appropriate to the size of the child. 2. Fit the cuff comfortably over the upper arm. 3. Place the stethoscope over the brachial artery in the cubital fossa. 4. Correlate your recordings with normal values for the age of child.*

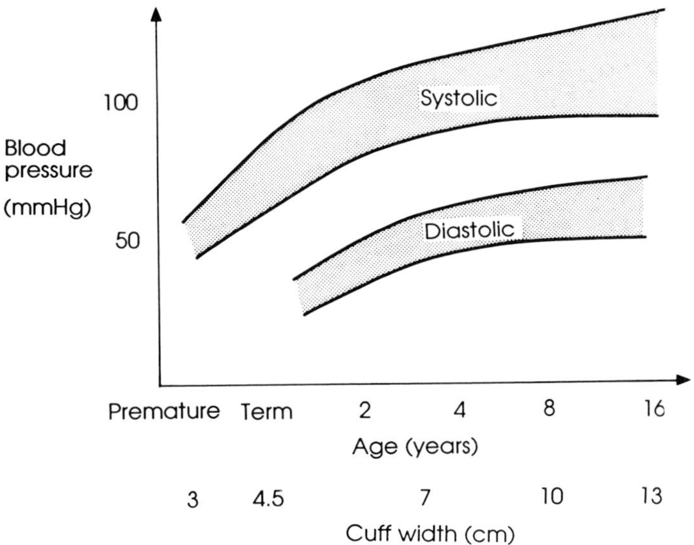

Fig. 14.9: *Normal blood pressure in children.*

Table 14.2 CAUSES OF HYPERTENSION

1. RENAL DISEASE (commonest)
   (i) Transient:
   - acute post-streptococcal glomerulonephritis
   - haemolytic uraemic syndrome
   - Henoch-Schönlein purpura

   (ii) Persistent:
   - chronic glomerulonephritis
   - chronic pyelonephritis
   - vesico-ureteric reflux
   - urinary tract obstruction
   - collagen disease

   (iii) Wilms' tumour
   (iv) Renal trauma
   (v) Renal artery stenosis
   (vi) Renal artery aneurysm, arteriovenous fistula
   (vii) Renal transplant
2. COARCTATION OF THE AORTA
3. ENDOCRINE DISEASE
   (i) Phaeochromocytoma
   (ii) Neuroblastoma
   (iii) Cushing's syndrome
4. CENTRAL NERVOUS SYSTEM DISEASE
   (i) Brain tumour
   (ii) Abscess
   (iii) Haemorrhage
   (iv) Encephalitis

inadequate to permit control of bladder function until the age of one to five years. When physiological control is achieved, the child can learn to be socially continent. Continuous dribbling of urine is always pathological. Wetting may occur both day and night, only during the day, or only at night (enuresis). In practice, those who wet only at night do not have an organic lesion (Table 14.3).

Causes of wetting

The most useful clues to the cause of 'wetting' come from the history.

Psychological

Most normal children have an occasional accident and there is no identifiable psychological reason for it. A few children wet in response to anxiety and stress, or regress to an earlier stage in their development of urinary continence when they become ill or have a disturbing emotional experience, such as admission to hospital or family break-up. Continence returns at a variable period after the initiating factors have gone. The wetting has an acute onset and there is a history of previous continence. The symptoms are rarely present during sleep.

Table 14.3 CAUSES OF WETTING

Cause	Main points
Psychological	Acute onset, previously continent, emotional upset, continent during sleep
Infection	Acute onset ± general signs of infection
Neurological	Continuous wetting since birth
Ectopic ureter	Continuous dribbling since birth in a girl with a normal micturition pattern
Urethral obstruction (including phimosis)	Poor flow of urine
Bladder exstrophy (including epispadias)	Continuous wetting since birth
Sphincter damage	History of perineal trauma

Infection

Infection of the urinary tract can cause wetting, which usually resolves dramatically with appropriate treatment of the infection. A second episode of infection may present as recurrence of wetting after a period of normal control. Dysuria, frequency and malodorous urine add further support to a diagnosis of infection.

Neurological

Children with no neurological control of bladder function have a characteristic pattern of wetting. During bladder filling in the normal child, the detrusor muscle relaxes so that the bladder can fill with little increase in pressure until its capacity is reached, while the urinary sphincters prevent the bladder emptying. To void, the sphincters relax and the detrusor contracts until the bladder is completely empty. In the paralysed or neurogenic bladder, there is no control of bladder filling or micturition, so that urine entering the bladder from the ureters passes into the urethra in an uncontrolled manner. This may be apparent clinically as dribbling which occurs every few minutes. The dribbling starts at birth and occurs every day without exception. Urine in the bladder at any time can be expressed by increasing the intra-abdominal pressure. Thus straining, coughing or exertion by the baby, or the deliberate application of pressure over the suprapubic area, will result in expression of urine from the bladder. On the other hand, when the infant is relaxed or asleep, the rate of dribbling may decrease.

Ectopic ureter

The ureter normally enters the bladder proximal to the bladder neck. In some instances, an ectopic ureter may open into the urethra (or rarely, the vagina) distal to the sphincter. Urine emanating from the ectopic ureter, which is often part of a duplex system, is not subject to normal sphincteric control and produces dribbling, whereas the normal ureters drain into the bladder and are subject to normal sphincteric control with a normal pattern of micturition. The function of the subservient renal moiety is often poor, and only small volumes of urine arise from the ectopic ureter. The characteristic pattern in girls is of normal micturition occurring independently of constant dribbling. The longer male urethra precludes this presentation in boys.

Phimosis

In a boy who has phimosis, there may be a history of ballooning of the foreskin during micturition, after which there is slight dribbling of urine for one to two minutes. The stenotic foreskin obstructs urine flow leading to accumulation of urine between the foreskin and glans, which slowly leaks through the narrowed opening after micturition is completed. The diagnosis is obvious on examination.

Urethral obstruction

Lesions which obstruct the urethra (e.g. posterior urethral valves, bladder diverticula and ureteroceles) cause an inadequate stream with poor flow, after which continued leakage of urine may occur. Urine retained in the dilated prostatic urethra continues to drain after micturition. Once the entire urethra is empty, no further dribbling occurs until the next void. In many of these patients, infection is superimposed.

Bladder exstrophy

Wetting occurs in bladder exstrophy and in severe cases of epispadias, but the cause is immediately apparent.

Sphincter damage

Penetrating perineal injuries (see Chapter 12) which cause damage to the sphincters directly, or to the pelvic parasympathetic nerves supplying them, may result in wetting. Operations for Hirschsprung's disease and for high anorectal anomalies, also may damage the pelvic parasympathetic nerves during dissection of the pelvis. Damage to the urinary sphincters has been caused by over-enthusiastic resection of posterior urethral valves.

Clinical diagnosis

The history will provide substantial clues to the likely diagnosis. The extreme variability and apparent inconsistency of the functional group, and the obvious external manifestations of spina bifida, bladder exstrophy, epispadias, phimosis and trauma to the spine or perineum, can be identified readily and separated from those with a less obvious structural cause. The time of onset of symptoms is important, since it enables acute problems (e.g. psychological or infection) to be separated from chronic structural or congenital anomalies.

If the child dribbles without periods of dryness, the lesion is likely to be neurological in origin, 'neurogenic', or in girls, an ectopic ureter opening distal to the internal sphincter of the bladder. Examination is directed towards demonstrating an expressible bladder by pressing firmly on the lower abdomen. Care must be taken to avoid excessive pressure because the 'spastic' bladder may be ruptured. A spastic bladder is seen occasionally with spina bifida, spinal tumours and traumatic transection of the spinal cord. Where a neurogenic bladder is present, the anus may be seen to be patulous with poor anal tone. The natal cleft is shallow, and perianal anaesthesia can be demonstrated (see Chapter 18). The lower back should be examined carefully for evidence of sacral agenesis which can be determined by palpation of the spinous processes of the sacrum. In sacral agenesis, a variable number of sacral segments are absent, and with them the sacral nerve roots supplying the bladder. Sacral agenesis and spina bifida occulta can be confirmed by x-rays. If the wetting is caused by an ectopic ureter, the perineum should be examined carefully for evidence of a ureteric orifice between the urethra and vagina.

In patients with chronic but intermittent wetting, the problem is likely to be structural. Management involves the identification and treatment of infection, if present, and investigation of the urinary tract. In most situations, the upper urinary tract is visualized by ultrasound or intravenous pyelogram (IVP) and the lower urinary tract by micturating cystourethrogram (MCU). Further investigation and treatment is dependent on the findings of these investigations.

HAEMATURIA

Haematuria, or blood in the urine, can be macroscopic or microscopic. In macroscopic haematuria, the colour of the urine ranges from a pink tinge to bright red, and may involve the passage of clots of blood during voiding. In microscopic haematuria, the urine appears normal, but blood is detected on biochemical analysis.

Children will present to the doctor if there is visible haematuria, although by the time that they are seen, the urine has often returned to normal. Analysis of the urine will show microscopic haematuria or no blood.

There are numerous causes of haematuria (Table 14.4) of which a proportion can be identified from the history and clinical findings. The remainder become apparent on microscopy and culture of the urine, and with specialized radiological techniques. Occasionally endoscopy, renal biopsy or other specialized investigations are required.

Clues from the history

Evenly blood-stained urine throughout micturition suggests the problem resides at, or proximal to, the bladder. Spots of blood passed at the end of micturition indicate an abnormality of the lower urinary tract, and a meatal ulcer or preputial pathology is likely. Recent circumcision points to a meatal ulcer and may be associated with splaying of the stream or a thin stream and pain at the tip of the penis on micturition (see Chapter 5). The pain is sharp and occurs at the commencement of micturition, leading to the passage of urine in short painful spurts. Characteristically, the child screams when he attempts to pass urine. In an uncircumcised boy, attempts at forced retraction of the foreskin in the presence of phimosis or congenital adhesions of the under surface of the prepuce to the glans, may cause spots of bleeding.

Table 14.4 CAUSES OF HAEMATURIA

1. PENILE
   - Meatal ulcer
   - Trauma
   - Trauma to the foreskin
2. INFECTION
   - Urinary tract infection
     - cystitis
     - pyelonephritis (often secondary to obstruction or stasis)
3. TUMOUR
   - Wilms' tumour
4. OBSTRUCTION AND STASIS
   - Pelviureteric obstruction
   - Urinary calculi
   - Vesico-ureteric obstruction
   - Vesico-ureteric reflux
   - Ureterocele
   - Polyp, diverticulum
5. TRAUMA
6. 'MEDICAL' DISEASE
   - IgA nephropathy
   - Glomerulonephritis
   - Bleeding diathesis
   - Henoch-Schönlein purpura
   - Hereditary haematuria
7. MISLEADING 'HAEMATURIA'
   - Vaginal bleeding
   - Ingested dye and pigments

Fever, malaise, anorexia and vomiting indicate infection of the urinary tract. The older child may describe urinary frequency with dysuria and abdominal pain. The pain may be located in the suprapubic region, loin or back depending on the site and extent of inflammation.

A history of recent weight loss and lethargy with vague abdominal discomfort points to a renal malignancy.

A history of a sore throat or impetigo preceding the onset of haematuria by two or three weeks, puffiness of the face, generalized oedema, anorexia and malaise in a child aged five to 12 years, strongly suggests acute post-streptococcal glomerulonephritis. There is often oliguria and either obvious haematuria or dark brown urine.

Haemolytic uraemic syndrome should be considered in the sick child under three years of age who has diarrhoea (sometimes bloody) or bruising of the limbs, who develops low urine output with blood.

Henoch-Schönlein purpura involving the kidneys results in haematuria. Interrogation will reveal migratory joint pain commonly involving the wrists, elbows, ankles and knees, abdominal pain and a rash over the buttocks and legs.

When trauma is responsible for haematuria, the history is usually obvious, In child abuse, however, there may be no story of physical injury.

A history of excessive bruising or prolonged bleeding after minor trauma provides a clue to the existence of a bleeding disorder. In the majority of patients, the nature of the bleeding diathesis will have been determined already.

Clues from the examination

In circumcised boys with a history of painful voiding, the meatus must be inspected for a meatal ulcer. The external urethral meatus appears small with a tiny scab at its entrance. After micturition, a small drop of blood appears at the site of the ulcer.

A number of systemic, non-infective causes of haematuria can be identified on clinical grounds. In acute post-streptococcal glomerulonephritis, there is generalized oedema most usually recognized as puffiness of the face and overlying the sacrum. The blood pressure is often raised, but must be related to the normal values for the age of the patient. In Henoch-Schönlein purpura, the elevated purpuric rash over the buttocks and legs is evident. There may be tenderness of the abdomen and joints which are painful on movement. Bruising and petechiae of varying stages of resolution can be seen in the bleeding diatheses.

If the child looks toxic and unwell, infection must be considered. The temperature and pulse should be recorded: pyrexia and tachycardia are likely. The cause of infection is not usually apparent on clinical examination, but where obstruction is present, the distended proximal urinary structures may be palpable. Tenderness of an affected loin and suprapubic region may indicate the area infected.

A mass in the abdomen may also be a Wilms' tumour (see Chapter 15). Further radiological investigation clarifies the nature of the pathology.

Pseudohaematuria

Ingestion of beetroot, dye-stuffs and some medications may give red-coloured urine in the absence of blood. Bleeding from the vagina or introitus may be confused with haematuria. Where no clear association with menstruation or perineal trauma is given by the child or parents, child abuse or a vaginal foreign body need to be considered.

GOLDEN RULES

(1) Urinary infection should be suspected in all unwell children where there is no obvious cause.
(2) Urinary anomalies should be excluded in all children with proven urinary tract infection.
(3) The blood pressure should be taken in every child with a suspected urinary tract problem.
(4) Acute onset of wetting which occurs only during the day, is likely to be caused by emotional upset.
(5) Continuous dribbling or wetting from birth is the hallmark of a congenital abnormality, such as neurogenic bladder or ectopic ureter.
(6) The cause of wetting can be determined by the history of its onset, duration and relationship to sleep.
(7) Evenly blood-stained urine is caused by disease in, or proximal to, the bladder.
(8) Clear urine followed by bright blood indicates pathology in the urethra or tip of the penis.
(9) Beware vaginal bleeding presenting as haematuria: this may be caused by sexual abuse or a retained foreign body.

Further Reading

Jones P.G., Woodward A.A., eds. (1986). *Clinical Paediatric Surgery*, 3rd edn. Oxford: Blackwell Scientific Publications.

15 Abdominal masses

There are numerous organs in the peritoneal cavity and retroperitoneal space which can produce an abnormal mass. Neoplastic or hamartomatous enlargements of the organs may be solid or cystic, while mechanical obstruction to the hollow tubes in the abdominal cavity produces cystic dilatation.

THE QUESTIONS TO BE ANSWERED

A mass may be found within the abdomen by accident or by design. In either event, the physician should adopt the same approach to diagnosis as would be followed elsewhere in the body (Fig. 15.1). First, the *age* of the child should be considered, since nearly all diseases in children occur at specific ages. In particular, malignant tumours of childhood which present commonly as incidental abdominal masses are much more common in pre-school children.

The second question to be answered is: '*From which organ does the mass arise?*' Knowledge of the organ of origin will eliminate numerous possibilities from any list of differential diagnoses. The third question is: '*What are the features of the*

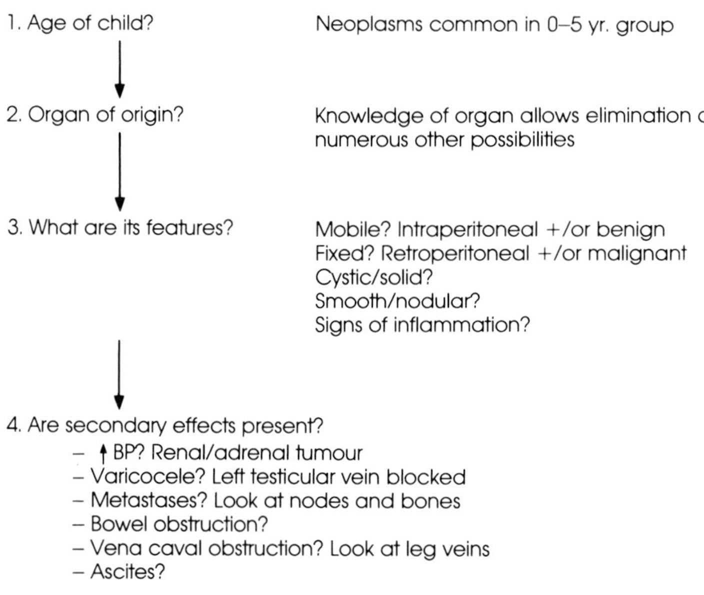

Fig. 15.1: *The systematic approach to adopt when an abdominal mass is found.*

mass?' This is answered by careful examination to elicit whether it is mobile or fixed, cystic or solid, smooth or nodular, or whether there are signs of inflammation. These features assist in the determination of which pathological process has produced the mass. The mobility of an abdominal mass is a key feature in the diagnosis, since mobile masses must be within the peritoneal cavity itself, rather than in the retroperitoneal tissue. In addition, mobile lumps usually are benign.

The last question to be answered is: '*What secondary effects does the mass cause?*' The blood pressure may need to be measured, particularly if a Wilms' tumour, neuroblastoma or renal disease is suspected. A varicocele may be present if the left renal vein is obstructed. Metastases may be present in distant lymph nodes or bones. Secondary effects, such as bowel obstruction, vena caval obstruction or ascites, may be present within the abdomen itself.

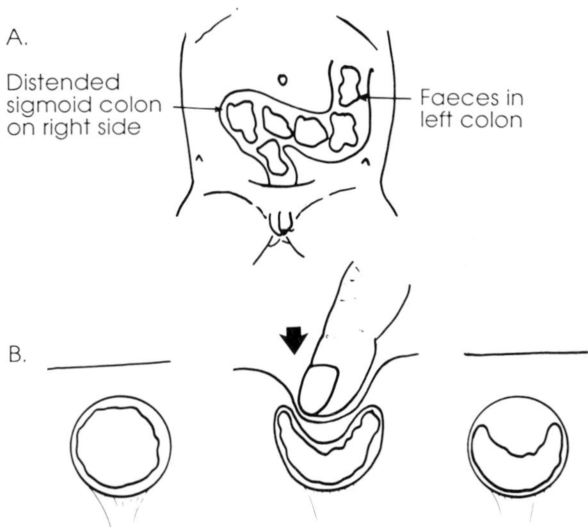

Fig. 15.3: *Hard faeces as an 'abdominal mass'. A. When the sigmoid is distended, hard faeces may be palpable on the right side of the abdomen. B. The pathognomonic sign of a faecal mass is indentation on compression.*

NORMAL MASSES

When an abdominal mass is discovered, either by the parent or the attending physician, it is important to determine whether the mass is normal (Fig. 15.2). The liver and spleen usually are palpable in the neonatal period and in early infancy, when their haemopoietic function is active. They become impalpable later in childhood, when they no longer produce red cells, and when the shape of the costal margin changes with growth to conceal the organs of the upper abdomen. In small or thin children, the lower poles of the kidneys are palpable in the paravertebral gutters.

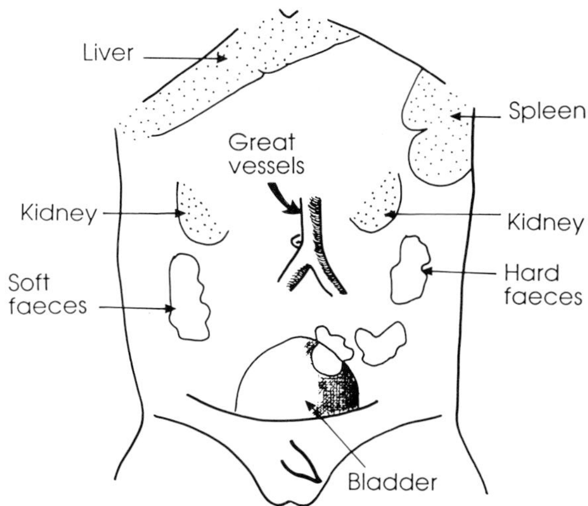

Fig. 15.2: *Normal structures which are palpable in the abdomen.*

When the infant is relaxed, the great vessels are palpable behind and to the left of the umbilicus. The aortic pulsation can be felt in infants and small children, since the lumbosacral promontory is relatively anterior. In both iliac fossae, and especially on the left, faeces may be palpated within the colon. On the right side, the colonic contents are pultaceous and relatively soft. In contrast, in the left descending and sigmoid colon, hard rock-like faeces may be palpable in the presence of constipation. In the middle of the lower abdomen, the bladder may be demonstrated on percussion or palpation, since in small children the bladder is not obscured by the pelvis.

Hard faeces are the commonest abdominal masses (Fig. 15.3). Usually, the faeces are palpable in the left side of the colon, and may vary in consistency from pultaceous to stony hard. In chronic constipation, the sigmoid may be so enlarged that firm faeces are palpable in the right side of the abdomen. In severe cases of constipation, faeces will be palpable in the right colon as well. To determine whether a mass is present within the colon, an attempt should be made to indent the mass by compression through the abdominal wall. The pathognomonic sign of faeces is the indentation produced on compression.

The bladder is misdiagnosed commonly as a pathological abdominal mass (Fig. 15.4A). Bladder enlargement will cause protuberance of the lower abdomen. In addition, palpation will be tender and is likely to induce the urge to void. If there is doubt as to whether a mass is the bladder, the child should be re-examined after voiding or catheterization.

COMMON ABNORMAL ABDOMINAL MASSES

Two common masses, described elsewhere in this volume, are the inflammatory mass of appendicitis (Chapter 3), and the sausage-shaped mass of intussusception (Chapter 8). The appendix mass (Fig. 15.5) is caused by inflammation or perforation which is walled off by adjacent bowel and great omentum. The mass is palpable in the right iliac fossa or pelvis and exhibits signs of inflammation, including loss of mobility. There may be associated signs of bowel obstruction. In a child over 10 years of age, a rare differential diagnosis includes inflammatory bowel disease. In addition, a malignant lymphoma of the small bowel may mimic an appendix mass.

The mass of intussusception may be difficult to feel (Fig. 15.6). The child may be crying and restless, which makes the mass difficult to palpate behind the rectus muscles. It is further concealed by voluntary guarding. The intussusception mass is more medial than the usual position of the right colon because of telescoping of the mesentery (see Chapter 8 for details).

Urinary obstruction produces different types of cystic dilatation of the kidney according to the time of obstruction in relation to renal development (Fig. 15.7). In ureteric atresia, early fetal obstruction prevents normal nephron development and results in dysplastic cysts. This leads to a multicystic kidney in the neonate. The cysts are of different sizes and the kidney feels like an irregular bunch of grapes. In late fetal or postnatal obstruction, the nephrons have had time to develop

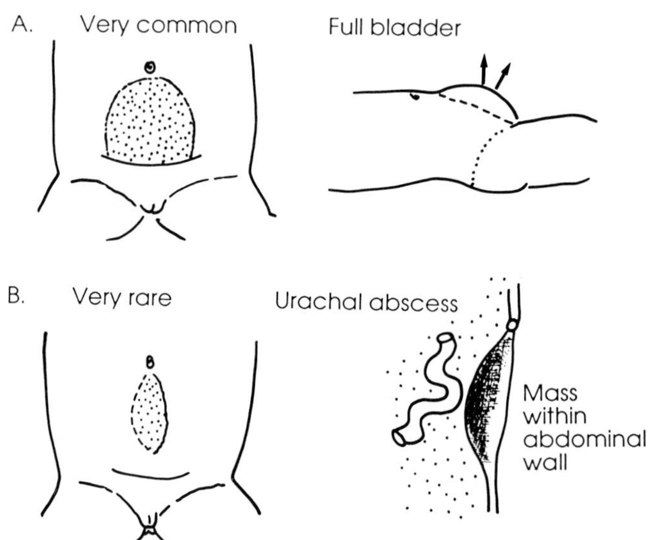

Fig. 15.4: *The bladder as an 'abdominal mass'.* A. *A full bladder is very common: it is tender on palpation and disappears on voiding or aspiration of urine.* B. *A urachal abscess is very rare: it is tender on palpation, but remains after voiding. Careful examination reveals its location within, rather than behind, the abdominal wall.*

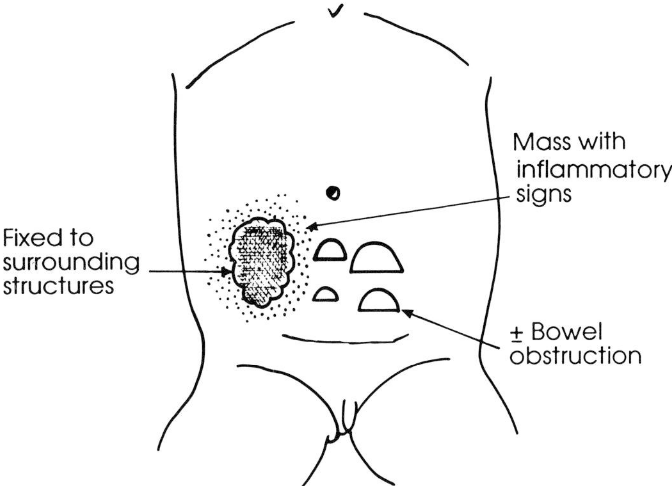

Fig. 15.5: *The appendix mass – appendix, bowel loops, omentum ± abscess cavity – is an intraperitoneal benign lesion which is not mobile. The differential diagnosis should include inflammatory bowel disease and the rare lymphosarcoma of the bowel.*

normally before obstruction occurs, and the more usual hydronephrotic kidney is produced. If the obstruction is in the distal urinary tract, a dilated ureter also may be palpable. Hydronephrosis produces a smooth cystic enlargement of the kidney which retains its shape. Gerota's fascia confines the kidney so that it does not cross the midline, and it may be felt to move downwards on inspiration. A loin or flank mass should be ballotable (Fig. 15.8). Bimanual palpation with the lower hand pushing the kidney forwards from behind should allow the hand at the front of the abdomen to feel the mass. A mass anterior to the plane of the kidney cannot be pushed forward by a hand in the loin. Finally, a large cystic kidney in an infant with little body fat can be transilluminated provided that the room is dark and the torch is bright (Fig. 15.9).

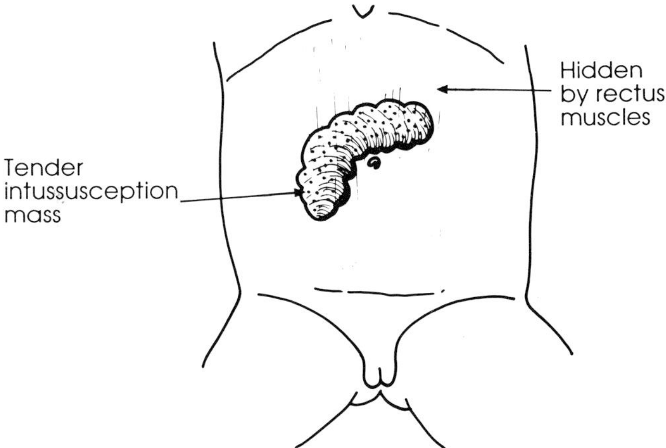

Fig. 15.6: *Intussusception producing an abdominal mass: the tender 'sausage' is hidden by voluntary guarding of the rectus abdominis muscles. The intussusception is more medial than the normal colon because of 'telescoping' of the mesentery.*

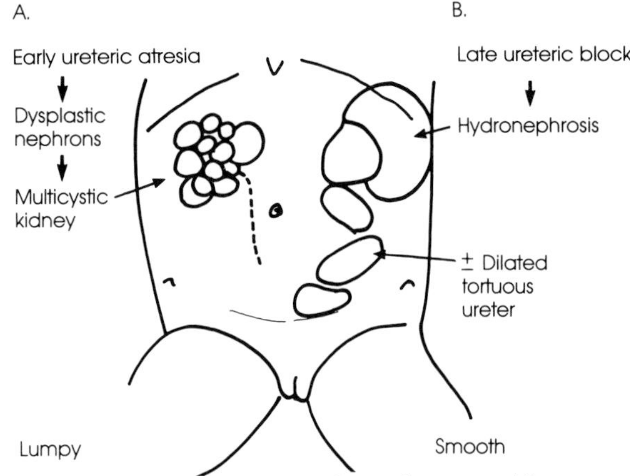

Fig. 15.7: *The clinical features of a renal cyst caused by obstruction depend on the stage of renal development. A. Early obstruction (ureteric atresia) causes a multicystic kidney. B. Late obstruction produces hydronephrosis. Both lesions are cystic and soft, and may transilluminate. In addition, both are ballotable and move downwards on inspiration.*

TUMOUR PRESENTING AS AN ABDOMINAL MASS

The embryonic tumours – neuroblastoma, Wilms' tumour and hepatoblastoma (Fig. 15.10) – are relatively common in the first five years of life. Leukaemias and lymphomas are the common neoplasms which present as an abdominal mass later in childhood. Hepatosplenomegaly, with enlargement of lymph nodes in other parts of the body, in association with fever, weight loss or night sweats, should arouse suspicion of an underlying haematological neoplasm.

Neuroblastoma is an embryonic neoplasm of the neural crest cells which arises most commonly from the adrenal medulla, but is also found anywhere along the sympathetic chain. The protuberant upper abdomen of the infant may conceal the tumour until it is quite large (Fig. 15.11). There is significant malaise, perhaps related to metabolic effects of the tumour, with fever, weight loss and anorexia. The tumour is non-cystic, feels stony hard and, since it grows without a significant capsule, its surface is irregular and nodular to palpation. When it arises from the adrenal or adjacent sympathetic chain, it displaces the kidney downwards and spreads rapidly to the para-aortic nodes, the liver, the cervical nodes and, occasionally, to more distant sites such as the bones and skin. Neuroblastoma commencing *in utero* may spread to the skin before birth, producing multiple bluish skin nodules which have been described as 'blueberry muffins'. Clinical characteristics caused by the invasiveness of the tumour are its extension across the midline and its immobility. Examination is not complete without a

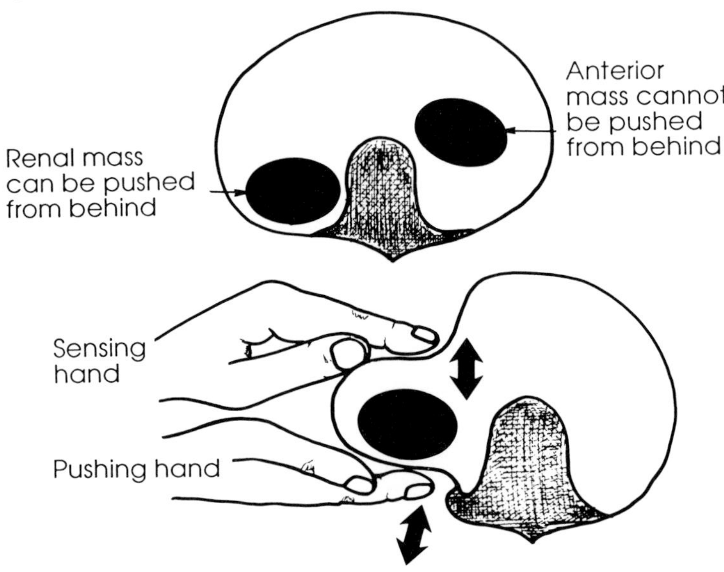

Fig. 15.8: *Balloting a renal mass: the posterior hand pushes the kidney forward to enable it to be felt by the anterior hand.*

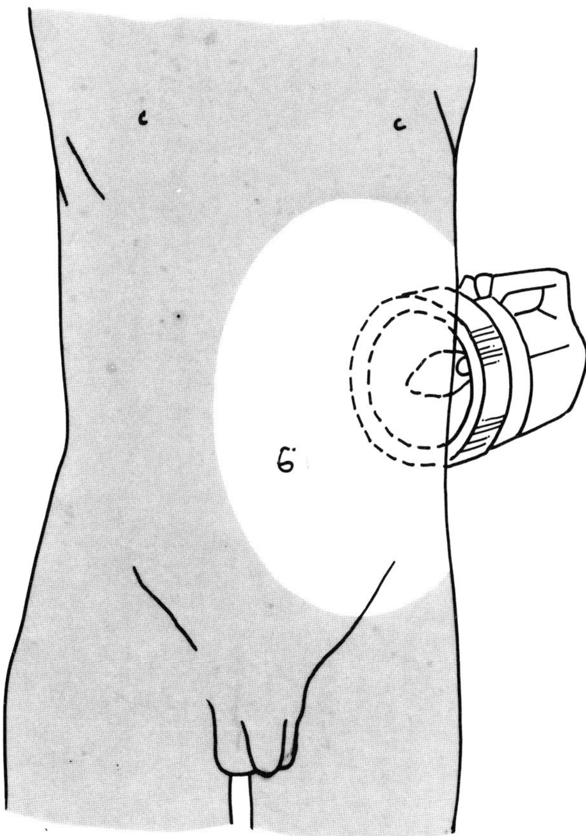

Fig. 15.9: *Transillumination of a renal mass to distinguish a solid tumour from hydronephrosis. A dark room and a bright torch are required.*

search for distant metastases and measurement of the blood pressure, since the tumour may produce noradrenaline or adrenaline and may directly compress the renal arteries.

The physical signs and symptoms of a Wilms' tumour often allow it to be distinguished from a neuroblastoma. Commonly, the loin mass is an incidental finding because the tumour has grown to a large size before producing symptoms. The mass is non-cystic and firm, and has a smooth surface because it expands without infiltration, creating a pseudocapsule (Fig. 15.12). Except in advanced disease, the tumour remains confined by Gerota's fascia, moves downwards on inspiration and does not cross the midline. An attempt should be made to ballot the tumour since this is good confirmatory evidence that it arises from the kidney. Unlike the child with neuroblastoma, a child with Wilms' tumour appears reasonably well. The urine is examined for evidence of haematuria, even if this has not been noted by the parents. The scrotum is examined with the boy standing, to look for a varicocele. The testicular vein, particularly on the left side, may be obstructed by the enlarging renal tumour. A Wilms' tumour may spread by direct growth into the renal vein and obstruct the left testicular vein. Hypertension is a common sequel of this tumour because of renal artery compression and production of renin.

UNCOMMON ABNORMAL MASSES

Two relatively uncommon renal masses which may confound the examiner are the horseshoe kidney and the pelvic kidney (Fig. 15.13). Fusion of the lower poles of the kidneys prevents ascent during embryogenesis because the isthmus of the horseshoe kidney is arrested by the inferior mesenteric artery. The kidney remains anterior to the lumbosacral promontory, and is palpable behind the rectus abdominis muscles at, or below, the umbilicus. The pelvic or dysplastic pancake-like kidney has failed to ascend to the normal renal position and usually is found overlying the iliac vessels. It may be confused with an abdominal

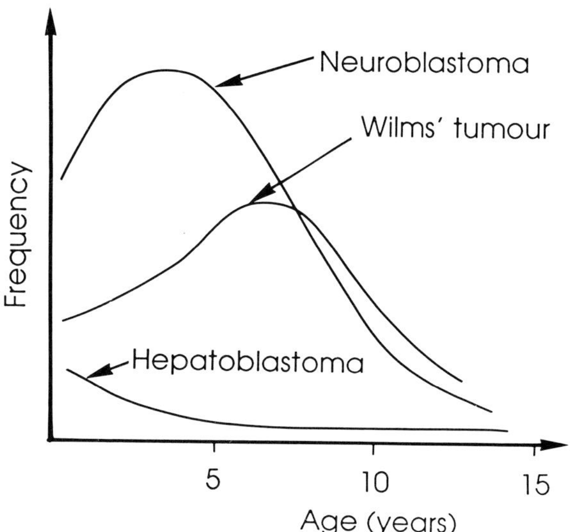

Fig. 15.10: *The frequency of the common embryonal tumours relative to age.*

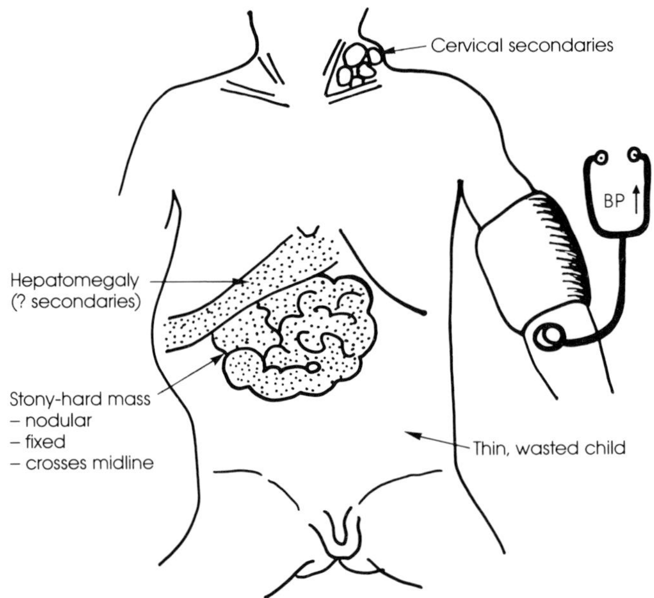

Fig. 15.11: *The clinical features produced by an adrenal neuroblastoma.*

tumour or an appendix mass when it is present on the right side. Both masses are quite superficial in the abdomen because of the proximity of the sacral promontory to the anterior abdominal wall, causing them to be detected on incidental palpation. Diagnosis is confirmed by ultrasound or intravenous pyelogram.

Rare causes of pathological masses near the bladder include cysts or abscesses of the urachus – the embryological connection between the bladder and the allantois. In some vertebrates, including man, the allantois is a vestigial structure in the umbilical cord, and the urachus is of little practical significance. Where some part of the urachus

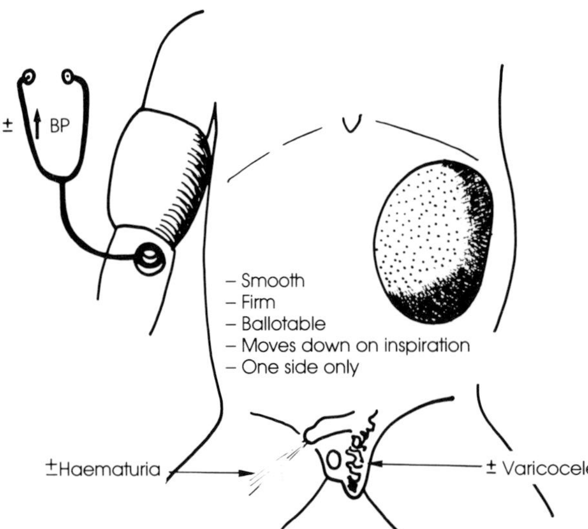

Fig. 15.12: *The clinical features of a Wilms' tumour (nephroblastoma).*

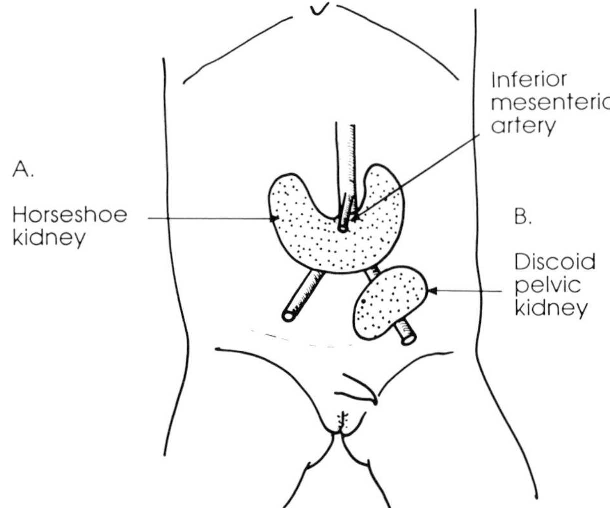

Fig. 15.13: *Uncommon renal masses. A. The horseshoe kidney is anterior to the lumbosacral promontory because the inferior mesenteric artery prevents further ascent. B. The pelvic kidney is a discoid mass overlying the iliac vessels.*

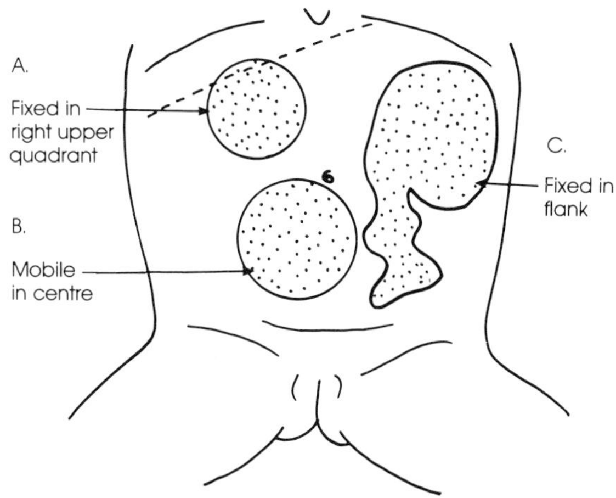

Fig. 15.14: *The cystic masses in the abdomen at birth.* A. *Choledochal or hepatic cysts are fixed and in the right upper quadrant* (RUQ). B. *Mesenteric, duplication or ovarian cysts are mobile and in the middle of the abdomen.* C. *Dilated kidneys and ureters are fixed in the flank.*

remains patent, it produces an isolated cyst, sinus or abscess (see Fig. 15.4B). The transitional epithelium which lines the urachus is an effective barrier to the spread of infection, such that a urachal abscess presents as localized chronic disease. There may be minor systemic symptoms of infection in association with a mass and tenderness in the lower abdomen. Characteristically, the mass is within the abdominal wall rather than deep to the abdominal wall. The tenderness is superficial and may be exquisite, without the child appearing unwell. Radiological examination may reveal ectopic calcification in the suprapubic region, caused by chronic inflammatory change and calcium deposition within the cavity.

NEONATAL ABDOMINAL MASSES

There are a large number of masses which may be palpable at, or shortly after, birth – but fortunately most of these are rare (Table 15.1). The three common areas in which masses are found are shown in Fig. 15.14. In the middle of the abdomen, there may be mesenteric, duplication or ovarian cysts, all of which have considerable mobility. In the flank, there may be cystic enlargement of the kidneys or ureters which are fixed by the retroperitoneum. In the right upper quadrant, there may be choledochal or hepatic cysts immobilized by the attachments of the liver and the porta hepatis. In addition, abdominal masses may be caused by neonatal tumours or bowel obstruction (Chapter 21). The neonatal pelvis is so narrow and shallow that any large pelvic mass tends to be displaced into the abdominal cavity.

An algorithm can be used to approach the assessment of an abdominal cyst in the neonate (Fig. 15.15). The most important criterion is mobility of the cyst, which will distinguish intraperitoneal from retroperitoneal masses. Cystic lesions in the retroperitoneal plane arise from obstructed or dysplastic kidneys. Less common masses, which are usually solid, include a swollen kidney from renal vein thrombosis, or an adrenal haemorrhage. Current high standards of obstetric care result in these conditions now being seen rarely. Benign or malignant renal tumours, along with neuroblastoma, can occur in the neonate but their clinical presentation is similar to that described already in this chapter. Intraperitoneal masses can be diagnosed by the associated physical signs, including partial or complete bowel obstruction, jaundice and, occasionally, by the characteristics of the cyst itself, i.e. whether it is unilocular or multilocular.

Intestinal duplication causes cystic dilatation within the peritoneal cavity. This is a rare abnormality of gut development in which two intestinal tubes have been formed. The more common sites for duplication are the duodenum and ileum. The duplication may be tubular or a simple cyst (Fig. 15.16). Tubular duplications may open into the normal bowel and hence do not cause obstruction or even a palpable mass. On occasions, they present with bleeding secondary to ulceration from acid produced by ectopic gastric mucosa within them. Cystic duplications do not communicate with the bowel but enlarge in size with accumulation of secretions. The cyst is in the mesentery and is very mobile. As the cyst enlarges, the normal bowel is stretched across its surface and obstructed.

'Mesenteric' cysts are usually lymphangiomata arising in the mesenteric lymphatics (Fig. 15.17). As with the cystic hygroma in the neck, they are

Table 15.1 PART A CLINICAL CHARACTERISTICS OF ABDOMINAL MASSES

Mass	Symptoms	Location	Mobility	Transillumination	Characteristics
Hydronephrosis	± abdominal pain	Flank	Little Down on inspiration Ballotable	Yes	Smooth Soft/firm
Multicystic kidney	± renal failure	Flank	Little Down on inspiration Ballotable	Yes	Irregular cysts
Wilms' tumour	± BP ↑ Fever, pain ± haematuria	Flank	Little Down on inspiration Ballotable	None	Firm Smooth
Bowel duplication	± intestinal obstruction ± bile-stained vomit	Centre	Mobile (if in the small bowel mesentery)	Not usually	Round firm cyst or tubular + soft
Mesenteric cyst	Rarely obstruction	Centre	Mobile	Yes	Soft/multilocular + firm
Neuroblastoma	± BP ↑ Malignant malaise Pain, fever	Along the sympathetic chain/adrenal ± across midline	None	None	Hard, irregular or nodular
Hydrometrocolpos	± imperforate anus	Pelvis → centre	Little	None	Smooth, cystic
Ovarian cyst	Female	Centre	Very mobile unless too big	Yes	Smooth, cystic
Choledochal cyst	Jaundice, pain	RUQ	Little	None	Small, smooth cyst
Hepatoblastoma	± ascites	RUQ	Little	None	Hard, smooth

Adapted from Filston and Izant (1978).
BP = blood pressure; RUQ = right upper quadrant

Table 15.1 PART B: IMAGING CHARACTERISTICS OF ABDOMINAL MASSES

Mass	X-ray	Ultrasound
Hydronephrosis	Obstruction on IVP	Dilated kidney
Multicystic kidney	No function on IVP	Multicystic
Wilms' tumour	Distorted calyces on IVP	Solid mass arising from kidney
Bowel duplication	± bowel obstruction ± extra fluid levels	Mobile cystic lesion with bowel
Mesenteric cyst	–	Multilocular cyst with bowel
Neuroblastoma	Displacement of kidney on IVP Calcification on plain abdominal x-ray	Solid mass not in kidney
Hydrometrocolpos	Displaced ureters on IVP	Cystic, arising from pelvis
Ovarian cyst	Displaced bowel on abdominal x-ray	Single cyst with 'sludge'
Choledochal cyst	Displaced duodenum on abdominal x-ray and barium meal	Cystic, in porta hepatis
Hepatoblastoma	Enlarged liver outline	Solid mass in liver

IVP = intravenous pyelogram

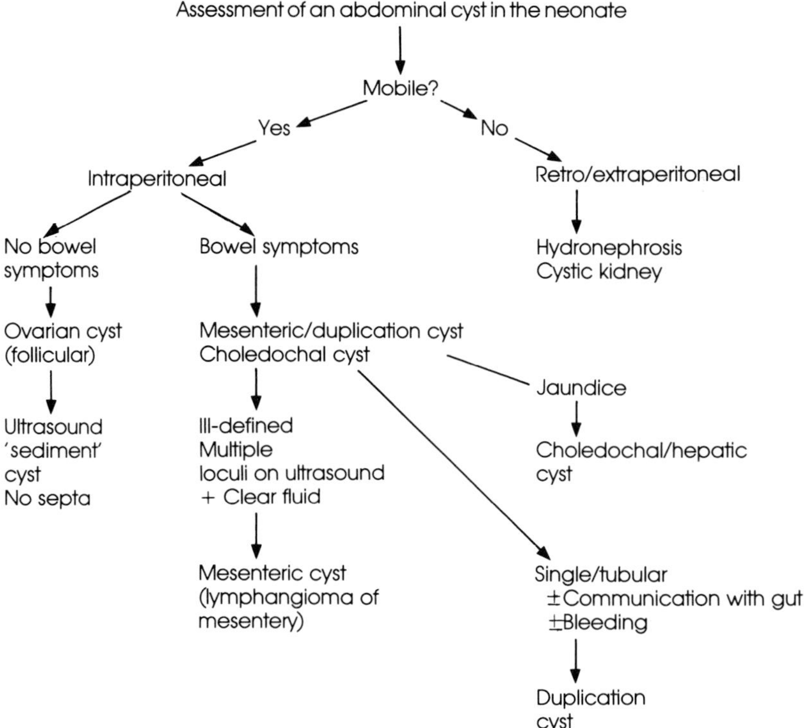

Fig. 15.15: *Assessment of an abdominal cyst in the neonate.*

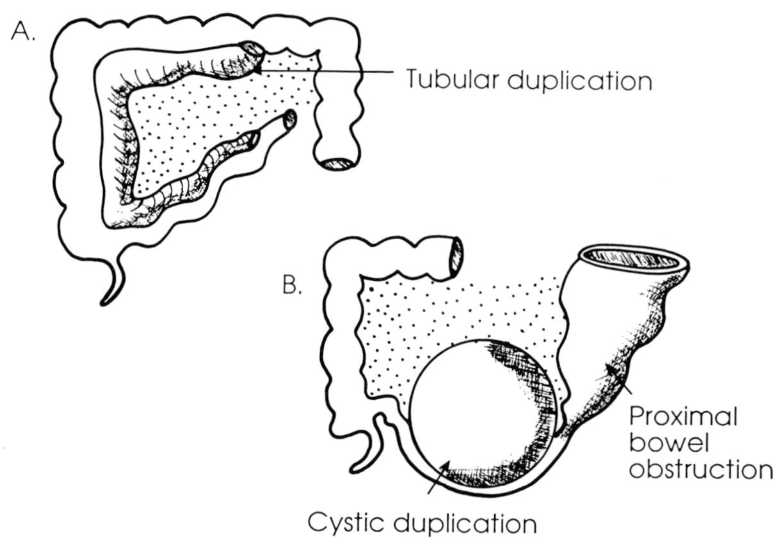

Fig. 15.16: *The two types of duplication of the intestine. A. Tubular duplications may be impalpable if they communicate with the normal bowel. They will form a sausage-shaped cyst if there is no communication. B. Simple duplication cysts expand with secretions in the mesentery and compress the normal bowel.*

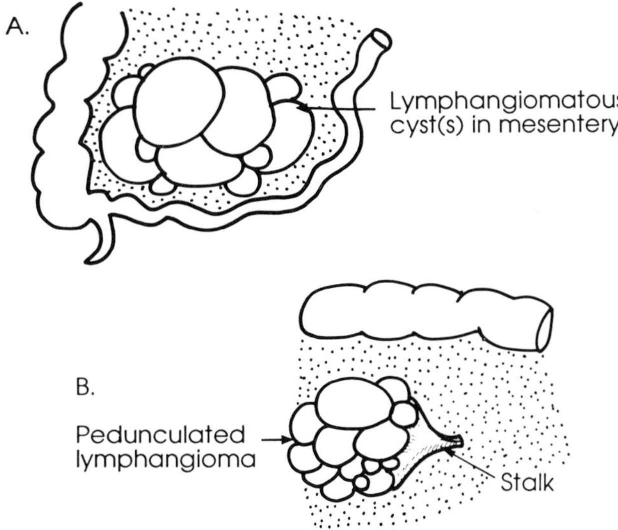

Fig. 15.17: *Mesenteric lymphangiomata may form simple or multiple cysts within the mesentery (A), or on a pedunculated stalk (B). Large cysts are lax and filled with clear fluid, and may mimic ascites.*

lax, fluid-filled cysts which may be so ill-defined that the fluid collection mimics ascites. Occasionally, the lymphangioma is pedunculated, containing cysts of varying diameters, but still arises from the mesentery. It may undergo torsion and produce acute symptoms.

The aetiology of choledochal cysts, or dilatation of the bile ducts, is unknown. One explanation is that the choledochal cyst forms as a 'blow-out' of the bile duct secondary to inflammation. Partial destruction of the duct wall produces cystic dilatation. Choledochal cysts may be caused by the same pathological process which leads to biliary atresia. They present as an incidental right upper quadrant mass, or are associated with intermittent pain and jaundice (Fig. 15.18). The firm and spherical mass is immobile on account of its location in the porta hepatis. The diagnosis can be confirmed on abdominal ultrasound or endoscopic retrograde cholangiopancreatography (ERCP).

PELVIC LESIONS

Palpable masses in the pelvis are common, although many may be felt only on rectal examination. Benign lesions are particularly common, as shown in Fig. 15.19. Excluding a full bladder and palpable faeces, the most frequent mass found in the pelvis is an appendix abscess, which has obvious signs of inflammation, including pain, heat and tenderness. A clinical diagnosis following rectal examination is straightforward (see Chapter 3). Cystic lesions in the pelvis may be more difficult to diagnose. Rare but significant cystic lesions include the anterior sacral meningocele and the presacral teratoma. These lesions are characterized by their palpation on the posterior wall of the rectum, in front of the bony sacrum or coccyx.

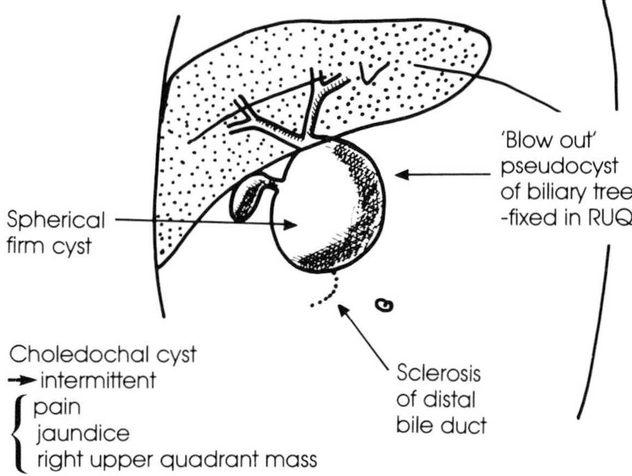

Fig. 15.18: *The features of a choledochal cyst, which can present at any time in childhood.*

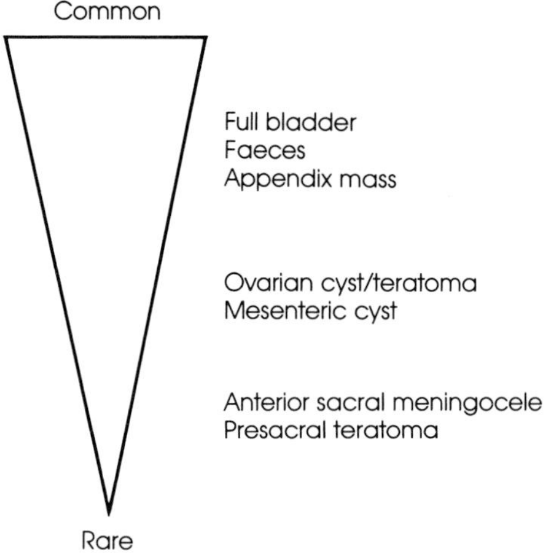

Fig. 15.19: *The relative frequency of benign pelvic masses.*

This is in contrast to most other pelvic masses which, on rectal examination, are palpable anteriorly or laterally.

An algorithm for distinguishing benign from malignant pelvic masses is shown in Fig. 15.20. The four important features, as for abdominal masses, are (1) the age of the child, (2) the organ of origin of the mass, (3) the mobility and other characteristics of the mass, and (4) the secondary effects of the lesion elsewhere in the patient. The commonest benign lesion in a pre-adolescent girl is an ovarian cyst, which is very mobile. The secondary effects include pain and vomiting from torsion of the cyst, and these may mimic appendicitis. Diagnosis is confirmed by rectal examination. Malignant pelvic masses usually occur in much younger children and in infants. Often the mass is fixed to the pelvic wall by direct extension of the tumour and feels hard or stony. There may be direct extension of tumour to produce a nodular mass in the introitus. This is known as sarcoma botryoides, and is caused by a rhabdomyosarcoma of the bladder or vagina. The secondary effects of this tumour include urinary and bowel obstruction, or vaginal bleeding. The important malignant tumours which may arise in the pelvis are ovarian carcinoma, rhabdomyosarcoma, malignant sacrococcygeal teratoma and neuroblastoma.

The common clinical presentation of benign ovarian teratomas or dermoids is shown in Fig. 15.21. The girl is prepubertal with a mean age of 11 years. The mass may be asymptomatic, but commonly causes acute colic or severe pain when torsion occurs. The diagnosis of a teratoma can be confirmed by the presence of ectopic bone or dysplastic teeth on abdominal x-ray. Torsion of an

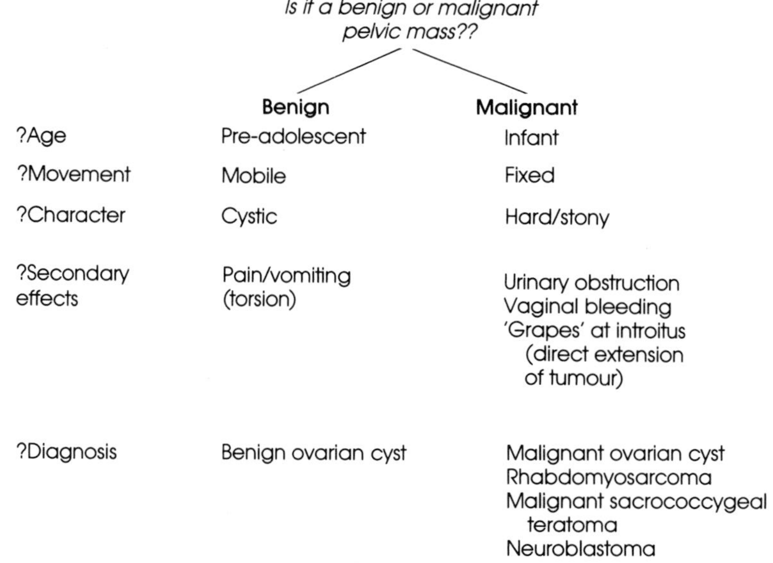

Fig. 15.20: *The criteria for distinguishing benign from malignant pelvic masses.*

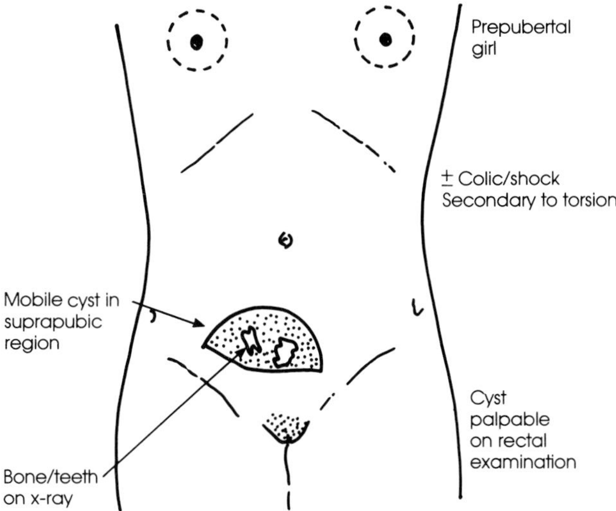

Fig. 15.21: *The clinical features of a (benign) ovarian teratoma ('dermoid').*

ovarian cyst usually indicates that it is benign, since fixation to surrounding structures prevents malignant, infiltrating tumours from twisting.

GOLDEN RULES

(1) The key to the diagnosis of an abdominal mass is finding out the organ of origin and the pathological characteristics of the mass.
(2) Mobile lesions are usually benign, unless there is acute inflammation which causes secondary fixation.
(3) Fluctuant/cystic masses are usually benign (e.g. cysts or hydronephrosis).
(4) A lower abdominal mass with calcified regions on x-ray is likely to be a benign ovarian teratoma.
(5) All abdominal masses must be assumed to be potentially serious until a definite diagnosis is established.
(6) Rectal examination should be performed in all patients presenting with a mass in the lower half of the abdomen.

Further Reading

Filston H.C., Izant R. (1978). *The Surgical Neonate.* New York: Appleton-Century-Crofts

Jones P.G., Campbell P.E., eds. (1976). *Tumours of Infancy and Childhood.* Oxford: Blackwell Scientific Publications.

Jones P.G., Woodward A.A., eds. (1986). *Clinical Paediatric Surgery*, 3rd edn. Oxford: Blackwell Scientific Publications.

16 Gastro-intestinal bleeding

Gastro-intestinal bleeding is a relatively common symptom in childhood, but only rarely does it signify serious disease. This is because most children with gastro-intestinal bleeding have an anal fissure or gastro-enteritis, rather than the more dramatic bleeding of the Meckel's diverticulum or oesophageal varices.

When a child presents with bleeding from the gut, the history is of paramount importance, since the cause often may be determined by careful questioning.

THE APPEARANCE OF THE STOOL

Blood entering the alimentary tract, unless vomited, will appear ultimately on or within the stools. The longer it stays in the bowel, the more it is broken down and the darker it becomes. Therefore, it can be seen that the appearance of the blood in the rectum is a function of its point of entry (i.e. how far it has to travel) and of its transit time (i.e. how long it takes to traverse the alimentary tract). As a general rule, bleeding from the oesophagus, stomach and duodenum appears as black and tarry stools (melaena), from the small bowel as dark red-brown stools, and from the colon as red 'altered blood' mixed with the stools. Bleeding from the anorectal region itself appears as bright red streaking on the surface of the stool or on the toilet paper, because the stool has been formed already at the time of contact with the blood.

Blood mixed with diarrhoea is seen in inflammatory conditions of the bowel, particularly colitis and proctitis, which may be caused by acute infection. Bleeding with chronic diarrhoea is more suggestive of inflammatory bowel disease.

THE APPEARANCE OF THE VOMITUS

Rapid bleeding from the oesophagus, stomach or duodenum may cause a child to vomit bright red blood (haematemesis), which will be observed in association with pallor and signs of shock. With slower bleeding from the upper gastro-intestinal tract, the blood becomes altered by the gastric acid to appear as 'coffee-ground' vomitus. However, bleeding may occur from these organs without vomiting.

MINOR BLEEDING IN THE HEALTHY NEONATE

In the neonate, the most common cause of bleeding is an anal fissure, which may result from the passage of a stool or may be iatrogenic and sustained during introduction of a rectal thermometer. Small, bright red streaks of blood can be seen on the stool or as spots on the nappy. The child is otherwise well, feeds normally and has a soft, non-tender abdomen.

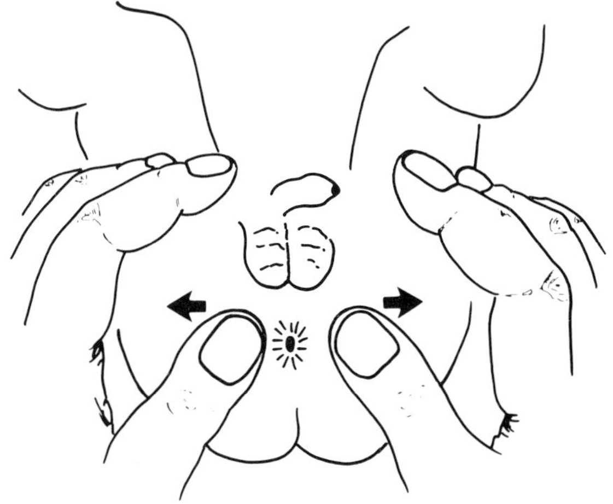

Fig. 16.1: *Examination of the anus in a neonate to look for an anal fissure.*

The anus should be examined carefully for evidence of a fissure by parting the perianal skin in a lateral direction (Fig. 16.1) with the baby lying supine. It may be helpful to use an assistant to support the legs. A fissure appears as a breach in the mucosa running longitudinally within the anal canal. It is unusual for the examination to make the fissure bleed and there is rarely evidence of inflammation around it. Therefore, it is easily overlooked unless the perianal skin is stretched well apart and the anal canal inspected carefully. Where a fissure has not been demonstrated adequately, gentle digital examination of the rectum should be performed using the little finger of the right hand, while the left hand supports the legs (Fig. 16.2). The finger should be gloved and lubricated to avoid further trauma to the anal canal. Slow withdrawal of the slightly flexed little finger, at the same time as the opposite thumb applies traction to the perianal skin, may further evert the skin and mucosa of the anal canal to expose the anal fissure (Fig. 16.3). The fissure cannot be palpated because it is acute, with little inflammation or induration around it, and no fibrosis. It is located most commonly in the midline, posteriorly or anteriorly. The appearance of faeces or blood on the glove should be noted. Introduction of the little finger into the anal canal dilates the canal, and in anal fissure, is therapeutic.

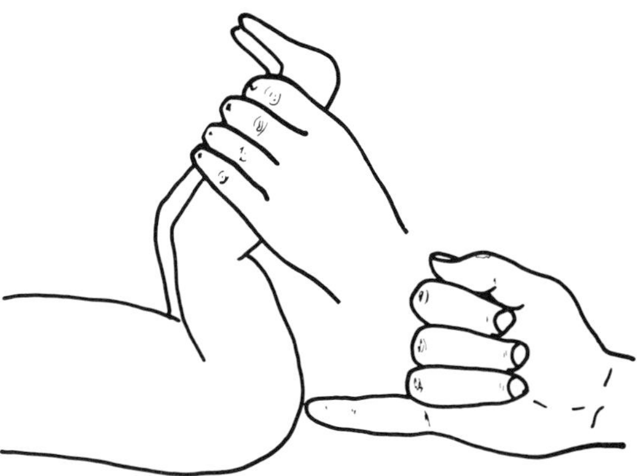

Fig. 16.2: *The technique of rectal examination in a neonate, using the little finger and holding up the legs of the baby with the other hand.*

BLEEDING IN THE SICK NEONATE

Necrotizing enterocolitis is an acquired disease of the newborn where a variable length and distribution of bowel becomes ischaemic and gangrenous. One manifestation of the disease is the passage of blood *per rectum* (see Chapter 21). In the early stages of enterocolitis, reducing substances may be detected in the stools because absorption of sugars is impaired. Soon, obvious blood is passed rectally. The infant often is premature and has experienced major physiological stress in the perinatal period. The symptoms appear between three and 14 days of age. The child rapidly becomes unwell, lethargic and refuses feeds; vomiting may occur. Abdominal distension, if not already present, will develop over the ensuing hours. The abdomen becomes tender, and where there is gangrenous bowel present, the abdominal wall becomes tight, oedematous and red, reflecting the underlying peritonitis. Often, the first indication of necrotizing enterocolitis is the onset of apnoeic spells and bradycardia. The diagnosis is confirmed on plain radiology. In severe cases of necrotizing enterocolitis, frank blood and even blood-stained tissue can be passed rectally.

Mid-gut volvulus is another life-threatening condition which may present with gastro-intestinal bleeding in the neonate. When the mid-gut returns to the abdominal cavity in the 10-week-old embryo, it undergoes rotation and fixation to the posterior abdominal wall. Failure of this

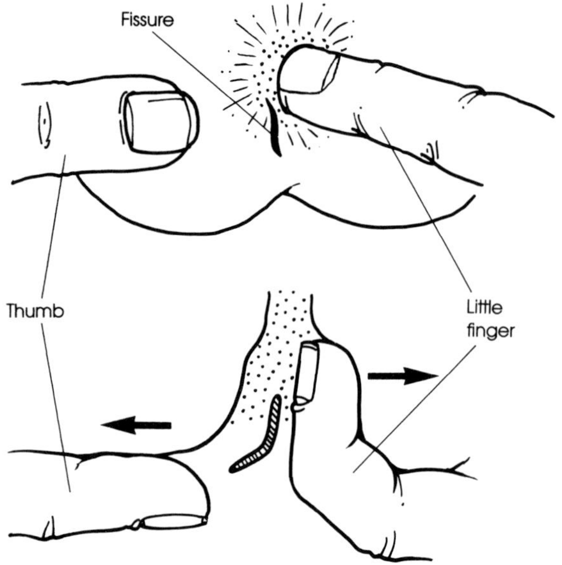

Fig. 16.3: A *manoeuvre to expose the skin and anal mucosa during digital examination of the rectum.*

process makes it vulnerable to subsequent twisting and ischaemia (see Chapter 21). The sudden onset of blood-stained stools in association with bilious vomiting in an infant is strongly suggestive of malrotation with volvulus. This may occur in the absence of abdominal distension. Malrotation with volvulus is a surgical emergency if the entire mid-gut is to be saved. Examination of the abdomen may be unremarkable or may demonstrate some tenderness. Abdominal distension in malrotation with volvulus is a late sign and suggests that the blood supply to the mid-gut has become severely compromised with gangrene impending. As the bowel becomes increasingly ischaemic, it dilates and fluid transudate leaks into the peritoneal cavity. Diagnosis can be confirmed with barium studies or at immediate laparotomy.

Now that vitamin K is administered routinely at birth, haemorrhagic disease of the newborn is rare, but nevertheless should be suspected in all cases of neonatal gastro-intestinal bleeding.

SMALL AMOUNTS OF RECTAL BLEEDING IN A WELL CHILD

Small amounts of bleeding in a well child suggest benign pathology of the anorectum. Often, it follows an acute episode of diarrhoea or constipation. The passage of a hard stool may cause a small tear in the mucosa of the anus, producing a painful anal fissure. Further defaecation is avoided, and the faeces become hard and more difficult to pass. When they are passed eventually, further trauma to the anal canal causes a small amount of bleeding which can be seen as red streaks on the stool or spots of blood on the nappy or toilet paper. In severe cases, there is build-up of faeces in the rectum (faecal impaction) and fluid escapes around the mass (spurious diarrhoea). Continuous leakage of fluid from the anus is highly irritating to the perianal skin, which becomes severely excoriated and bleeds (Fig. 16.4). Rectal examination is exquisitely painful and not mandatory where an anal fissure is seen, but if it is performed will provide information on the amount and hardness of faeces within the rectum.

In rectal prolapse, part or all of the rectum protrudes through the anal canal. The part prolapsed may involve the mucosa alone or the entire wall of the rectum. Rectal prolapse is seen sometimes in association with other conditions, e.g. myelomeningocele (paresis of the pelvic floor), exstrophy of the bladder (disturbance of the structural support of the rectum), cystic fibrosis (chronic cough with increased abdominal pressure) and chronic diarrhoea, but most often occurs without an obvious underlying cause. It occurs rarely after the age of three years and is usually seen in boys during the second year of life.

Prolapse occurs after straining at stool and may follow either constipation or an episode of acute diarrhoea. The rectal mucosa is normal in appearance and has a pink-red, glistening surface. With chronic prolapse, it may become congested and ulcerated but almost never becomes gangrenous. The mucosa bleeds readily on contact with nappies or dressings. Frequently, the prolapse reduces spontaneously after straining is ceased, but sometimes the rectum remains prolapsed and requires gentle manual reduction. It can be distinguished from a prolapsing intussusception in that the child is otherwise well, and that there is no sulcus between the prolapse and the anal margin (Fig. 16.5). At first glance, a rectal polyp may be similar in appearance, but this will be distinguished by demonstration of a sulcus and its pedunculated

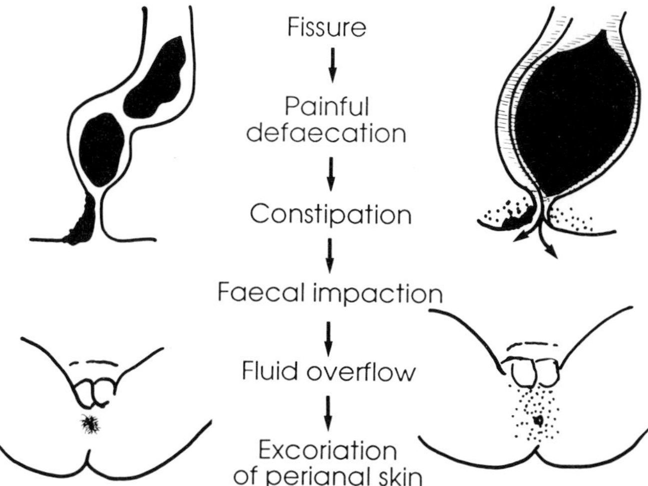

Fig. 16.4: *The mechanism by which an anal fissure leads to progressive constipation and eventual impaction with overflow, which causes excoriation of perianal skin.*

stalk. A rectal prolapse can be reduced by gentle pressure on the exposed rectum.

BLEEDING WITH AN ACUTE ABDOMEN

Outside the neonatal period, the most common cause of rectal bleeding in association with an acute abdomen is intussusception. Intussusception can occur at any age, but 75% of cases involve children between three and 12 months of age. Usually, episodic abdominal pain and vomiting are present, but there may be only lethargy and pallor. The pain is colicky and lasts a minute or

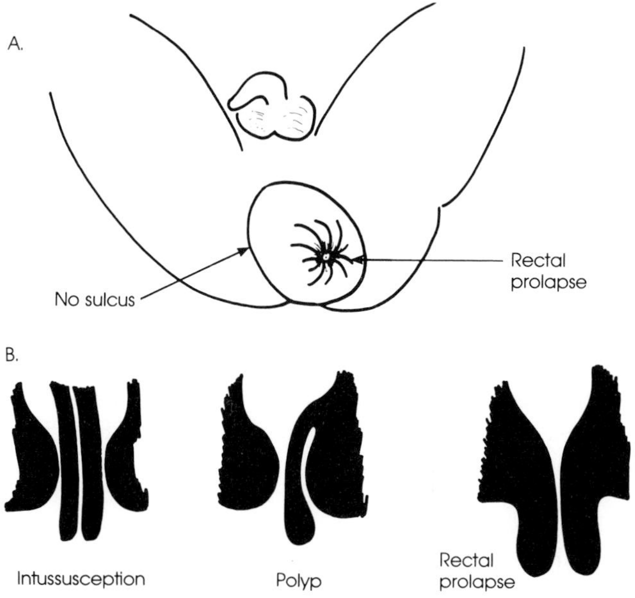

Fig. 16.5: *The external appearance of rectal prolapse* (A), *and the comparison between rectal prolapse and intussusception or rectal polyp* (B).

two, with a longer period without pain between episodes. As the intussusception progresses, the pain becomes continuous and less colicky. A small child is unable to communicate pain except by crying or by drawing up his legs. Between attacks, the child is lethargic and feeds are refused. Pallor is often pronounced and probably caused by a reflex autonomic response to pain. Palpation of the abdomen may reveal a tender mass (see Chapter 8). Where intussusception is suspected, a rectal examination will identify whether there is blood in the rectum or whether the lead-point has advanced as far as the rectum. The small amount of blood is dark red and has the appearance of red currant jelly because it is mixed with excessive mucus and poorly formed stool. Rectal bleeding in intussusception is a late sign, and one should not wait for its appearance before making the diagnosis.

A less common, but extremely important, cause of small volume rectal bleeding is ischaemia of the bowel with impending gangrene. In small children, this is caused by volvulus, which may be secondary to malrotation and failure of fixation, a Meckel's diverticulum and band, or by a closed loop obstruction from postoperative adhesions. The child is anorexic, unwell and vomits, and with progression of symptoms, becomes toxic and dehydrated. The abdomen is distended, and one or more dilated loops of bowel may be palpable. There is abdominal tenderness with guarding if peritonitis is present. These children require vigorous resuscitation and early laparotomy.

A rare cause of rectal bleeding with an acute abdomen is Henoch-Schönlein purpura. Its characteristic rash and arthralgia may be absent initially. There may be either localized or generalized abdominal tenderness and the passage of blood within the stools. The abdominal pain and rectal bleeding are the result of (1) vasculitis with bleeding into the peritoneal cavity and lumen of the bowel, or (2) intussusception (usually of the small bowel).

MAJOR GASTRO-INTESTINAL HAEMORRHAGE

The commonest causes are a bleeding Meckel's diverticulum and haemorrhage from juvenile polyps. Upper gastro-intestinal haemorrhage, although less common, is often major and results from peptic ulcer disease or bleeding oesophageal varices. Oesophageal varices are a manifestation of portal hypertension and are seen in association with features of liver disease (see Chapter 17).

A Meckel's diverticulum causes haemorrhage because it contains ectopic gastric mucosa. Hydrochloric acid from the gastric mucosa causes an ulcer in the adjacent ileal mucosa. The blood loss may be profound and rapid and, while usually painless, is associated sometimes with cramping or colicky abdominal pain localized to the periumbilical region. The blood is brick-red in colour, and there may be a history of several previous episodes of bleeding. With major blood loss, the child is pale and has a tachycardia. The haemoglobin falls after some hours. The diagnosis is confirmed by performing a ^{99m}Tc sodium pertechnetate scan.

CHRONIC DIARRHOEA AND BLEEDING

Bleeding associated with persistent diarrhoea may be caused by certain organisms, such as *Campylobacter* or *Salmonella*. Where there is no history of prior gastro-enteritis, chronic bloody diarrhoea in older children is suggestive of inflammatory bowel disease. Explosive bowel movements of loose, mucousy stools preceded by cramping abdominal pains, may be the first indication of ulcerative colitis. There may be associated growth failure and weight loss, anaemia and arthritis. Insidious mild diarrhoea with occasional mucus or blood and intermittent pain in a pre-adolescent is more common in regional enteritis (Crohn's disease).

Examination of the abdomen may reveal an inflammatory mass in the right iliac fossa, or there may be a chronic anal fissure which antedated the onset of diarrhoea. Alternatively, there may be no specific signs with either form of inflammatory bowel disease, and diagnosis is confirmed on barium studies, colonoscopy and histology.

GOLDEN RULES

(1) Major bleeding can occur from the oesophagus, stomach and duodenum without vomiting (haematemesis).
(2) The appearance of blood in the rectum is related to the distance travelled and the time taken by the red cells to get from the point of bleeding to the rectum.
(3) Beware haemorrhagic disease of the newborn: check that the infant received vitamin K.
(4) The commonest cause of rectal bleeding in the neonate is an anal fissure.
(5) A fissure-in-ano is usually in the midline anteriorly or posteriorly.
(6) Bleeding may have stopped by the time a child presents to a medical practitioner.
(7) Malrotation with volvulus is a surgical emergency which requires immediate laparotomy.
(8) Do not wait for the appearance of rectal bleeding before making a diagnosis of intussusception: it is a late sign which indicates that the blood supply to the intussusceptum has been compromised.
(9) A chronic, painless and lateral anal fissure may indicate chronic inflammatory bowel disease.

17 Jaundice

Jaundice is a common sign in the first two weeks of life. It is usually 'physiological', in that it is due to the functional immaturity of the normal liver, which matures rapidly after birth. Deep jaundice or the development of jaundice within 24 hours of birth, implies that additional factors such as haemolysis, infection or inborn metabolic errors may be present, and demands urgent investigation and treatment. An unconjugated bilirubin level above 300 μmol/l (250 μmol/l in premature infants) may damage the brain (kernicterus).

Jaundice which appears later than, or persists into, the third week of life, is not likely to be benign 'physiological' jaundice, and should be treated as requiring urgent investigation, as rapid diagnosis and prompt treatment may prevent death or permanent damage to the infant (Table 17.1). Jaundice at this stage, accompanied by pale grey (acholic) stools, dark urine and an elevated serum bilirubin which is largely conjugated bilirubin, may have a 'surgical' cause. Biliary atresia (or a choledochal cyst) causes an obstructive jaundice in the first months of life (Fig. 17.1). Severe hepatic damage associated with cholestasis may show a similar clinical picture. Neonatal hepatitis of unknown cause or hepatic damage secondary to septicaemia, viral infections (e.g. cytomegalovirus) or inborn errors of metabolism (e.g. galactosaemia) need to be considered also. Jaundice without obstructive features (i.e. normal stool and urine colour) may follow less severe hepatic injury without cholestasis, or be due to impaired bilirubin uptake and conjugation (e.g. hypothyroidism, haemolysis, breast milk jaundice or rare congenital enzyme defects).

Table 17.1 POTENTIAL CAUSES OF PERSISTENT JAUNDICE AFTER BIRTH

Surgical	Non-surgical
Biliary atresia	Breast milk jaundice
Choledochal cyst	Primary hepatitis
	Secondary hepatitis
	Galactosaemia
	Cretinism
	Congenital enzyme defects

ASSESSMENT OF A PATIENT WITH PERSISTENT NEONATAL JAUNDICE

When jaundice persists beyond the second week after birth, biliary atresia must be considered, although the diagnosis is usually one of exclusion. Rhesus incompatibility, other forms of haemolytic disease of the newborn and congenital infections of the fetus, such as rubella, herpes, cytomegalovirus, syphilis and toxoplasmosis, present with jaundice in the first day or two of life (Table 17.2). In the haemolytic diseases, the Coombs' test is positive.

The common causes of jaundice between the first day and the first week are produced by immature enzymes, so-called physiological jaundice. The bilirubin is unconjugated and there are no anti-red cell antibodies (Coombs' test negative). The children are often premature, but otherwise well. In the first week, septicaemia with secondary hepatic dysfunction may also cause jaundice and will be confirmed when septic screening tests show a positive blood culture.

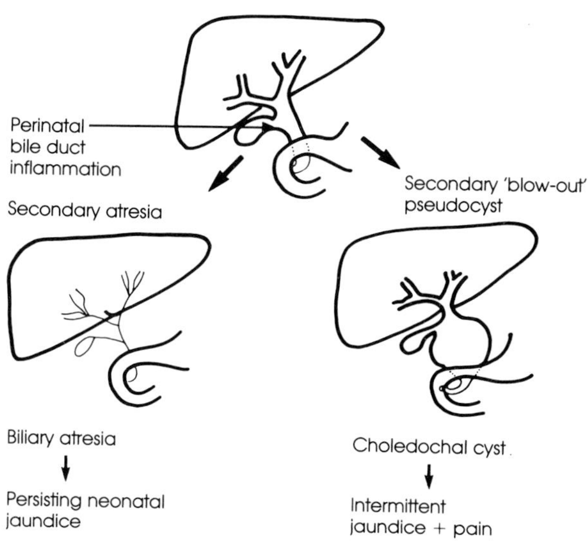

Fig. 17.1: *The suspected common aetiology of biliary atresia and choledochal cyst.*

After the first week, jaundice still may be caused by a number of congenital disorders which must be excluded. Hypothyroidism, or neonatal cretinism, may be difficult to diagnose clinically and is best excluded by thyroid function screening tests. The bilirubin is unconjugated because the maturation of this function of the hepatocytes is suppressed in the absence of thyroxin. In galactosaemia, hepatic damage is produced by abnormal sugars in the blood stream. The bilirubin may be unconjugated, but there are non-glucose sugars in the urine, and the galactose screen test is positive. The high level of sugar in the blood and urine may predispose to sepsis, which itself may mask the underlying diagnosis. In breast milk jaundice, the bilirubin is unconjugated because of suppression of glucuronyl transferase by substances in the milk. The baby is an otherwise healthy, breast-fed infant. Alpha-1-antitrypsin deficiency is an uncommon cause of jaundice that produces cholestasis and a conjugated hyperbilirubinaemia, which may mimic obstruction of the bile duct. It can be excluded by estimation of the α-1-antitrypsin concentration in the blood. In cystic fibrosis, there may be high concentrations of conjugated bilirubin secondary to cholestasis. Other features of cystic fibrosis, such as delayed passage of meconium or meconium ileus, may be present. A positive sweat test is diagnostic.

When the above abnormalities have been excluded, the diagnoses remaining are either biliary atresia or persisting neonatal hepatitis. Biliary atresia presents with signs of outlet obstruction of bile and high levels of conjugated bilirubin in a well baby. The stools are clay-coloured, but not always white since some bile may enter the stools

Table 17.2 NEONATAL JAUNDICE

Day of onset	Clinical questions	Useful investigation/results
Day 1	Haemolysis?	Unconjugated bilirubin, Coombs' test positive
	Congenital infection?	Unconjugated bilirubin, Coombs' test negative; positive serology (toxoplasmosis)
Day 2–3	Immature enzymes? ('Physiological')	Unconjugated bilirubin, Coombs' test negative; premature but well baby
	Sepsis?	Septic screening tests positive; sick baby
Day 7–8	Hypothyroidism?	Unconjugated bilirubin; thyroid function down
	Galactosaemia?	Unconjugated or mixed conjugated/unconjugated; non-glucose sugar in urine; galactoscreen positive often with associated sepsis
	Breast milk jaundice?	Unconjugated bilirubin; breast-fed, healthy baby
	α-1-antitrypsin deficiency?	Conjugated bilirubin; α-1-antitrypsin down (cholestasis)
	Cystic fibrosis?	Conjugated bilirubin (cholestasis); delayed meconium; sweat test positive
	Biliary atresia?	Conjugated bilirubin; well baby
	Persisting hepatitis?	Conjugated bilirubin; well baby

through the colonic mucosa. The urine contains a high level of urobilinogen which gives it a characteristic dark colour (Fig. 17.2). The baby is jaundiced and has a slightly enlarged liver and spleen. The examiner needs to be aware of a potential pitfall in the examination of the very large liver. If hepatomegaly is pronounced, the lower edge of the liver may be missed altogether, and the firmness of the right upper quadrant may be incorrectly interpreted as rigidity of the muscles. Percussion of the right chest and upper abdomen will reveal the upper and lower borders of the liver at their margin with the air-filled lung superiorly and the gas-filled bowel inferiorly (Fig. 17.3). Once the lower margin of the liver is determined by percussion, it is readily palpated, particularly if the examining hand starts well below it in the abdomen and works upwards. The anterior surface of the liver exposed below the costal margin can be palpated to determine its hardness and nodularity, which are signs of developing cirrhosis. If the diagnosis of biliary artresia is delayed, other physical signs which indicate portal hypertension may appear (*vide infra*). One of these, enlargement of the spleen, is detected in a way similar to that of the enlarged liver (Fig. 17.4). Initial percussion of the left upper quadrant determines an area of dullness: the edge of the spleen is then felt by commencing palpation in the right lower quadrant and working towards the left upper quadrant. Palpation of the notch in the anteromedial border of the spleen, and the movement of the spleen downwards and to the right on inspiration, are the two features which confirm the enlarged organ to be the spleen.

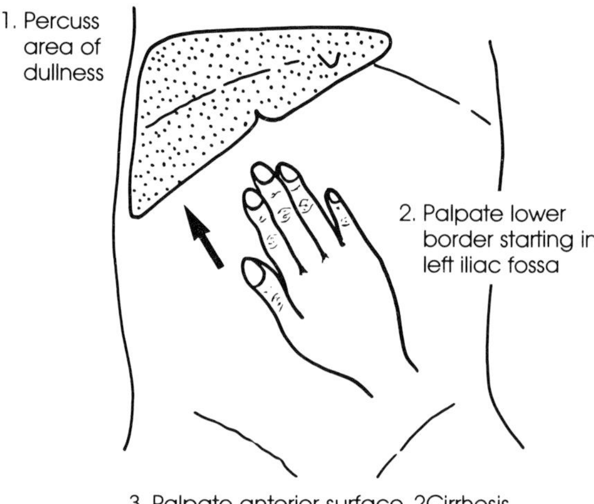

Fig. 17.3: *Determination of liver size and characteristics in infants.*

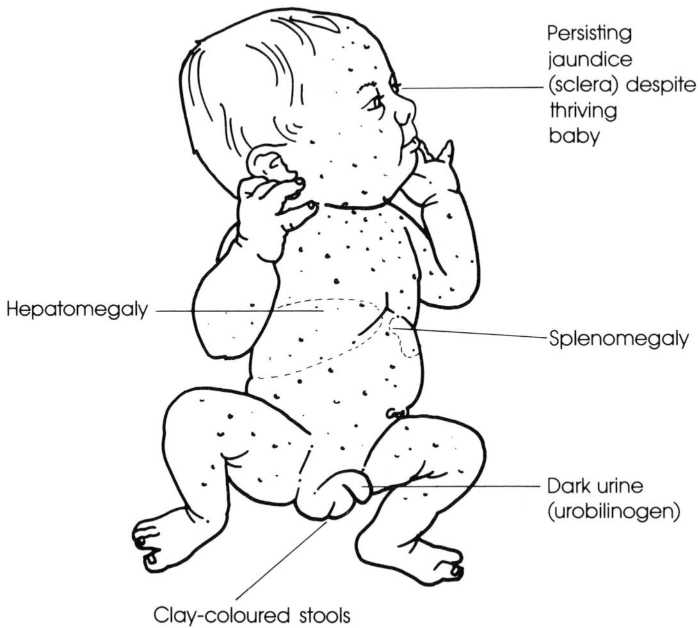

Fig. 17.2: *The clinical features of biliary atresia.*

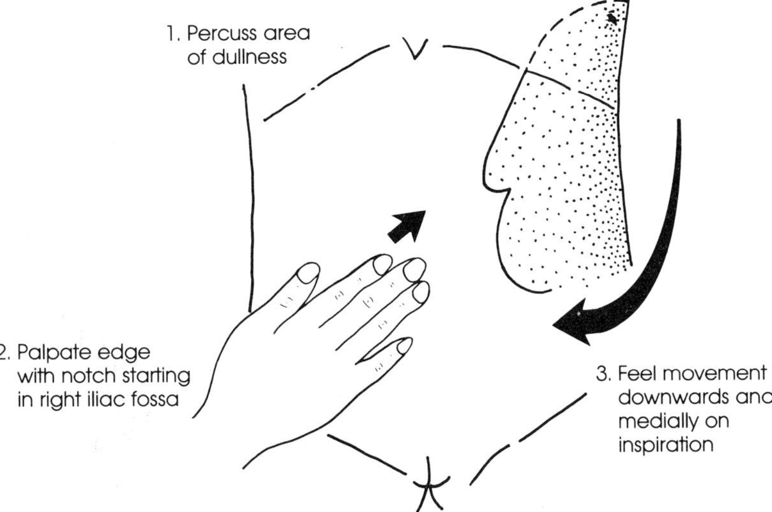

Fig. 17.4: *Estimation of splenic size in children.*

In the first few weeks after birth, it is difficult to distinguish biliary atresia from persisting neonatal hepatitis. Jaundice with minor enlargement of the liver and spleen is present in both, and the only difference may be the higher level of unconjugated bilirubin in the hepatitis patient. Since neonatal hepatitis and biliary atresia may be part of a spectrum of inflammatory disease of the biliary tract, this similarity in physical presentation is not surprising. It is essential that any child with apparent neonatal hepatitis be submitted urgently for further investigation to determine whether biliary atresia is present. Investigations include liver biopsy, along with the new modalities of radionuclide liver function tests and conventional or computed tomographic radiology. If any doubt persists following investigation, laparotomy is indicated since early diagnosis, before sclerosis of the biliary duct has progressed too far, makes treatment more likely to be successful.

PORTAL HYPERTENSION

Cirrhosis is the common sequel to biliary atresia and some inherited metabolic disorders where liver cells are damaged by accumulation of toxic substances. Thrombosis of the portal vein secondary to neonatal umbilical sepsis may also cause portal hypertension. High pressure in the portal circulation causes dilatation of collateral veins which connect with the systemic vessels. These are particularly apparent in the gastro-oesophageal region, where oesophageal varices may enlarge; in the umbilical region, where veins in the falciform ligament communicate with those of the abdominal wall to produce a 'caput Medusae'; and to a lesser degree, in the inferior rectal veins where haemorrhoids may be produced (Fig. 17.5).

The child with full-blown features of cirrhosis and secondary portal hypertension is shown in Figure 17.6. There is wasting and inhibition of growth, obvious jaundice and a distended abdomen. The spleen is palpable, and the liver may or may not be palpable depending on whether its size has decreased because of the cirrhosis. The abdomen is distended because of hepatosplenomegaly or associated ascites (Figs. 17.7 and 17.8). The increase in intra-abdominal pressure may be manifested by an umbilical hernia. Symptoms or signs of dilated collateral veins include blood-stained vomitus from bleeding oesophageal varices, or fresh blood or melaena in the stool from the haemorrhoidal veins or major oesophageal variceal bleeding. Dilated veins which radiate from the umbilicus may be visible on the abdominal wall, the so-called 'caput Medusae'. These dilated superficial veins resemble the arms of an octopus (Fig. 17.9). Blood reaches the umbilicus from the high pressure portal system through the falciform liga-

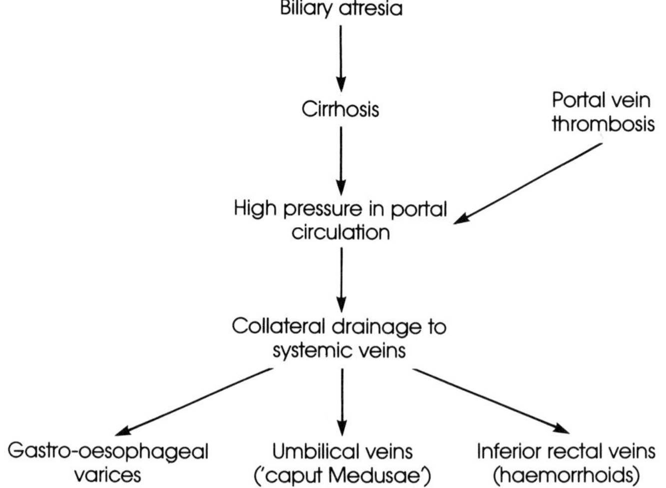

Fig. 17.5: *Common causes and consequences of portal hypertension.*

ment, and drains centrifugally to the axillary and inguinal veins. Compression and release of the veins will demonstrate that the direction of flow is away from the umbilicus. By contrast, in diseases which produce obstruction of the inferior vena cava (e.g. neuroblastoma, Wilms' tumour or lymphoma), flow in collateral veins is from the groin to the axilla.

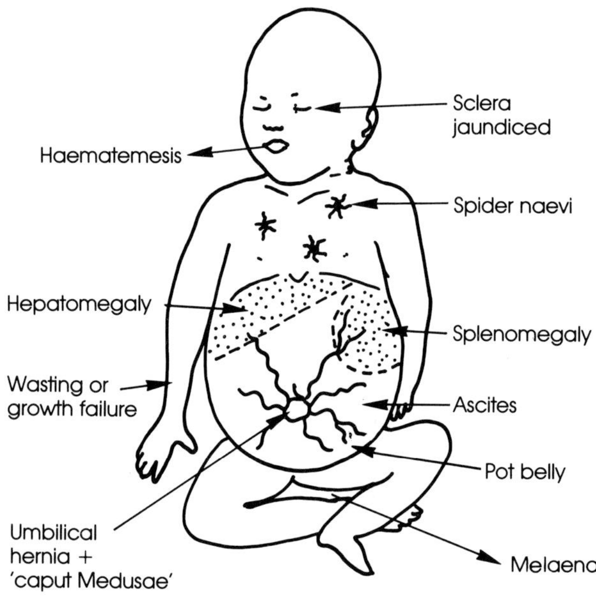

Fig. 17.6: *The clinical features of advanced cirrhosis in childhood.*

Systemic signs of liver failure are uncommon in children with hepatic cirrhosis, although minor abnormalities, such as cutaneous telangiectasia or spider naevi, may be seen. Spider naevi usually are present on the upper half of the body and appear as tiny red spots of vessels radiating from a central arteriole. The lesion can be blanched by finger-tip compression, following which the vessels refill from the centre (Fig. 17.10).

CHOLELITHIASIS

Gall-stones are un uncommon problem in childhood, except in adolescence and/or in association with diseases which cause chronic haemolysis. Stones caused by accumulation of bile pigments occur in haemolytic disorders such as thalassaemia and spherocytosis. Should a child with these underlying conditions present with a gall-stone obstructing the bile duct, the underlying diagnosis will almost certainly have been made some years previously. Therefore, the presentation is usually of a child with a known haemolytic anaemia who suddenly develops jaundice and abdominal pain. General examination of the child and local examination of the abdomen should indicate a gall-stone in the bile duct and prompt appropriate further investigation.

Cholelithiasis may occur in late childhood and is

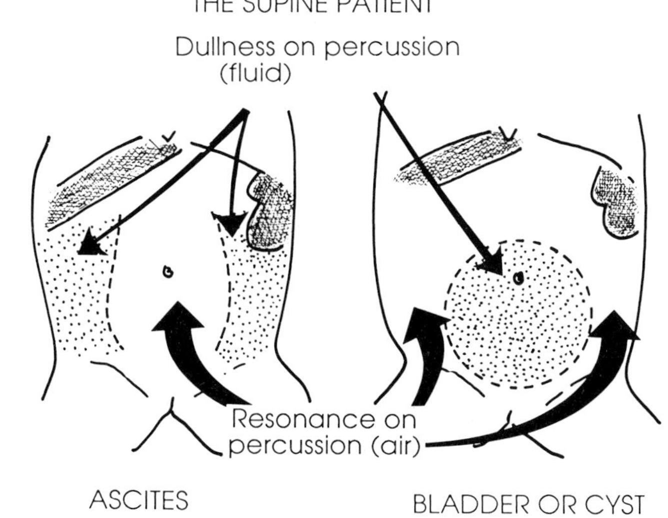

Fig. 17.7: *Comparison of ascites and fluid-filled cysts in examination of the abdomen.*

an example of a common abnormality of adults presenting at an earlier age. Gall-stones in this situation are usually cholesterol stones, rather than pigment stones, and are related more to diet and genetic predisposition. Epigastric pain in a child more thn 10 years of age should alert the examiner to the possibility of cholelithiasis. The area where maximum tenderness or a mass can be felt is in the angle between the costal margin and the right rectus abdominis muscle. This can be demonstrated with the child supine or sitting forwards (Fig. 17.11). In the latter situation, the examiner is positioned behind the child who is bent forward to relax the abdominal muscles. The examiner's hand feels for tenderness in the angle between the costal margin and the right rectus, and for the gall

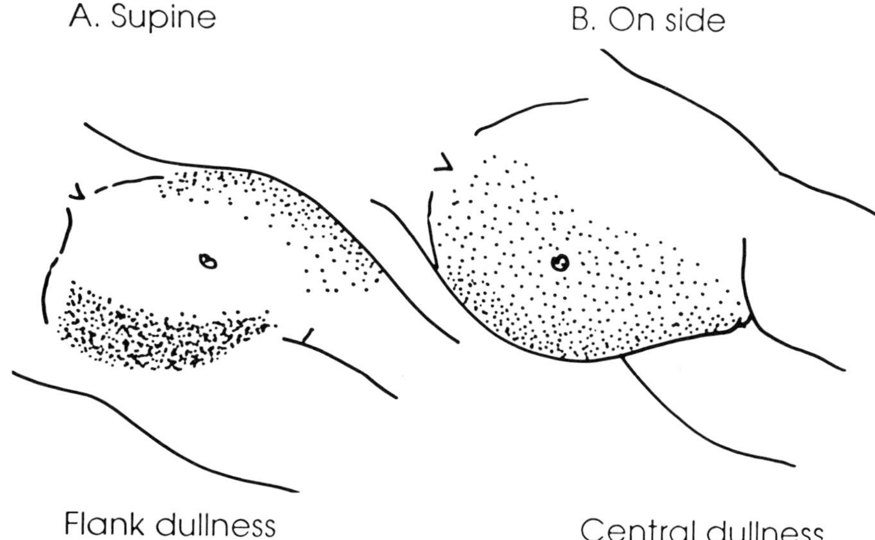

Fig. 17.8: *Demonstration of shifting dullness as a sign of ascites.*

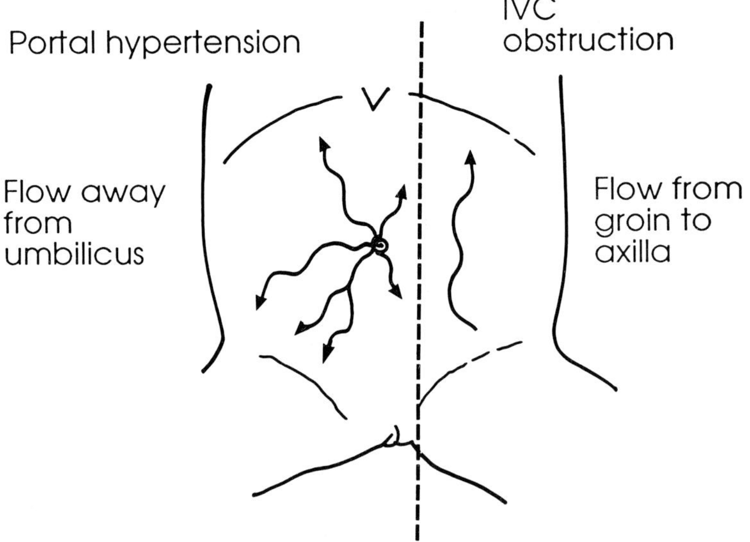

Fig. 17.9: *Examination of dilated veins of the abdominal wall.*

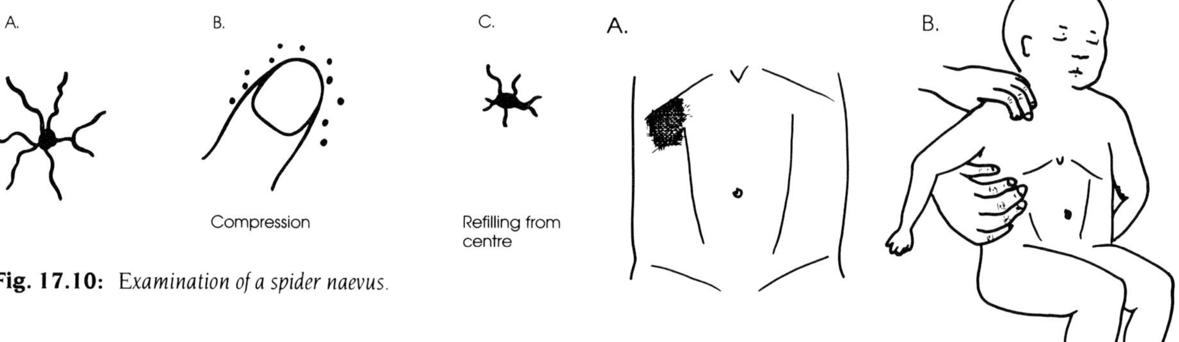

Fig. 17.10: *Examination of a spider naevus.*

bladder itself which may be felt as the liver descends on inspiration. In cholecystitis, movement of the inflamed gall bladder against the parietal peritoneum causes pain (Murphy's sign). This is positive when palpation in the angle between the right costal margin and the rectus abdominis muscle causes pain on inspiration.

Fig. 17.11: *Examination of the gall bladder can be achieved with the child lying supine or sitting forwards as shown here. Figure* 17.11(A) *show the site of maximal tenderness.*

GOLDEN RULES

(1) Jaundice which fails to resolve within one month of birth must be referred immediately to a specialist centre to exclude biliary atresia.
(2) Diagnosis of biliary atresia is urgent because delay in operative correction beyond 10 weeks significantly worsens the prognosis.

18 Spina bifida

Defects caused by failure of fusion of the neural tube may present as posterior midline swellings anywhere from the bridge of the nose to the tip of the coccyx. Many are associated with severe neurological deficit or related malformations of the central nervous system such as hydrocephalus. One of the most common neural tube abnormalities is anencephaly, in which the cephalic part of the neural tube has failed to close. The vault of the skull is absent, exposing the deficient cerebrum with only the brain stem and cerebellum remaining. The abnormality is not compatible with life, and fortunately most fetuses with this abnormality are stillborn. Meningoceles and encephaloceles are discussed further in the chapter on cranial abnormalities (Chapter 10).

In this chapter, the various presentations of spina bifida are described so that an adequate initial assessment can be made at birth or whenever the abnormality is diagnosed. These anomalies require highly specialized neurosurgical, orthopaedic and urological management, but the primary physician needs some knowledge of the clinical problems so that initial management and referral can be performed correctly.

EMBRYOLOGY

The neural tube forms as a thickening of the dorsal ectoderm two weeks after conception, with complete fusion of the neural tube 8–10 days later. Hence, neural tube defects represent a very early and fundamental abnormality of embryogenesis. In the severe abnormality of myelomeningocele, the neural tube remains completely unfused and incompletely covered by skin exposing the meninges to the outside. In the less severe meningocele, there is protrusion of the meninges through a defect in the spinous processus, but the swelling is competely covered by skin (Fig. 18.1). In the least severe form of spina bifida, spina bifida occulta, there is a defect of the dorsal arches of the vertebrae, but no protrusion of the meninges.

The cystic form of spina bifida, including myelomeningocele, is readily apparent at birth, while occult spina bifida may not present until

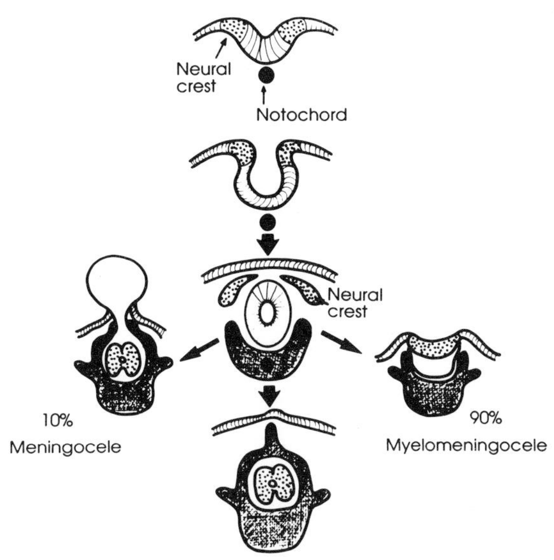

Fig. 18.1: *The aetiology of meningocele (10%) and myelomeningocele (90%); the different clinical states are produced by defects at different stages of neural tube fusion.*

adolescence. In the latter abnormality, a posterior defect in the spinal canal is associated frequently with either a dermal sinus connecting with the subarachnoid space, a haemangioma, lipoma, hairy patch or hairy naevus. These abnormalities represent dysplasia of the ectoderm overlying the neural tube defect.

NEONATAL ASSESSMENT OF SPINA BIFIDA

When a new baby is seen with obvious cystic spina bifida, the primary physician must assess:

(1) the neurological deficit, including motor and sensory loss and bladder and bowel function;
(2) the presence or absence of hydrocephalus;
(3) orthopaedic deformities of the spine, hips and feet;
(4) other coexisting abnormalities.

There may be some features in the obstetric history which have pointed to the abnormality, although once the child is born the lesion is very obvious. Antenatal ultrasound in the second trimester may have detected the abnormality, and there may be a record of high serum and amniotic fluid concentrations of alphafetoprotein. This protein escapes into the amniotic fluid and maternal circulation from the exposed surface of the myelomeningocele. When a meningocele is covered by normal skin, the alphafetoprotein concen-

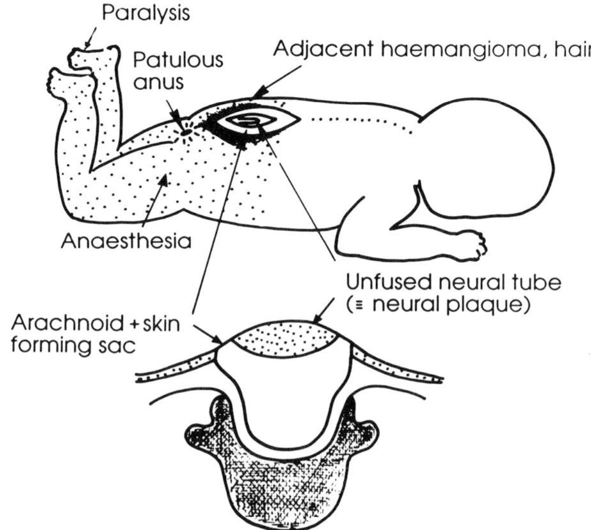

Fig. 18.3: *The common lumbar type of myelomeningocele.*

trations remain normal. The prenatal diagnosis of myelomeningocele may be an indication for caesarean section.

Examination of the lesion

The first step in the clinical examination is to determine the level of the neural tube defect in relation to the bony landmarks of the spinal column. The level of the lesion is important since the degree of neurological deficit depends on the segment of spinal cord involved. Lumbosacral lesions are the most frequent (Fig. 18.2)

After estimating its level, the lesion should be examined carefully to determine whether there is a complete covering of skin or whether the unfused neural tube is exposed. When a myelomeningocele is not covered by skin, it is almost invariably associated with paralysis. Commonly, the unfused neural tube is present in the middle of the lesion (Fig. 18.3), and may leak cerebrospinal fluid or tissue fluid from the exposed neuro-epithelium. Once physical abrasion and bacterial contamination stimulate the production of granulation tissue, the fluid weeping from the open lesion is more likely to be transudate from the granulations.

If the spinal cord is not visible on the surface of the lesion, its position within the sac can be

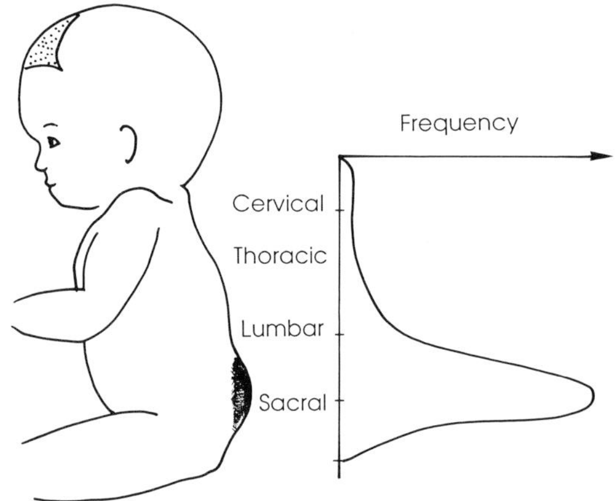

Fig. 18.2: *The frequency of spina bifida in relation to the level of the spine. Lumbosacral lesions are by far the commonest.*

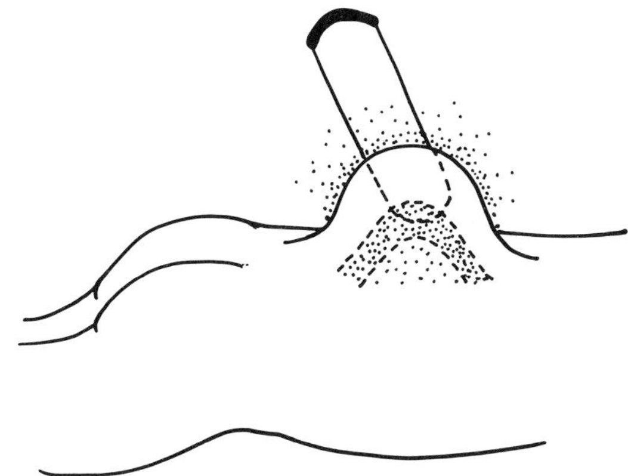

Fig. 18.4: *Transillumination of a skin-covered sac will determine whether it contains the spinal cord.*

determined by transillumination (Fig. 18.4). The adjacent skin commonly shows evidence of dysplasia with abnormal hair production, capillary haemangioma or a lipoma. After the myelomeningocele has been examined, the surface should be covered with a protective, non-stick dressing to reduce physical trauma and diminish the risk of infection.

The appearance of a meningocele is different, since the skin overlying the cystic lesion is likely to be intact. Meningoceles have a more even distribution along the vertebral column than myelomeningoceles, which are most commonly found in the lumbosacral region. A communication with the subarachnoid space can be determined by direct pressure on the skin-covered lesion which will cause the fontanelle to bulge. Conversely, during crying when the intracranial pressure is elevated, the lesion will become more tense (Fig. 18.5). The posture and spontaneous movement of the child usually indicates no serious neurological anomaly (Fig. 18.6).

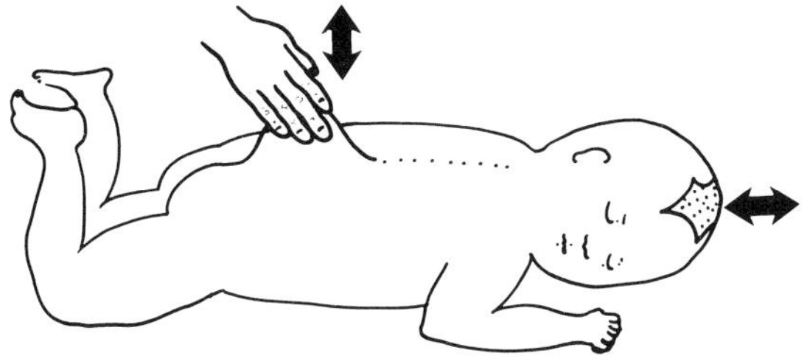

Fig. 18.5: *When the neck of the sac communicates with the cerebrospinal fluid, pressure on the sac will make the fontanelle bulge.*

Before completing the examination of the lesion itself, the bony defect should be palpated to document its size and spinal level: the size of the bony defect is related to the degree of neural tube abnormality, and hence, to the severity of the underlying neurological deficit.

Neurological deficit

In the neonate, the degree of paralysis is difficult to determine because of the lack of patient cooperation. The spontaneous movement of the hips, knees and ankles should be observed without external stimulation, since reflex spinal movements following painful stimuli may simulate conscious control. The motor deficit can be determined by observing the joints about which active movement occurs (Fig. 18.7)

For the common lesions in the lumbosacral region, paralysis falls into one of four groups (Fig. 18.8). When the myelomeningocele includes nerves up to and including the third lumbar segment (L3), the legs are totally paralysed. If the third lumbar segment is functioning, as occurs with lesions affecting the fourth and fifth lumbar segments (L4,5), the baby has a characteristic posture with flexion of the hip and extension of the knee, but essentially no other limb movement. When L4 and L5 spinal segments are preserved, there is movement of the hip and the knee, and the foot can dorsiflex but cannot plantarflex. The imbalance in the muscles around the ankle may manifest itself by a talipes calcaneovalgus deformity, or may only be obvious on close inspection of conscious movement. When the first and second sacral segments (S1,2) are preserved, leg movements are essentially normal but bowel and bladder incontinence is likely to persist. This is usually the case in low sacral lesions. The common appearance of infants with lumbosacral myelomeningoceles is shown in Figure 18.9, where the straight legs are flexed at the hips and the feet are commonly deformed by malposition *in utero*.

Assessment of the sensory deficit

Determination of the level of sensory deficit will complement the assessment of motor loss, but

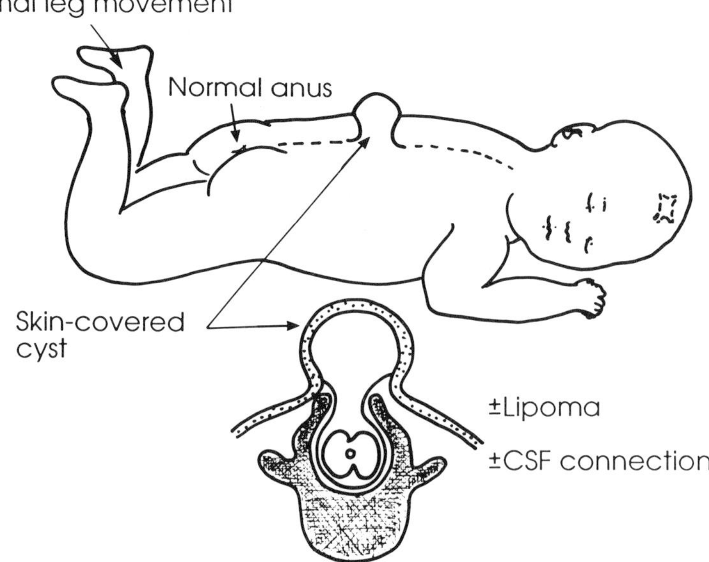

Fig. 18.6: *The less common abnormality of thoracic meningocele.*

sensory deficiency is usually found to be slightly less than the motor loss. The pattern of dermatomes in the neonate is similar to that seen in adults (Fig. 18.10), with thoracic dermatomes (T10–12) supplying the lower abdomen, and the lumbar segments (L1–5) innervating the skin from the groin down to the lateral side of the calf. The first and second sacral segments (S1,2) innervate the lateral side of the foot and the dorsum of the leg from the heel to perineum. The third and fourth sacral segments (S3,4) supply the perianal region (Fig. 18.11). By holding the baby's legs in the air, the level of sensory loss should be tested by beginning with a painful stimulus in the perianal region. A blunt-ended safety-pin should be sufficiently sharp to elicit a painful stimulus without harming the child. Starting around the anus, test the fourth and third sacral segments, and then proceed down the back of the leg following the second sacral segment to the heels (Fig. 18.12). From the heel, the first sacral segment can be tested on the lateral side of the sole, proceeding to the medial side of the sole to include L5 and L4 segments. By continuing up the anteromedial side of the leg from the medial malleolus to the groin, the fourth, third, second and first lumbar segments can be tested in succession. The sensory level should never be elicited by commencing in a normal area, but should always begin in the anaesthetic region and proceed upwards. This will enable separation of spinal reflex movements from conscious responses to pain.

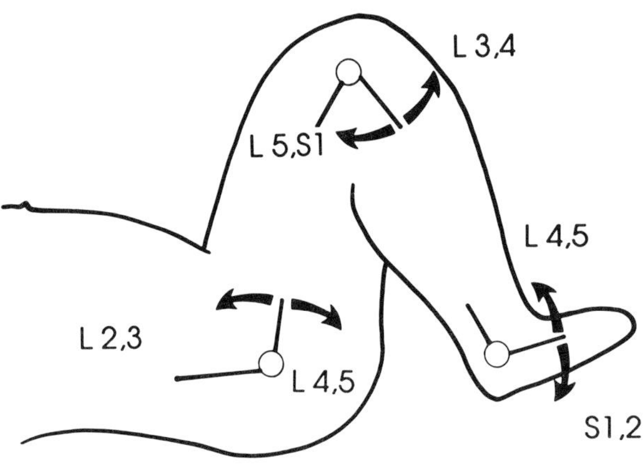

Fig. 18.7: *The segmental innervation of the muscles controlling the hips, knees and ankles.*

Bowel and bladder function

The perineum is a critical area for examination since the likely function of the bowel and bladder can be predicted from the appearance and sensation elicited in the perineum. The appearance of

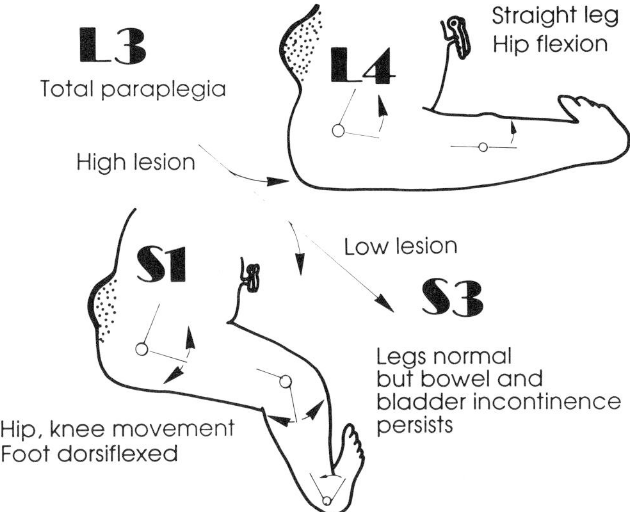

Fig. 18.8: *The four common presentations of weakness in the legs, depending on the upper level of the spinal defect.*

a rectal prolapse or absence of a natal cleft indicates paralysis of the pelvic floor muscles and adjacent bowel and bladder sphincters (Fig. 18.13). This can be confirmed by testing for anaesthesia in the perianal region (Fig. 18.14). The legs of the baby should be held up in one hand, while the other hand scratches the perianal skin with a blunt-ended pin. Reflex contraction of the external anal sphincter and gluteal muscles will occur if the low sacral segments are intact. The demonstration of perineal anaesthesia indicates that bladder function will be abnormal, and this can be confirmed by manual compression of the lower abdomen to produce incontinence of urine.

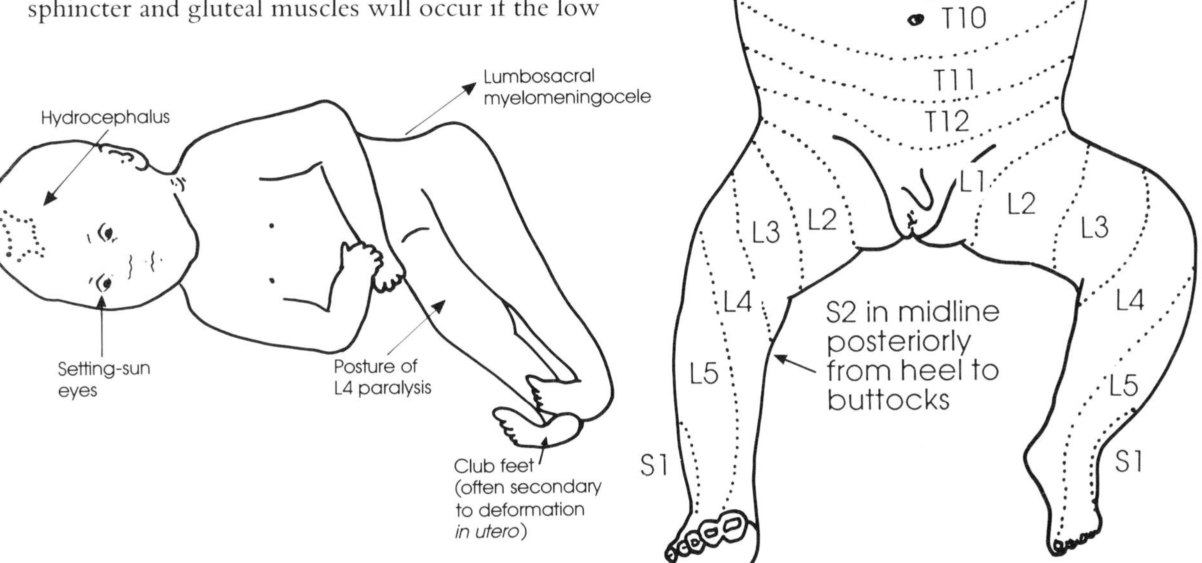

Fig. 18.9: *The usual physical signs of lumbosacral myelomeningocele in the neonate.*

Fig. 18.10: *Lower dermatomes in the neonate.*

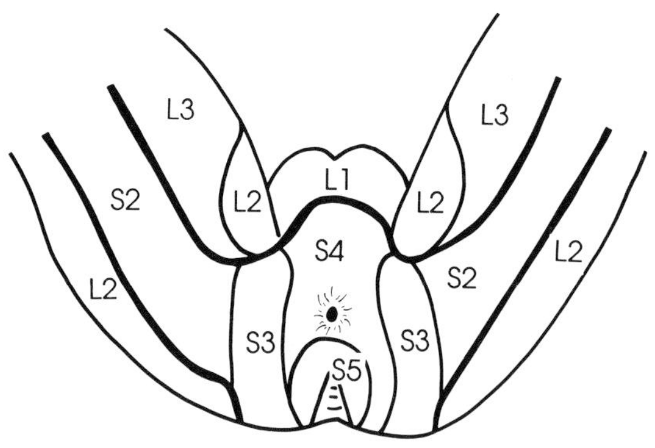

Fig. 18.11: *Perineal dermatomes.*

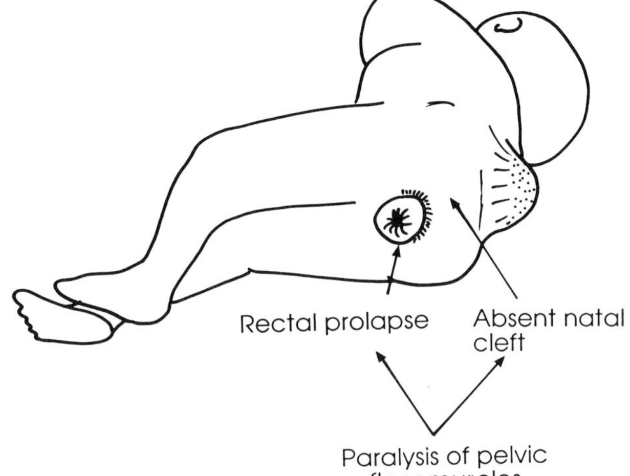

Fig. 18.13: *Physical signs indicating paralysis of the perineal muscles.*

Presence of hydrocephalus or meningitis

Once the neurological deficit has been determined, the child should be examined carefully for signs of hydrocephalus and for meningitis, which are described in Chapter 10.

Orthopaedic deformities

The spine, hips and feet need to be assessed carefully for secondary or associated anomalies. Paralysis and the absence of the dorsal arches of the spinal canal over a large number of segments will destabilize the posture of the spine. The secondary kyphoscoliosis caused by these abnormalities, and by associated hemivertebrae, may be present at birth. Such spinal deformity is a poor prognostic sign because of the high level of the abnormality. The lumbosacral myelomeningocele commonly produces imbalance of the hip muscles and secondary congenital dislocation of the hip. The position of the hips, therefore, should be determined by Ortolani's test, as described in

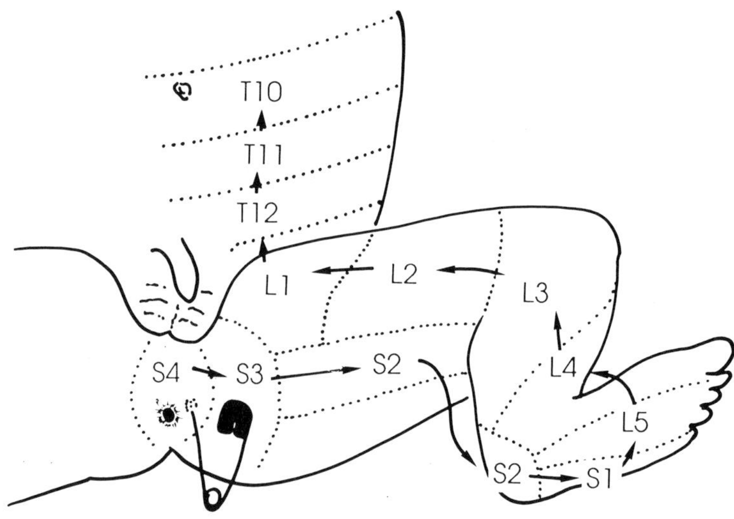

Fig. 18.12: *Testing the level of sensory loss. Start in the perineal region, proceed down the back of the leg to the heel, test the sole from lateral to medial, then proceed up the anteromedial side of the leg from the malleolus to the groin.*

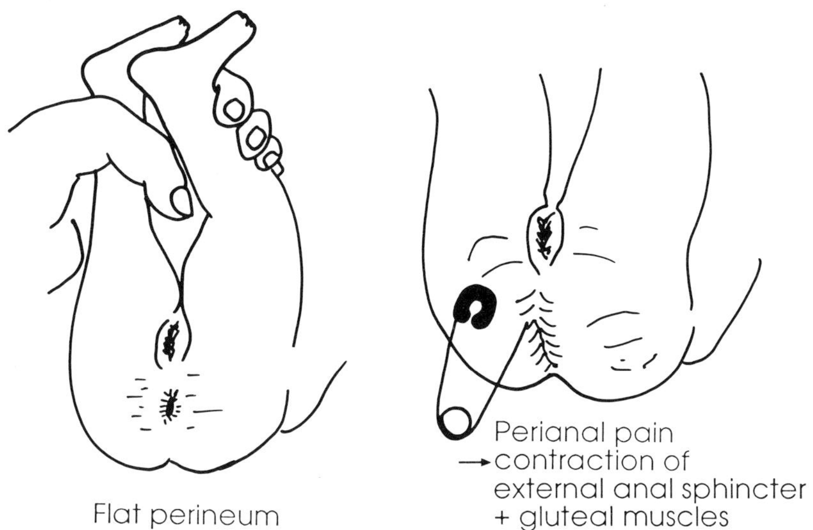

Fig. 18.14: *Testing the perianal reflex. Hold up the legs and examine whether the perineum is flat. Prick the perianal skin with a pin to see whether this induces reflex contraction of the external anal sphincter and gluteal muscles. A normal response requires intact S4 and S5 nerves and pelvic floor muscles.*

Chapter 13. Deformity of the feet may be caused by imbalance of the muscles when the lesion affects the fifth lumbar and first sacral segments, or may be caused by deformity *in utero* of a completely paralysed foot. This latter variety is common in high lumbar lesions.

Coexisting anomalies

Failure of neural tube closure is a severe and early deformity in embryogenesis, and therefore is commonly associated with other major abnormalities. In addition to the skeletal abnormalities already described, there may be partial or complete sacral agenesis. The most important abnormalities in terms of long-term management are those affecting the urinary tract, since the risk of infection will be exacerbated by any abnormalities of urinary anatomy in the presence of incontinence or urinary retention.

SPINA BIFIDA OCCULTA

Occult spina bifida is an extremely common condition; on x-ray, it is present in one fifth of the population. Usually, there is a gap in the dorsal arches of the fourth and fifth lumbar vertebrae and the first sacral vertebra, without any other abnormality. However, in a small number of patients, there may be important symptoms or signs (Table 18.1). A lesion on the skin overlying the spine (haemangioma, hairy patch, naevus or lipoma), or a narrow sinus connecting the skin with the subarachnoid space, signal that there could be a more widespread structural anomaly, involving all the germ cell layers. All children found to have one of these lesions should be

Table 18.1 THE PRESENTATIONS OF OCCULT SPINA BIFIDA

1. Asymptomatic
2. Lesion on the back – haemangioma
   – hairy patch
   – naevus
   – lipoma
   – sinus
3. Club foot
4. Short leg/limp
5. Dribbling urine (neurogenic bladder)
6. Recurrent meningitis

referred for a neurosurgical opinion, since associated tethering of the cord may cause neurological signs to develop later in childhood. The level of the lowest point of the spinal cord changes with age, ascending from the lower border of the third lumbar vertebra to the second lumbar vertebra (Fig. 18.15). This change in the relative position of the spinal cord to the vertebrae may impair the mobility of the cord and stretch it if the filum terminale or nerve roots are abnormally tethered in the region of the bony defect. This produces secondary neurological signs which appear during the period of rapid growth in late childhood, even in the absence of the cutaneous manifestations of spina bifida occulta.

Uncommon lesions which may be difficult to diagnose by examination of the back include the split spinal cord syndrome, or diastematomyelia, where the spinal cord is divided into two parts by a central bony spike in which the overlying spinous process is broader than those above or below. In some patients, the spinal lesion is first manifested by weakness of the lower limb, leading to progressive deformity of the foot believed to be secondary to nerve traction during growth. In a child with a discrepancy in shoe sizes, in which one foot is short with a high arch, the possibility of muscular imbalance from nerve traction should be considered. These children commonly present with the mother complaining that she is unable to buy shoes for the child. Occasionally, the growth of the foot is not significantly abnormal, but the whole leg may be slightly shorter or thinner than the contralateral normal leg. These children present with a minor limp or stumbling, which may be noticeable only during sports or other physical activity. Such children should be referred for careful neurological and orthopaedic opinion.

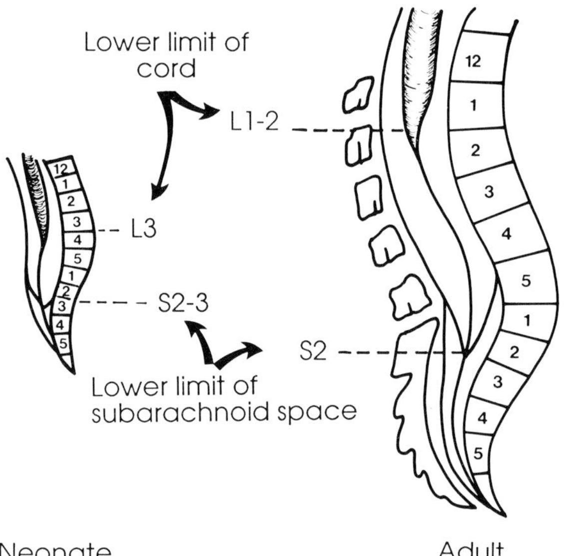

Fig. 18.15: *The relative change in the lower limit of the spinal cord with elongation of the vertebral column as the child grows.*

Two rare but important presentations of occult spina bifida include the gradual onset of neurogenic bladder and recurrent meningitis.

Frequent dribbling of small volumes of urine exacerbated by raising the abdominal pressure, and frequent infections, are both suggestive of a neurogenic bladder. In lesions affecting only the fourth and fifth sacral nerves, leg movements may be normal, yet examination of the perineum will reveal perianal anaesthesia. If the possibility of a neurogenic bladder is suspected – particularly if there is some abnormality of the skin over the sacral or lumbar spine – referral to a paediatric urologist is necessary for complete assessment.

When a sinus or dermoid cyst of the spinal canal has an external connection, meningitis may occur. Whenever meningitis is recurrent, or the causative organisms are found to be atypical or unusual, a communication with the subarachnoid space must be suspected. It may be present in the midline anywhere over the spine, or in the midline of the scalp. Such lesions require immediate referral to a neurosurgeon for complete investigation and excision.

GOLDEN RULES

(1) Paralysis and sensory loss nearly always occur with a myelomeningocele, except where it is low sacral.
(2) In myelomeningocele, the meninges are exposed to the air.
(3) Perianal anaesthesia means that bladder function will be abnormal.
(4) Motor loss is often higher than sensory loss.
(5) Children with meningoceles or occult spina bifida should be followed up until after

puberty since growth of the spine with cord-tethering may produce progressive neurological signs.

(6) Cervical or high thoracic meningoceles generally do not cause severe neurological deficits.

(7) Skeletal deformity progresses with age because of the imbalance in muscle strength.

(8) Paralysis leads to relatively shorter legs with age because the growth of the bones requires normal innervation and active movement.

(9) Paralysis and limb dependency lead to poor venous return and lymphatic oedema, producing puffy legs which, with sensory loss, make the feet susceptible to pressure sores.

(10) Beware recurrent meningitis: a sinus connecting with the subarachnoid space should be sought by careful examination of the entire back and midline scalp.

Further Reading

Smith E.D. (1965). *Spina Bifida and the Total Care of Spinal Myelomeningocele*. Springfield, Illinois: Charles C. Thomas.

19 Abnormalities of the chest wall and breast

There is a group of heterogeneous disorders which present as abnormalities of the shape of the chest wall or breast. Chest wall deformities include anterior lesions involving the ribs and sternum, such as 'funnel chest' and 'pigeon chest', and posterior lesions involving the vertebrae, such as kyphosis and scoliosis. Lesions of the breast include congenital abnormalities, as well as acquired infections and hormonally induced enlargement.

All these problems are discovered when the clothes covering the trunk are removed, and present because the parents have noticed an abnormality, or the child has become concerned about the way he or she looks.

THE ANTERIOR CHEST WALL

Anterior deformities of the ribs and sternum can be separated readily into three major groups (Table 19.1): (1) the common depression deformities (funnel chest or pectus excavatum); (2) the less common protrusion deformities (pigeon chest or pectus carinatum); and (3) the rare deficiency deformities of the chest wall (which in themselves may be associated with a high protrusion deformity). The term 'deficiency' denotes absence or hypoplasia of one or more of the constituents of the chest wall: pectoral muscles, breast, ribs or costal cartilages. In the depression and protrusion groups, deformity may be symmetrical or asymmetrical. The great majority are congenital or genetically determined and may increase or decrease in severity with growth. The importance of careful clinical appraisal relates to:

(1) identification of those with a protrusion deformity secondary to intrathoracic pathology (e.g. tumour or congenital cystic lung);
(2) recognition of those with deficiency deformities;
(3) accurate analysis of the components of the deformity to assist in planning surgical correction where this is required.

Chest wall deformities rarely cause symptoms but can be distressing from the psychological point of

Table 19.1 ANTERIOR CHEST WALL DEFORMITIES

Type	Name	Frequency
Depression	Funnel chest (pectus excavatum)	Common
Protrusion	Pigeon chest (pectus carinatum)	Less common
Deficiency (of bone/muscle)	Poland's syndrome	Rare

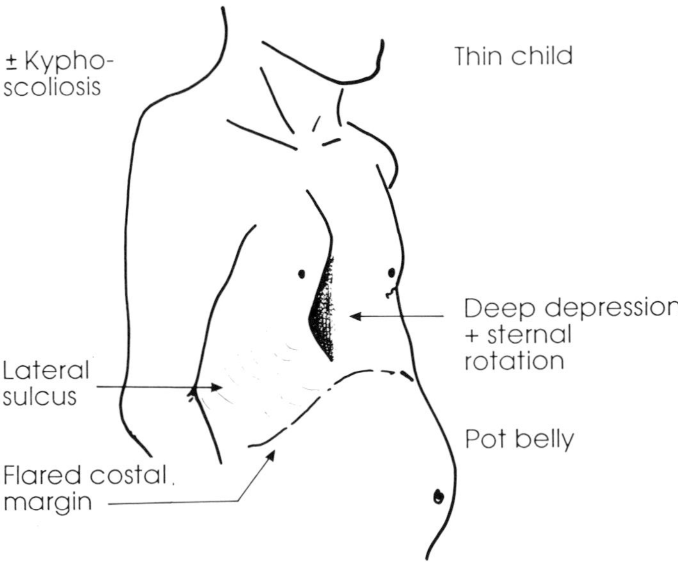

Fig. 19.1: *Depression deformity (funnel chest).*

view. Severe depression deformities may limit cardiac output with exercise in the erect position, but this is virtually never a clinical problem.

Clinical assessment

The initial clinical assessment is directed at establishing the type of chest wall deformity. This is achieved by determining the relationship of the sternum to its connecting costal cartilages. Where the sternum is posterior to the adjacent costal cartilages, the deformity is called a depression deformity (Fig. 19.1), and where it is anterior to them, it is described as a protrusion deformity (Fig. 19.2). In the latter case, one part of the sternum may be involved to a greater degree than the rest. Where it is angulated forwards in its upper part, it is termed a high protrusion. The sternum below this level may appear to produce a depression, but this is only relative as the sternoxiphisternal junction is placed normally. In other situations, the site of maximal protrusion is at the sternoxiphisternal junction, often with prominent adjacent costal cartilages on one or both sides and rotation of the sternum. Low sternal protrusion may be secondary to intrathoracic pathology, e.g. asthma, cystic fibrosis, cystic lung, congenital cardiac disease or intrathoracic malignancy, and these conditions should be ruled out on history, examination and chest x-ray. In other types, the chest wall deformity is the primary lesion, and there is no associated intrathoracic pathology, although in Marfan's syndrome there may be a mild coexisting depression deformity.

Once the type of deformity has been established, the following features should be more exactly defined: the vertical extent of the deformity; the level of its greatest extent; the degree of asymmetry; the rotation of the sternum; the prominence of the costal cartilages; the degree of

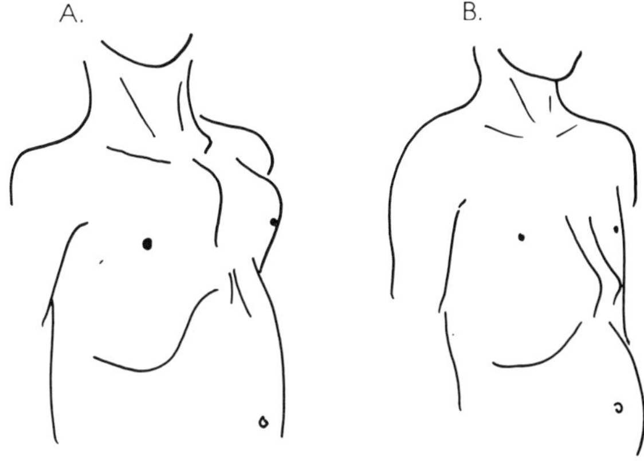

Fig. 19.2: *Protrusion deformities (pigeon chest). A. High protrusion. B. Low protrusion. Low protrusion deformities require limited investigation to exclude primary intrathoracic pathology.*

hollowing of the rib cage lateral to the sterno-xiphisternal junction; the flaring of the lower costal cartilages; and the degree of postural kyphosis and scoliosis. Asymmetry occurs when the sternum is rotated in its longitudinal axis to make the costal cartilages prominent on one side and recessive on the other (Fig. 19.3). In depression deformities, the sulcus lateral to the sternoxiphisternal junction is produced by the attachments of the diaphragm to the inner surface of the costal cartilages, and below this the costal margin is everted.

Most children with depression deformities are male, thin, have muscular and ligamentous laxity, and poor posture. In infants with severe depression deformities, there may be paradoxical sternal retraction on inspiration.

Progression of depression deformities with growth is unpredictable, whereas primary protrusion deformities have a tendency to spontaneous improvement. Where the deformity results from an intrathoracic lesion, treatment of the cause usually results in resolution of the deformity. Absence of breast, muscle, cartilage or bone indicates a deficiency deformity, such as Poland's syndrome (Fig. 19.4). In this condition, syndactyly and hypoplasia of the ipsilateral upper limb may be present as well.

An algorithm of the approach to a patient with a chest wall deformity is shown in Figure 19.5.

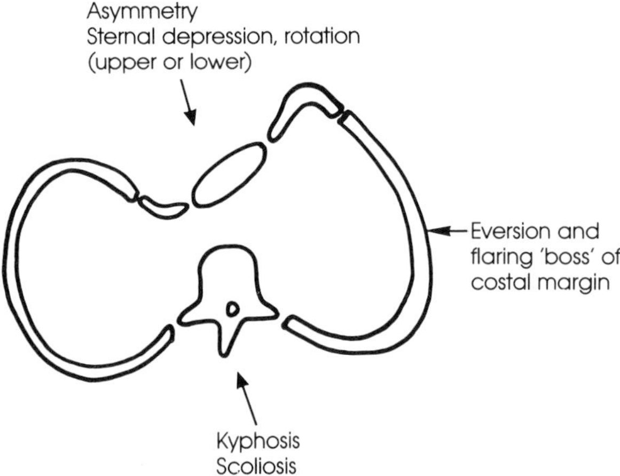

Fig. 19.3: *Features of chest wall deformities: asymmetry, sternal rotation, flaring of the costal margin and compensatory spinal deformities.*

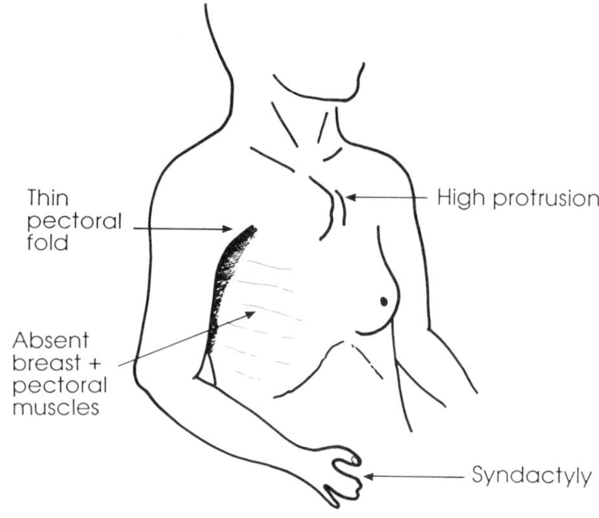

Fig. 19.4: *Deficiency deformities: Poland's syndrome.*

THE POSTERIOR CHEST WALL

An examination of the back requires all clothing to be removed to expose the back along its entire length. Footwear should be removed so that the length of the legs can be compared and to overcome the effect of high or unequal heels.

The key landmarks observed are the spinous processes, the angles of the scapulae and the iliac spines and crests. The contours of the back are observed. In the assessment of kyphosis and lordosis, it must be remembered that the shape of the back varies according to age and the attainment of the erect posture (Fig. 19.6).

The critical point to determine is whether or not the back deformity is postural or has some pathological basis.

Scoliosis

Scoliosis, or lateral curvature of the spine, is common in adolescent girls where there is a genetic defect in spinal structure. Scoliosis also may be compensatory or postural in origin, which can be distinguished from structural scoliosis on clinical examination (Table 19.2).

In assessing scoliosis, the child is examined first for evidence of compensatory scoliosis. In young children, compensatory scoliosis often is caused

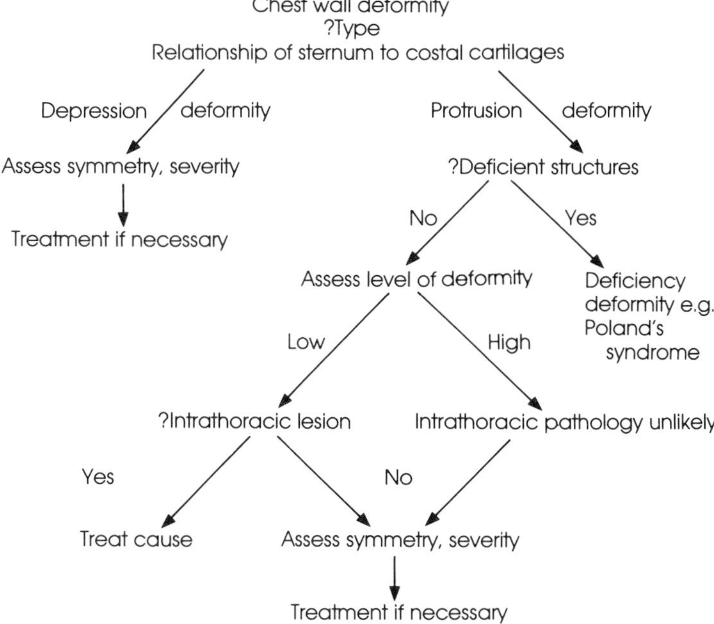

Fig. 19.5: *The clinical approach to chest wall deformities.*

by torticollis, following thoracotomy or when the legs are of unequal length. Torticollis is recognized on examination of the neck (see Chapter 9), and thoracotomy by a scar on the chest. To determine whether the legs are of equal length, the child stands with both feet on a firm, level surface, and the anterior or posterior iliac spines are palpated (Fig. 19.7). The bony landmarks are level if the legs are equal in length, but are at different heights when one leg is shorter than the other.

Table 19.2 THE CAUSES OF SCOLIOSIS

Type	Aetiology
Compensatory	Torticollis Post-thoracotomy Unequal legs Squint
Structural	Idiopathic (commonest) Hemivertebrae Neurological imbalance Fractured vertebrae von Recklinghausen's disease
Postural	Idiopathic

Once the legs have been shown to be equal in length, and other causes of compensatory scoliosis have not been found, postural scoliosis must be excluded. The child stands with her back to the examiner and then touches her toes. If the abnormal curve disappears during this manoeuvre, the scoliosis is postural (requiring no treatment), whereas if it persists, the scoliosis is structural (Fig. 19.8) and the girl will need further assessment by an orthopaedic surgeon. Structural scoliosis, which is associated often with some degree of kyphosis, has a number of causes and

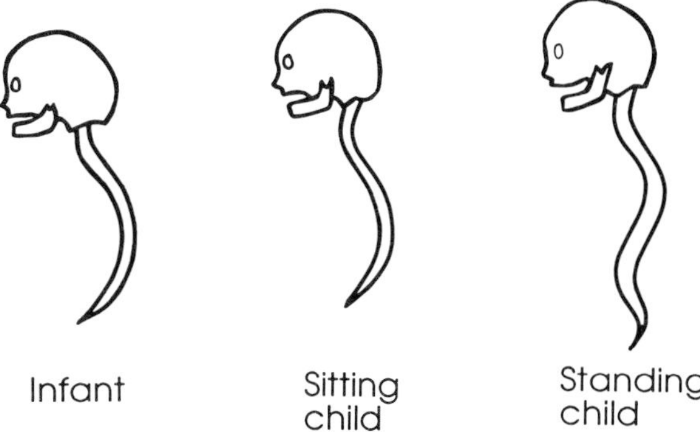

Fig. 19.6: *The three shapes of the spine.*

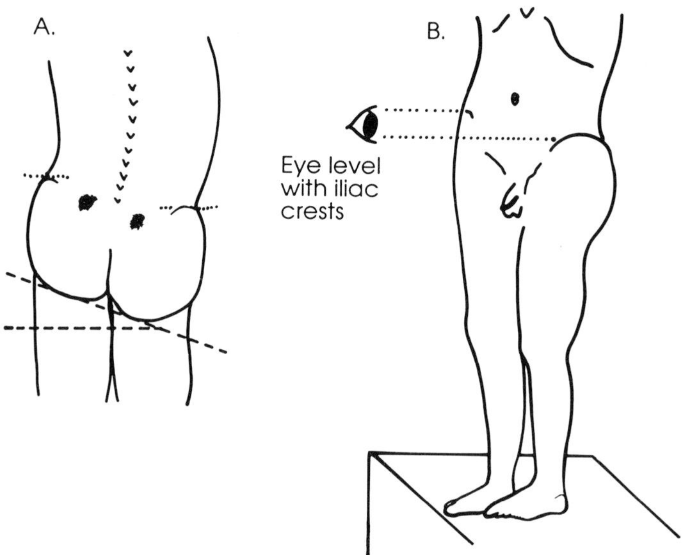

Fig. 19.7: *The assessment of pelvic tilt caused by unequal leg length.*
A. From behind: 1. Stand the patient on a firm surface with the buttocks level with the examiner's eyes. 2. Confirm that the heels are together and weight-bearing. 3. Observe the relative levels of (i) the posterior iliac spines, (ii) the dimples overlying the sacro-iliac joints, and (iii) the buttock folds.
B. From in front: 1. Stand the patient on a firm surface with the examiner's eyes level with the iliac crests. 2. Ensure that the patient's heels are together and weight-bearing. 3. Press the thumbs firmly on the anterior iliac spines and assess whether they are level.

demands careful examination of the nervous system and x-ray of the spine. The approach to diagnosis is outlined in Figure 19.9. Early diagnosis allows preventive treatment before the curvature increases during the adolescent growth phase.

Kyphosis

Kyphosis, or excessive rounding of the back common in adolescent boys, is caused by wedge compression of the growing vertebral bodies. It may be accompanied by a compensatory lordosis (Fig. 19.10). The curvature of mild postural kyphosis can be corrected by muscular control, whereas in structural kyphosis even strenuous muscular effort is unable to eliminate the deformity.

Scheuermann's disease is the common structural abnormality leading to kyphosis, which com-

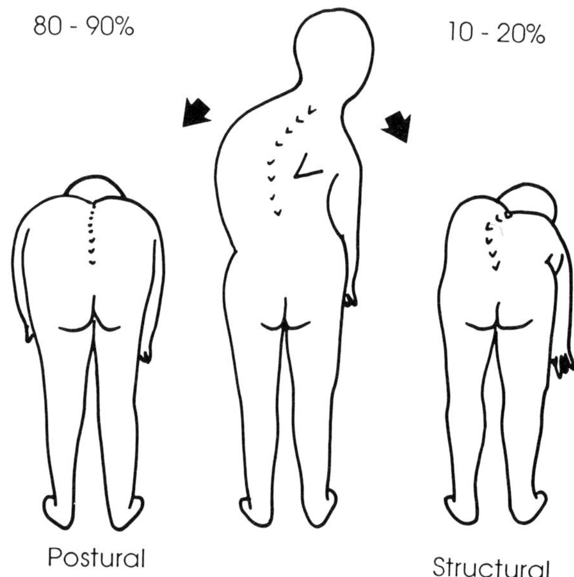

Fig. 19.8: *The effect of flexion on scoliosis.*

mences insidiously in early adolescence. It affects the upper thoracic spine with resultant limitation of flexion and extension. In more severe cases, there is a compensatory lordosis with decreased range of movement of the lumbar spine. As most flexion occurs through the lumbar spine rather than the thoracic spine, stiffness of the lumbar region has a pronounced effect on the boy's ability to touch his toes. Straight leg raising is reduced because the lordosis causes a relative tightening of the hamstrings. The patient is placed supine on a firm surface. The examiner's hand can be placed beneath the patient's lumber spine to assess the degree of compensatory lordosis. The right hand is then placed beneath the leg immediately above the ankle, and the leg elevated. Flexion of the knee is prevented by control of the thigh with the left hand (Fig. 19.11).

The angle to which the leg can be raised decreases with age, but in an adolescent should reach 90°. Early detection and treatment of Scheuermann's disease, with exercises or a brace, may prevent progression of the deformity and obviate the need for surgical fusion of the vertebrae.

Other causes of kyphosis are rare in children, but are important because they may need immediate treatment (Table 19.3). Fracture or collapse of a vertebral body from trauma or metastatic tumour may produce a kyphosis; the history usually provides the clue to the diagnosis. Deformity or disruption of the continuity of the spinous processes is assessed either visually or on palpation. One or more spinous processes may be tender. In trauma, one should look for supporting evidence such as superficial bruising and neurological deficit in the limbs, perineum and trunk.

Backache

Although the cause of backache may be difficult to diagnose in an adult, it is relatively easy in childhood. The likely cause is often determined from the history, since most conditions producing

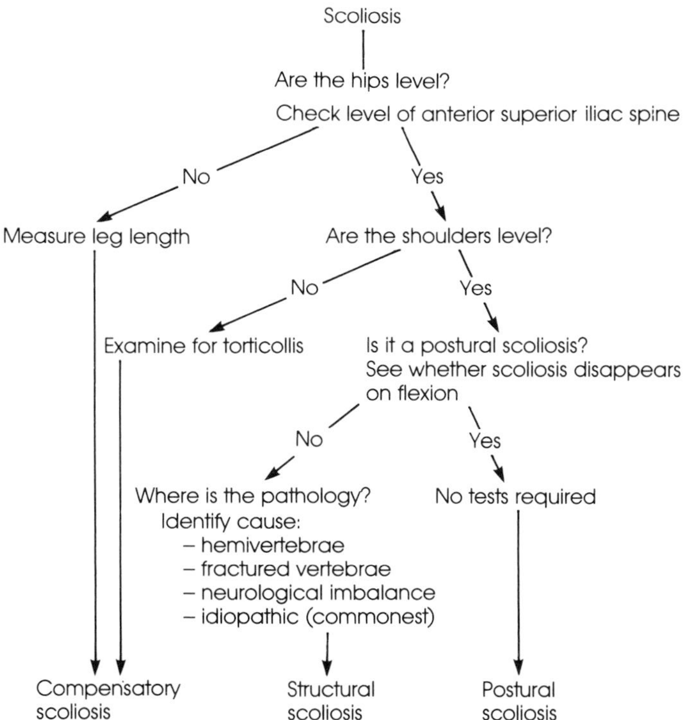

Fig. 19.9: *The clinical approach to scoliosis.*

Table 19.3 CAUSES OF KYPHOSIS IN CHILDREN

1. POSTURAL KYPHOSIS	Gentle curve Poor posture Straightened by muscular effort
2. ADOLESCENT KYPHOSIS (SCHEUERMANN'S DISEASE)	Appears in early adolescence Increasing deformity Unable to straighten a rigid back Back pain frequent Stiff lumbar lordosis Short hamstrings
3. LOCALIZED PATHOLOGY	E.g. fracture, tumour metastasis Localized abnormality Often tender

backache have characteristic features (Table 19.4). The exact location of the pain, its onset and duration, and whether it results in limitation of movement, all help to separate the causes. High thoracic pain in an adolescent is likely to be Scheuermann's disease, while low lumbar pain in a five-year-old child may be spondylolisthesis. Acute onset of pain suggests infection (osteomyelitis/discitis) or trauma (wedge fracture), while night pain is suspicious of a tumour. The presence of other abnormalities, such as fever (infection) or voiding difficulties (nerve compression), may be helpful. Limitation of general activity may indicate infection, while inability to bend forward as far as usual suggests kyphosis or spondylolisthesis, both of which may be associated with tight hamstring muscles.

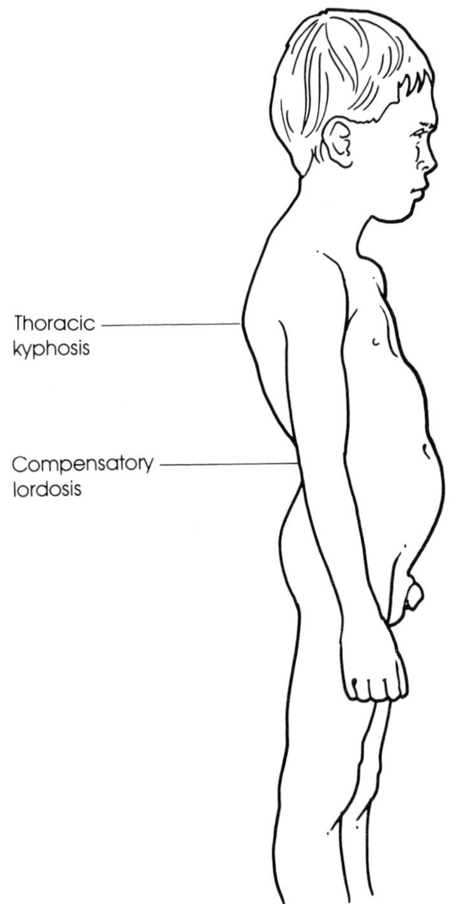

Fig. 19.10: *Adolescent kyphosis.*

THE BREAST

There are a number of congenital abnormalities of the breast which are easily recognized and harmless, but which may cause considerable anxiety and concern to both the parents and the patient (Table 19.5).

Likewise, most acquired conditions of the breast are not serious, but there is one situation where careful clinical examination is required: benign premature enlargement of the breast must be distinguished from precocious puberty, because the latter condition may be secondary to a hormone-producing tumour.

Primary breast tumours in children are exceedingly rare and are not considered further in this chapter.

Table 19.4 BACKACHE

Cause	Features
Scheuermann's disease	Adolescent High thoracic pain with kyphosis Pain worse after exercise/bending Tight hamstrings
Spondylolisthesis	Forward displacement of L5 on S1 Low back pain after a minor fall ≥ three years old Tight hamstrings
Vertebral osteomyelitis/discitis	Acute onset Day and night pain increasing Rigid back Fever and signs of infection
Prolapsed disc	Unusual Symptoms and signs similar to adults
Tumours (rare) – osteoid osteoma – osteoblastoma – eosinophilic granuloma	Night pain/day and night pain
Wedge fracture	Related to trauma

Congenital abnormalities

A common anomaly is multiple nipples. These may occur anywhere along the mammary or 'milk' line, which runs from the anterior axillary fold of the axilla through the normal nipple position to the groin (Fig. 19.12A). The accessory nipple may not be pigmented in infancy and early childhood, but becomes increasingly pigmented with age. Consequently, it may not be obvious at

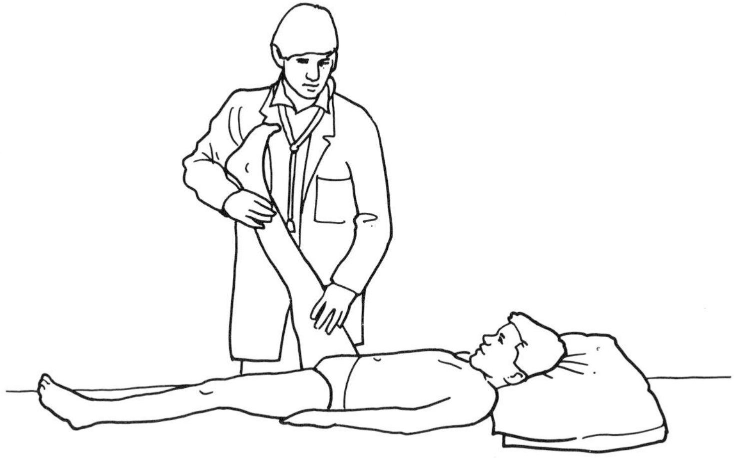

Fig. 19.11: *The assessment of straight leg raising. 1. Place the patient in a supine position with the head on a pillow. 2. Elevate one leg with the right hand behind the lower calf. 3. Prevent knee flexion by controlling the thigh with the left hand. 4. Estimate the angle from the horizontal plane at the limit of comfortable flexion.*

Table 19.5 BREAST LESIONS

CONGENITAL ABNORMALITIES	Absence of breast (amastia) Absence of nipple (athelia) Accessory nipples (polythelia) Accessory breast
BREAST ENLARGEMENT IN THE NEONATE	Neonatal hypertrophy (neonatal mastitis) Abscess
BREAST ENLARGEMENT IN SMALL GIRLS	Benign premature enlargement (premature hyperplasia, premature thelarche) Pathological precocious puberty Constitutional precocious puberty (idiopathic precocious puberty)
BREAST ENLARGEMENT IN BOYS	Pubertal mastitis Gynaecomastia

birth, which accounts for its frequent presentation in later childhood. Accessory nipples may occur bilaterally, and when they involve the axilla, breast tissue is often present; this breast tissue will enlarge during puberty, producing a soft swelling in the axilla (Fig. 19.12B).

A rare abnormality is complete absence of one breast and nipple, and when this occurs, it is usually associated with deficient development of the underlying pectoral muscles, the chest wall and ipsilateral upper limb ('Poland's syndrome' – see Fig. 19.4).

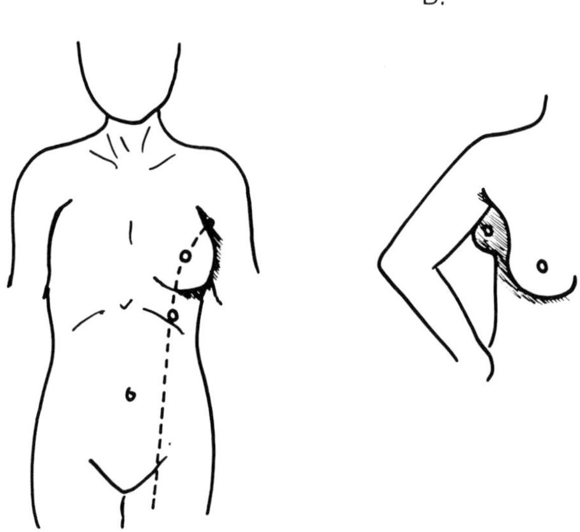

Fig. 19.12: *Congenital abnormalities of the breast. A. Absence of nipple and breast tissue on the right, obvious at birth, and a supernumerary nipple situated on the mammary line of the left, which is often not obvious until later in childhood. B. Axillary supernumerary breast and nipple, unnoticed until puberty.*

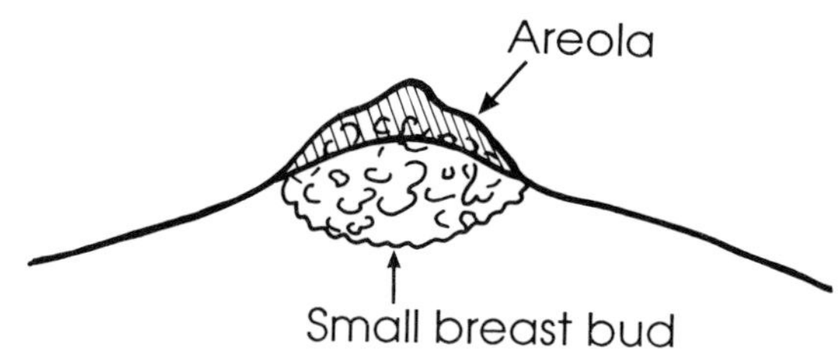

Fig. 19.13: *The discoid, well defined breast nodule – found in neonatal hypertrophy, male pubertal 'mastitis' and premature thelarche.*

Acquired abnormalities

Hypertrophy of the newborn breast ('neonatal mastitis')

This occurs in both sexes and is physiological in origin. Maternal oestrogens cross the placenta and cause enlargement of the fetal breast tissue. Lactogenic hormones in breast milk may even cause the secretion of the infant's own breast milk ('witch's milk'). The enlargement is most obvious between three and seven days of life and subsides within the first month. The swelling is firm and usually 1-2 cm in diameter, which is the diameter of the areola (Fig. 19.13).

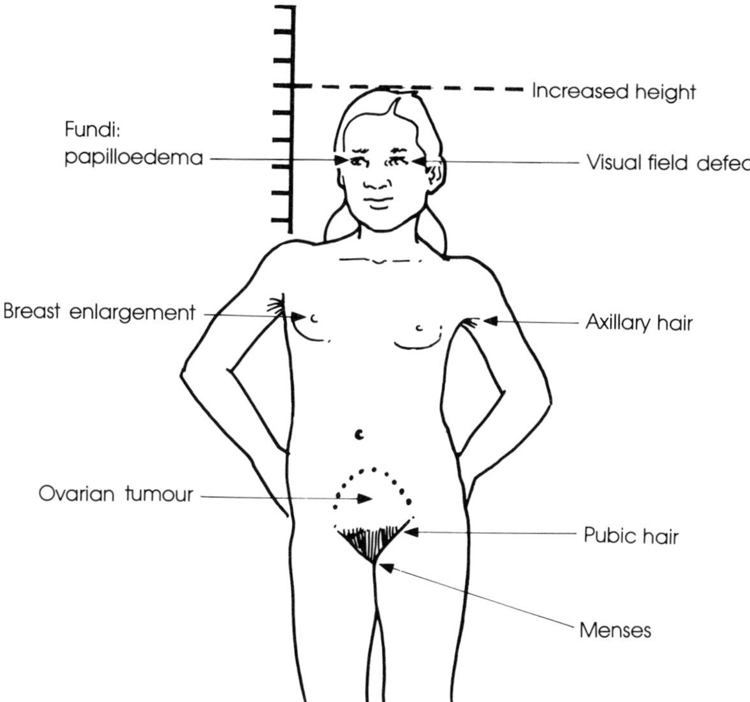

Fig. 19.14: *Examination of the girl with precocious puberty.*

The breast may become infected through the nipple, resulting in abscess formation, particularly if there have been repeated attempts at expression and massage. The swelling will be tender and fluctuant with a surrounding area of skin erythema. Neonatal breast abscess is an important condition since early diagnosis and treatment is essential to prevent damage to the breast, particularly if surgical drainage is required. Breast infection is extremely rare except in the neonate, since the breast is susceptible to infection only when it is secreting milk.

Breast enlargement in small girls

Benign, unilateral breast enlargement may occur in girls between five and 10 years of age. Frequently, the same changes appear in the other breast about one year later. There is a firm, well-defined lump up to 2 cm in diameter behind and attached to the nipple. It is usually non-tender. There is no axillary or pubic hair growth, menses, growth spurt or other signs suggesting the onset of puberty, and the changes remain static (until puberty commences) or may regress. The condition is known as benign premature enlargement, premature hyperplasia or premature thelarche. The significance of the condition is that it is completely harmless and biopsy of the breast is absolutely contra-indicated, as it would severely damage normal breast tissue.

Breast enlargement associated with other secondary sexual characteristics may occur from the age of one year and is termed 'precocious puberty'. It is usually idiopathic ('constitutional'), but may be a manifestation of an underlying cause such as ovarian, adrenocortical or hypothalamic dysfunction. Therefore, when confronted with a child with premature bilateral breast enlargement, one should proceed as follows:

(1) Look for other signs of sexual development (Fig. 19.14), i.e. pubic and axillary hair. Look at growth charts for evidence of a recent growth spurt, and ascertain whether menstruation has begun.
(2) Look for evidence of an underlying cause. Inspect the optic fundi for papilloedema indicating raised intracranial pressure, and test for

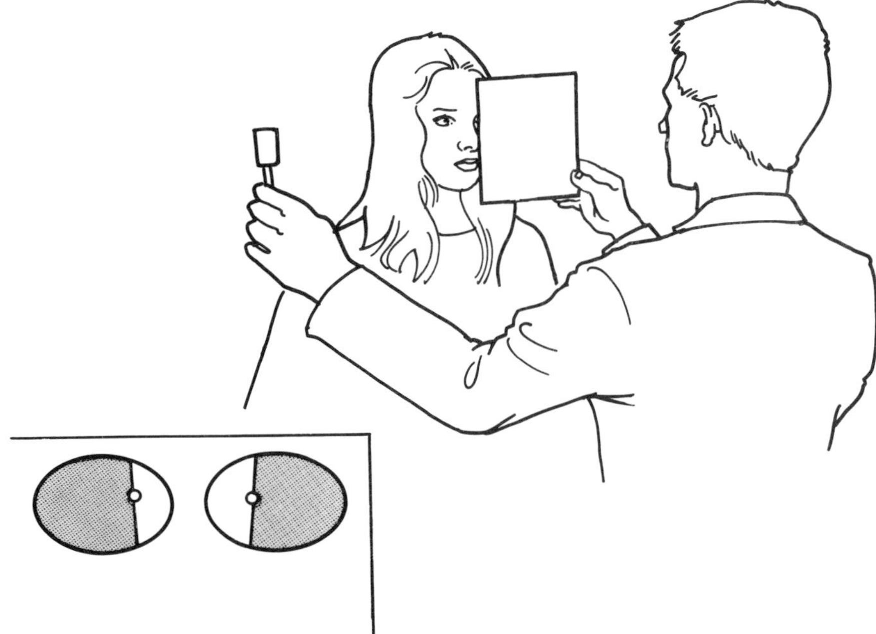

Fig. 19.15: *Examination for a visual field deficit. One eye is covered while the other is tested. Look for evidence of a bitemporal hemianopia (inset).*

visual field defects (Fig. 19.15), looking for temporal hemianopia caused by a pituitary tumour (Fig. 19.16). Palpate the abdomen for abnormal masses. Ovarian masses frequently are palpable on abdominal examination and often palpable on rectal digital examination. Where they are large, they may be ballotable between the examining finger and the fingers of the opposite hand placed above the pubic symphysis (Fig. 19.17).

True precocious puberty should be considered constitutional only after careful clinical examination and investigations fail to reveal an underlying cause.

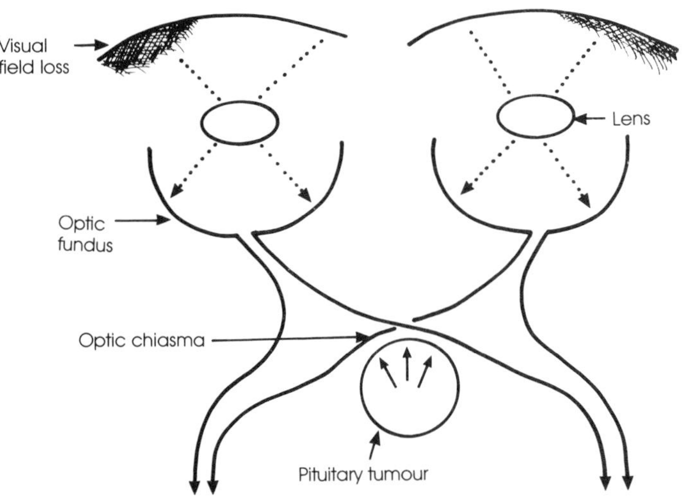

Fig. 19.16: *A defect in the peripheral field of vision from pressure on the optic chiasma, e.g. by a pituitary tumour.*

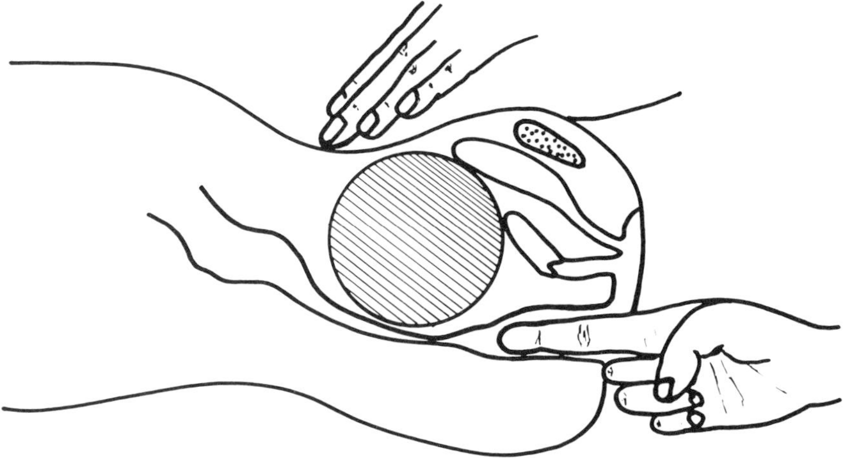

Fig. 19.17: *Bimanual palpation of an ovarian tumour in a child. The small shallow pelvis enables an intrapelvic mass to be felt easily.*

Pubertal 'mastitis' in boys

A minor degree of breast enlargement occurs in 70% of boys at puberty, with a firm, demarcated swelling appearing beneath the areola. This is believed to be caused by hormonal imbalance with an excess of, or increased sensitivity to, oestrogens. One side may be affected before or more than the other, and the swelling usually lasts up to two years. Occasionally, it causes discomfort and is tender. It should be distinguished from the swellings seen in fat boys (Fig. 19.18): in pubertal 'mastitis' the swelling is localized to the subareolar region and on palpation feels firm, whereas the breast in fat boys is less well localized and is part of generalized obesity. In these boys, there are often striae overlying the hips and lateral aspects of the thighs, and there is an apparently small penis as the result of considerable prepubic fat. They are of normal height and they experience a normal pubertal growth spurt.

Gynaecomastia

More significant breast enlargement in boys is called 'gynaecomastia'. It involves enlargement and hyperplasia of the glandular elements of the breast, although in common usage the term is often used to include fatty deposition producing the appearance of beast development in obese pubertal boys.

True gynaecomastia involves enlargement of breast elements and rarely is due to an underlying endocrine abnormality (Fig. 19.19). The child is usually of small stature. The external genitalia should be carefully inspected and the following questions answered:

(1) Is there evidence of ambiguous genitalia?
(2) Is the distribution of pubic hair normal?

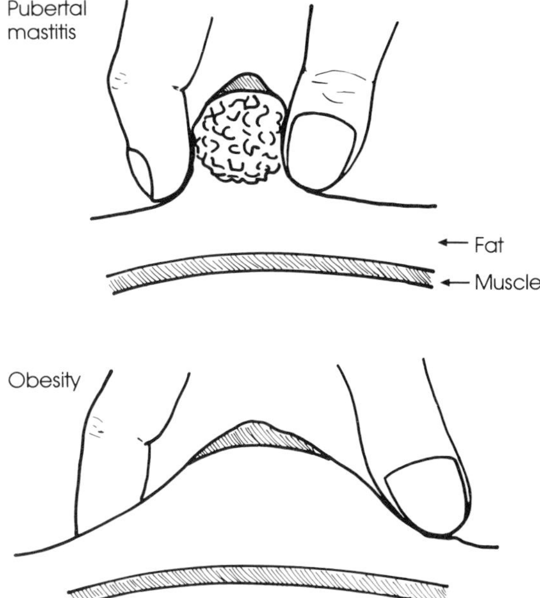

Fig. 19.18: *The differential diagnosis of pubertal mastitis and obesity in a boy.*

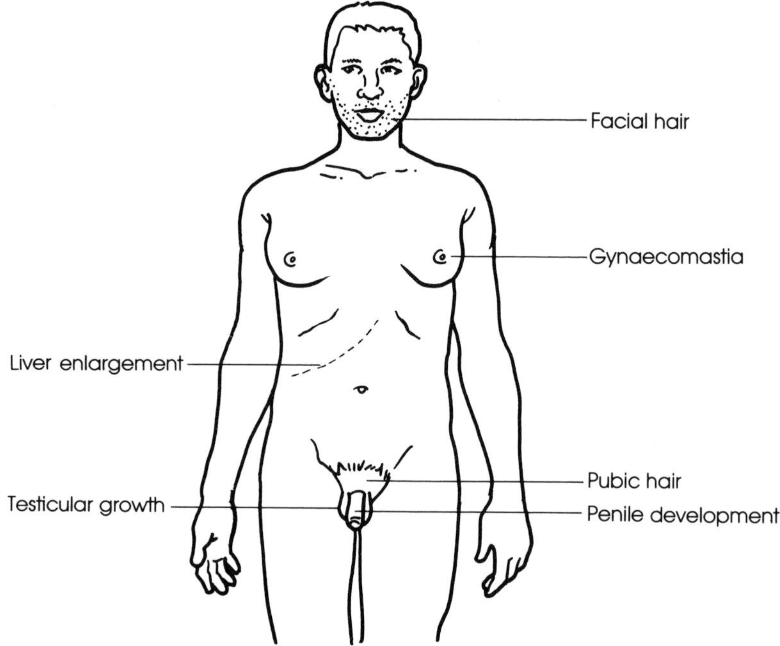

Fig. 19.19: *Examination of a boy with gynaecomastia: look for evidence of an underlying endocrine abnormality.*

(3) Has the penis shown normal pubertal enlargement?
(4) Are the testes present?
(5) If the testes are present, are they prepubertal or postpubertal in size?

Testes should be palpated carefully for a tumour. Rarely, the patient may have liver failure and be jaundiced, in which case hepatomegaly should be demonstrated. Liver failure leads to increased levels of circulating oestrogens because their excretion in the bile is impaired.

GOLDEN RULES

The anterior chest wall

(1) Determine whether the deformity is primarily protrusion or depression.
(2) Low protrusion deformities occasionally reflect intrathoracic pathology.
(3) Beware the chest wall deformity with symptoms: it suggests unrelated pathology.

Posterior chest wall

(1) Postural and adolescent kyphosis display a gentle curve; an angular deformity suggests significant localized pathology.
(2) Scoliosis (compensatory) can be caused by pathology above and below the back.

The breast

(1) Supernumerary nipples are located along the mammary line and may not be obvious at birth.
(2) When confronted with a patient with premature bilateral breast enlargement, look for other signs of puberty.
(3) Premature benign enlargement (premature hyperplasia) is common, is not associated with other signs of sexual development, and does not warrant biopsy.
(4) Beware precocious puberty: it may signify underlying ovarian, adrenocortical or hypothalamic pathology.
(5) Primary tumours of the breast in children are exceedingly rare.
(6) Neonatal 'mastitis' is a response to hormonal stimulation and, unless abscess supervenes, requires no treatment.
(7) The childhood breast is inactive except in the neonatal period. Breast abscess only occurs in the secreting neonatal breast because of duct patency and milk production.

20 Respiratory distress in the newborn

Oxygenation of the fetus is achieved through gas exchange in the placenta. At birth, this connection with the placenta is lost and the infant becomes dependent on the lungs which, within seconds of birth, fill with air and pulmonary blood flow increases. Respiratory distress in the newborn occurs if: (1) the lungs are unable to expand because of obstruction of the upper airways; (2) there is inadequate room within the thoracic cage for lung expansion to occur; or (3) the infant cannot produce sufficient negative intrathoracic pressure to inflate the lungs.

In the premature infant, lack of surfactant allows the alveoli to collapse and leads to respiratory distress (respiratory distress syndrome); this condition will worsen significantly the respiratory difficulties experienced by the newborn who has a coexisting anomaly which interferes with respiration. When respiratory distress is recognized in the newborn, its cause must be established promptly by careful examination and a chest x-ray.

Occasionally, antenatal ultrasound examination detects major congenital anomalies which cause respiratory insufficiency at birth. For example, the presence of bowel in the thorax with mediastinal shift is indicative of congenital diaphragmatic hernia and, in such a case, the mother should be transported to a major institution for the birth of her child. As soon as the child is born, the diagnosis can be confirmed and immediate resuscitation instituted.

CLINICAL FEATURES

The first sign of respiratory distress in the neonate is restlessness, (Table 20.1) which may be overlooked at first but is soon accompanied by tachypnoea. The relatively horizontal position of the ribs and lack of bucket-handle movement means that the neonate cannot increase the anteroposterior and transverse diameters of the thorax and relies almost entirely on diaphragmatic movement for effective inspiration (Fig. 20.1). Increase in respiratory effort is achieved by an increase in diaphragmatic effort and is manifested clinically by protrusion of the upper abdomen, grunting on expiration and flaring of the nostrils. The pliability of the ribs supporting the sternum results in the negative intrathoracic pressure during inspiration to cause retraction of the sternum. If the abdomen is distended already from air swallowing or the passage of air through a tracheo-oesophageal fistula, the diaphragm is pushed upwards and ventilation is compromised further (Fig. 20.2). In severe respiratory distress, oxygenation across the

Table 20.1 SIGNS OF RESPIRATORY DISTRESS IN THE NEONATE

1. Restlessness
2. Tachypnoea
3. Increased respiratory effort with sternal retraction
4. Cyanosis

lungs is impeded and cyanosis develops. Progression of respiratory distress results in respiratory failure and, subsequently, cardiovascular collapse.

The signs of respiratory distress are not specific for the cause. In some situations, the underlying abnormality is immediately apparent, although a chest x-ray may be required to make a diagnosis.

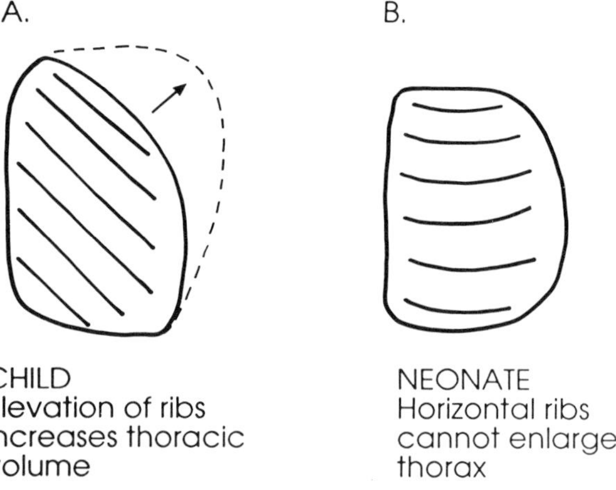

Fig. 20.1: *The effect of the shape of the rib cage on ventilation in the neonate.*

CAUSE OBVIOUS ON EXTERNAL EXAMINATION

Examine the face and neck. Look for a small undercut lower jaw (micrognathia). This may be seen in association with a cleft of the secondary palate (Pierre Robin syndrome), which can be detected by inspecting the roof of the mouth using a torch. Sometimes, the larger defects are palpable by running the little finger across the roof of the mouth, but this technique is less reliable and the diagnosis is made with greater certainty if seen directly. The small jaw confines the tongue to the back of the mouth where it may fill the cleft and cause obstruction of the nasopharynx (Fig. 20.3). The infant is nursed prone because in the supine position, the tongue falls backwards and exacerbates the obstruction. Persistence of respiratory distress in the prone position may necessitate additional manoeuvres, such as the insertion of a nasopharyngeal airway or a tracheostomy.

A large cystic hygroma involving the floor of the mouth or the pharynx may cause upper respiratory tract obstruction and demand early tracheostomy. The cystic hygroma may involve much of the neck and extend through the thoracic inlet into the anterior mediastinum, causing tracheal compression or distortion (Fig. 20.4). The swelling is ill-defined, fluctuant and composed of many cysts which transilluminate brilliantly. Haemorrhage or infection may cause the cysts to enlarge rapidly and obstruct the airway further (see Chapter 11 for further description).

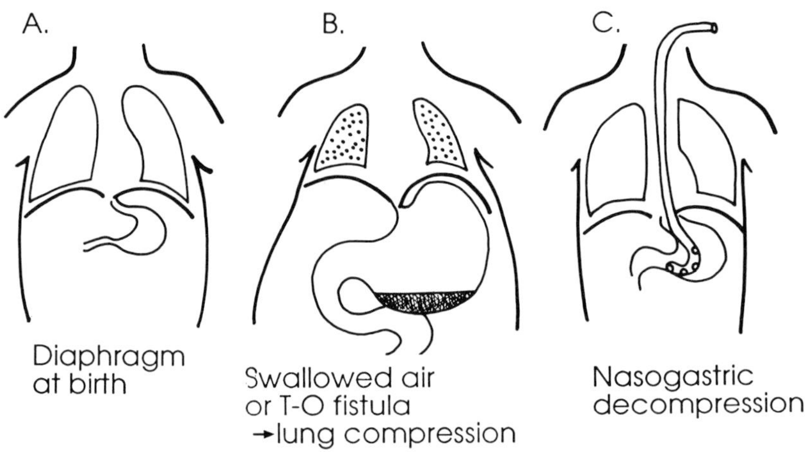

Fig. 20.2: *The effect of excess air in the stomach on neonatal ventilation.*

RESPIRATORY DISTRESS RELIEVED BY CRYING

The newborn infant is an obligate nose breather with little ability to breathe through the mouth, even where there is complete obstruction of the nasal passages. Choanal atresia is an uncommon anomaly where there is obstruction of the nasal airway and is important in that, if not recognized at birth, a fatal outcome may result. In complete bilateral choanal atresia, respiratory distress develops rapidly and is severe. The child becomes increasingly distressed and cyanotic, but rapidly turns pink when crying, with relief of the obstruction as air is exchanged via the mouth. The diagnosis of choanal atresia is suggested by the sudden improvement in the infant's condition on crying and the observation that the asphyxia is relieved by an oropharyngeal airway. The diagnosis is confirmed by inability to pass a small but firm nasogastric tube through either nasal passage. The tube should be directed posteriorly from the nostril in a horizontal plane beneath the turbinates (Fig. 20.5) and not upwards along the line of the nose. An alternative method of demonstrating complete nasal obstruction is to drip saline or Agarol into each nostril and note whether drainage occurs into the oropharynx. It is imperative that the oral airway remains in place until surgery has established a patent nasal passage on each side.

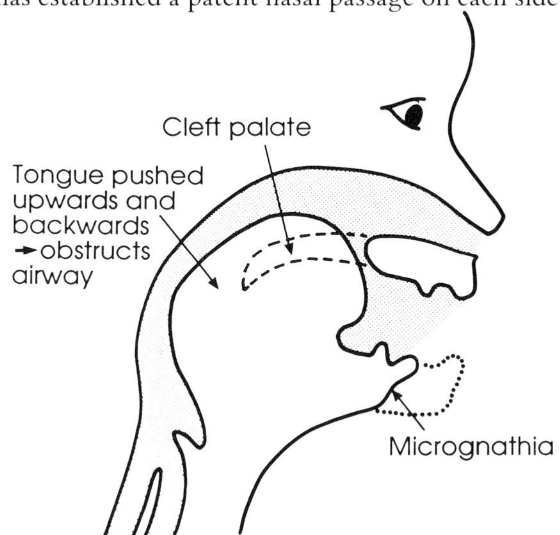

Fig. 20.3: *The cause of respiratory obstruction in Pierre Robin syndrome.*

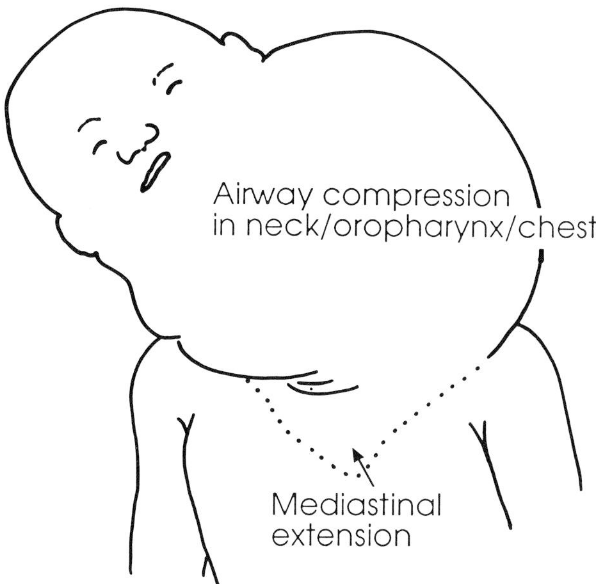

Fig. 20.4: *External compression of the airway with a congenital cervical hamartoma, e.g. cystic hygroma.*

Unilateral choanal atresia does not cause respiratory distress in the newborn and is detected in later years because of a persistent discharge from the obstructed nostril. It must be distinguished from a nasal foreign body which usually produces a purulent discharge.

A rare but potentially lethal cause of upper airway obstruction is a pedunculated hamartoma of the nasopharynx. It causes intermittent obstruction according to the posture of the infant and may be seen at the back of the mouth as it prolapses into the oropharynx. Early diagnosis permits surgical removal before asphyxia occurs.

THE FROTHY BABY IN RESPIRATORY DISTRESS

Oesophageal atresia is a relatively common congenital anomaly where there is interruption of the continuity of the oesophagus, associated in 85% with a fistulous communication between the lower trachea and distal oesophageal segment. The trachea and the oesophagus both form from the fore-gut tube, and the fistula represents persistence of this embryological connection.

Swallowed saliva fills the proximal oesopha-

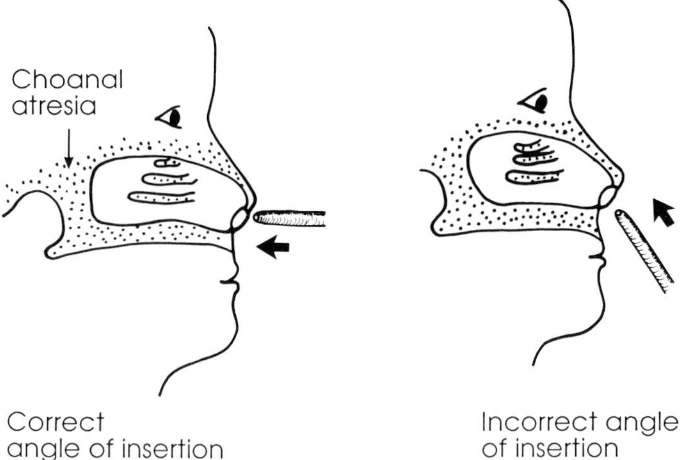

Fig. 20.5: *The technique for testing the patency of the nasal airway in choanal atresia. The stiff catheter needs to be passed horizontally below the inferior turbinate.*

gus, but the atresia prevents it from passing into the stomach. As a consequence, saliva accumulates in the pharynx and mouth, giving the appearance of excessive salivation. The babies are often described as being 'mucousy' or 'drooling', and frothy saliva is seen dribbling from the side of the mouth (Fig. 20.6). The fistula connecting the trachea with the lower oesophagus may interfere with effective ventilation if air passes preferentially down the fistula into the stomach. Accumulation of air in the stomach may cause abdominal distension with elevation of the diaphragm, and exacerbate the respiratory difficulty. In severe cases, cyanosis ensues. Frequently, there is a history of prematurity and maternal polyhydramnios.

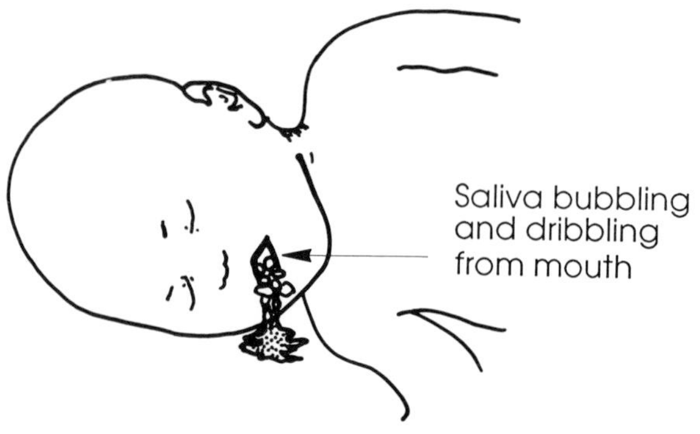

Fig. 20.6: *Excessive neonatal salivaton is highly suggestive of oesophageal atresia.*

The diagnosis of oesophageal atresia is confirmed easily using one simple clinical manoeuvre. A stiff 10 French gauge catheter is introduced through the mouth into the upper oesophagus. In oesophageal atresia, its progress is arrested between 9 and 13 cm from the gums (Fig. 20.7). A narrow catheter should not be used because it is likely to curl up in the dilated upper oesophagus giving a false impression of oesophageal continuity (Fig. 20.8). Once oesophageal atresia has been diagnosed using this test, the presence of abdominal distension and a resonant abdomen on percussion confirm the existence of a distal tracheo-oesophageal fistula.

If the diagnosis of oesophageal atresia has not been made at birth, it becomes apparent at the time of the first feed. The child gags and chokes and develops cyanotic respiratory distress with overflow of the milk from the oesophagus into the airway (Fig. 20.9). In oesophageal atresia, the pharynx should be suctioned frequently to remove excessive saliva and avoid aspiration.

Oesophageal atresia often (44%) is associated with other congenital anomalies, particularly cardiac, renal, anorectal, vertebral, radial and digital. The infant must be examined carefully for the presence of these anomalies. Oesophageal atresia is seen also in association with chromosomal trisomies, of which 13, 15, 18 and 21 are the most common.

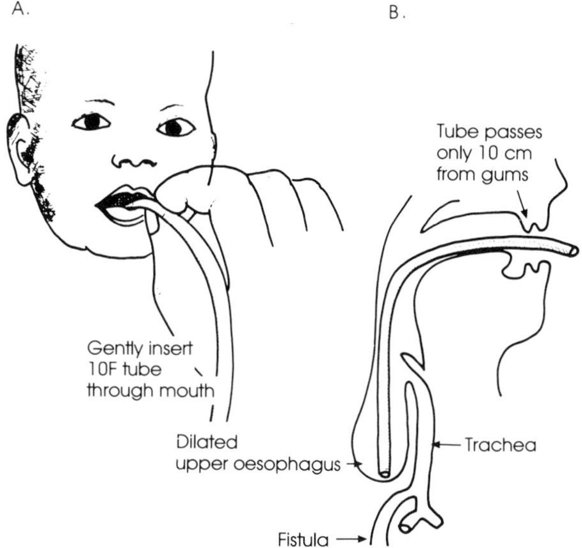

Fig. 20.7: *The diagnosis of oesophageal atresia.* A. *A* 10F *tube is inserted gently through the mouth.* B. *In oesophageal atresia, the catheter stops at* 10 *cm from the gums.*

A chest x-ray should be obtained in every case. This will often show the dilated upper 'pouch' of the oesophagus, and presence of air below the diaphragm suggests a distal tracheo-oesophageal fistula. A lateral film may show the lower oesophagus filled with air from the trachea. Absence of gas in the abdomen is indicative of the rare defects of atresia without fistula, or of atresia in association with a proximal tracheo-oesophageal fistula. Overflow of saliva, or reflux of gastric juice up the fistula into the trachea, may produce radiological signs of aspiration pneumonia. The vertebral column should be inspected for hemivertebrae or other anomalies. A contrast study is not needed to make the diagnosis of oesophageal atresia and should be avoided because of the high risk of aspiraton.

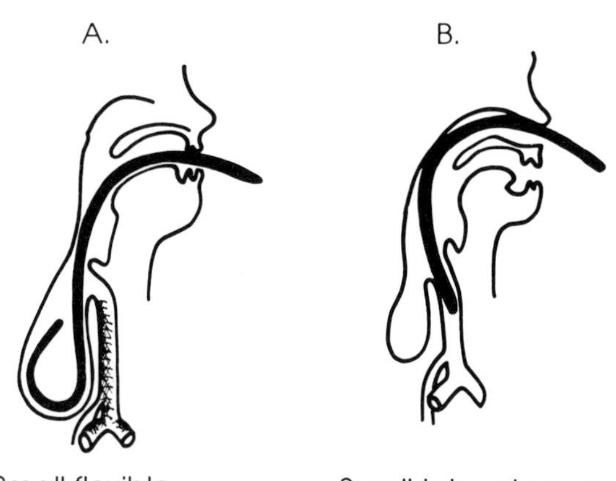

Fig. 20.8: *Pitfalls in the diagnosis of oesophageal atresia.* A. *A small, flexible catheter may roll up in the mouth or upper oesophagus.* B. *A small tube passed through the nose may enter the trachea.*

ONSET OF SEVERE OR PROGRESSIVE RESPIRATORY DISTRESS

Respiratory insufficiency shortly after birth in the absence of other conditions suggests a diagnosis of congenital diaphragmatic hernia. Development of the transverse septum between the chest and abdomen is defective, leaving a hole in the diaphragm – usually on the left side – through which the abdominal viscera herniate into the chest. This occurs before birth and inhibits pulmonary development by compressing the lung buds. At birth, this produces respiratory distress because of (1) lung hypoplasia, and (2) occupation of much of

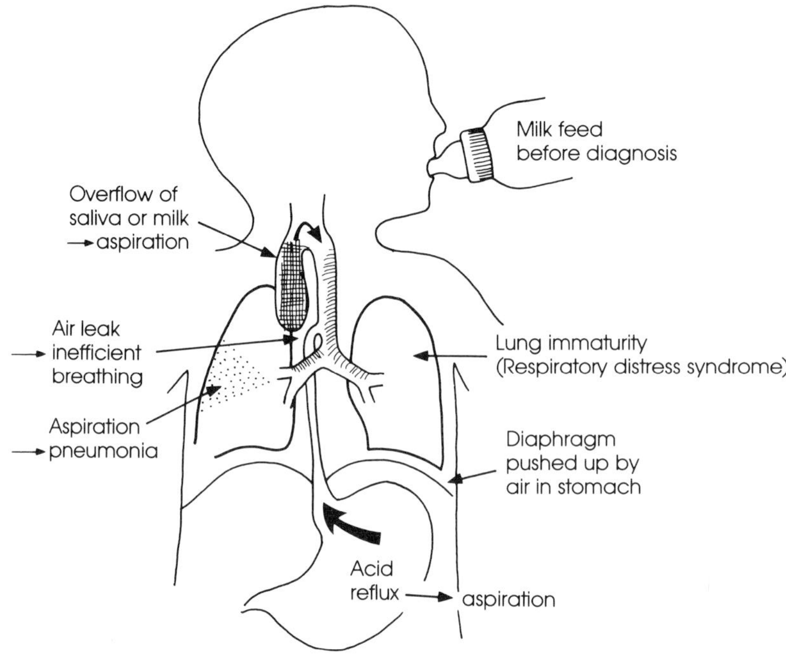

Fig. 20.9: *Causes of respiratory distress in oesophageal atresia.*

the thoracic volume by abdominal contents. The degree of lung hypoplasia is the ultimate determinant of survival.

Often, there is rapid development of respiratory distress with cyanosis. The age of onset and severity of symptoms vary with the degree of lung hypoplasia and the extent of interference with ventilation. In the most severe cases, poor peripheral perfusion and cardiovascular collapse occur within minutes of birth. Apgar scores remain low and, without immediate resuscitation, these infants die quickly. Lesser degrees of lung compression produce a less dramatic clinical picture, and a few children have no symptoms for days or months.

The chest is barrel-shaped and the abdomen is scaphoid because the bowel has herniated through the defect in the diaphragm into the pleural cavity (Fig. 20.10). However, once air is swallowed, this sign becomes less obvious. The presence of bowel and liver in the chest displaces the mediastinum to the contralateral side. Swallowed air makes this worse. In a left-sided hernia, this produces apparent dextrocardia (with the heart sounds most easily audible in the right chest) and poor breath sounds on the left side (Fig. 20.11). In the uncommon right-sided hernia, the signs are reversed. The classical sign of bowel sounds in one side of the chest on auscultation is not particularly reliable and may be difficult to elicit.

Where congenital diaphragmatic hernia is suspected on clinical grounds, an immediate plain chest x-ray must be obtained. The film should include the abdomen so that the distribution of bowel gas can be determined. The main radiological features include:

(1) loops of bowel in the chest on the side of the defect;
(2) hemidiaphragm not visible;
(3) mediastinal shift to the contralateral side;
(4) abnormal distribution of bowel gas within the abdomen.

There are a number of uncommon conditions which can have a similar radiological appearance to diaphragmatic hernia, e.g. cystic lung disease, lobar emphysema, staphylococcal pneumonia with pneumatocele, and other diaphragmatic defects, but these conditions are rarely a cause of such severe respiratory symptoms in the first few hours after birth.

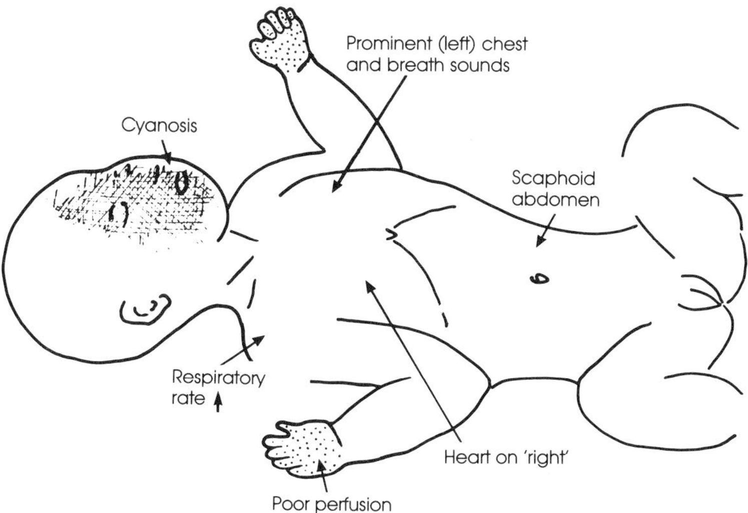

Fig. 20.10: *The clinical features of a left-sided congenital diaphragmatic hernia.*

SUDDEN ONSET OF RESPIRATORY DISTRESS

The sudden onset of severe and progressive symptoms of respiratory distress in an infant who has been asymptomatic or is stable following endotracheal intubation suggests the development of a pneumothorax. The respiratory rate increases with marked sternal retraction, diminished air entry on auscultation and increased resonance on percussion on the side of the pneumothorax. Shift of the mediastinum is difficult to detect in this condition. The diagnosis should always be considered in infants with a pre-existing condition known to predispose to the development of a pneumothorax. The most critical of these is diaphragmatic hernia, but a pneumothorax may also occur following a difficult delivery or in an infant with hyaline membrane disease, lung cyst and lobar emphysema. A plain radiograph of the chest confirms the diagnosis.

The development of a tension pneumothorax is particularly hazardous to the infant and is suggested by continued progression of symptoms as a result of further mediastinal shift, contralateral lung compression and interference of venous return. Cyanosis and cardiovascular collapse are later signs. The diagnosis of tension pneumothorax is confirmed on chest x-ray, but in some cases needle aspiration or tube thoracostomy are required as life-saving measures before an x-ray can be obtained. The best position in which to insert a chest drain is through the fourth or fifth intercostal spaces in the anterior axillary line.

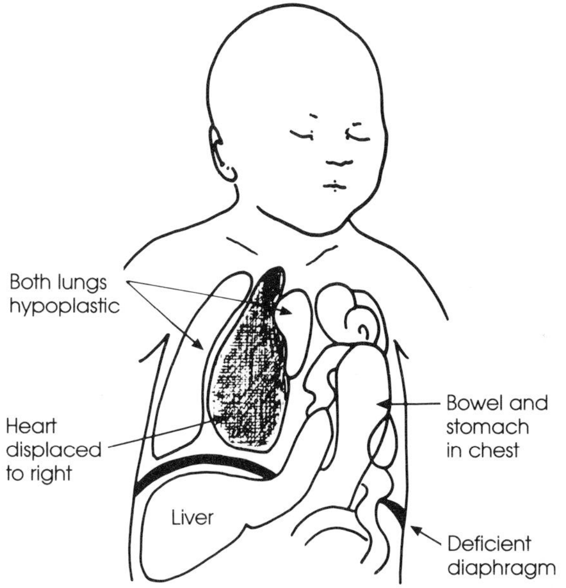

Fig. 20.11: *The intrathoracic anatomy in a left-sided congenital diaphragmatic hernia.*

GOLDEN RULES

(1) Beware excessive swallowed air in respiratory distress: it interferes with diaphragmatic breathing.
(2) Beware nasal obstruction: infants have difficulty breathing through the mouth.
(3) Cyanosis relieved by crying indicates nasal obstruction.
(4) A big tongue or small jaw may cause obstruction of the pharynx.
(5) Beware 'excessive' salivation in the neonate: this is likely to be due to inability to swallow saliva because of oesophageal atresia.
(6) Gas in the stomach in association with oesophageal atresia confirms the presence of a distal tracheo-oesophageal fistula.
(7) Oesophageal atresia is confirmed by gentle passage of a stiff 10F catheter through the mouth: the catheter is arrested at about 10 cm from the gums.
(8) An infant with oesophageal atresia requires careful examination for other anomalies.
(9) Diaphragmatic hernia or pneumothorax should be suspected where respiratory distress occurs soon after birth.
(10) Diaphragmatic hernia is the only common cause of respiratory distress where the abdomen is scaphoid (the bowel is in the thorax).

21 Neonatal bowel obstruction

Obstruction of the bowel at birth is a relatively common abnormality with a large number of possible causes, most of which are rare individually (Table 21.1). The common forms of obstruction in the neonatal period are Hirschsprung's disease and necrotizing enterocolitis. Less frequent conditions include small bowel atresia, either of the ileum or jejunum; malrotation or incomplete rotation of the bowel, with supervening volvulus (twisting of the bowel); duodenal atresia or stenosis; various abnormalities of the anorectal region, including imperforate anus; meconium ileus (as the first manifestation of cystic fibrosis); and perforation of the bowel, either prenatally (causing a sterile meconium peritonitis) or postnatally (causing septic peritonitis).

The pathological processes which lead to bowel obstruction at birth can be divided into three groups: an intrinsic abnormality of the bowel; an atresia secondary to occlusion of the blood vessels *in utero*; and a functional obstruction caused by inflammation, defective innervation or increased viscosity of the contents (Table 21.2). Such a classification has some use in the practical assessment since the symptoms and signs vary with the three groups, and the groups carry different prognostic implications for the baby.

Table 21.1 CAUSES OF NEONATAL BOWEL

Disease	Frequency
Hirschsprung's disease Necrotizing enterocolitis	More common
Small bowel atresia Malrotation with volvulus Duodenal atresia/stenosis Imperforate anus Meconium ileus	Less common
Prenatal perforation (meconium peritonitis)	Uncommon

THE CAUSES OF BOWEL OBSTRUCTION

Hirschsprung's disease

The ganglion cells of the intramural plexuses in the bowel control the coordination of contraction and relaxation of normal peristalsis. If these ganglion cells are missing, the bowel appears normal macroscopically, but it is obstructed functionally because of lack of coordinated peristalsis. The degree of resting contractility in the 'aganglionic' segment of bowel is variable, and it may be atonic or spastic. Meconium is unable to pass through the aperistaltic segment and leads to a functional obstruction with secondary proximal dilatation. The dilatation occurs in the normally innervated proximal bowel and, in the past, led to the term 'congenital megacolon' (Fig. 21.1). The length of colon affected by this deficiency of ganglion cells is variable, but in most patients extends from the

Table 21.2 CAUSES OF NEONATAL BOWEL OBSTRUCTION: PATHOLOGY

Pathogenesis	Disease
Failure of gut development	Oesophageal atresia
Failure of gut canalization	Duodenal atresia
Ischaemic involution (thrombo-embolus, volvulus, intussusception)	Small bowel atresia
Functional obstruction	
– inflammation	Necrotizing enterocolitis
– defective nerves	Hirschsprung's disease
– meconium viscosity	Meconium ileus (cystic fibrosis)

anus proximally as far as the rectosigmoid junction. Pathological confirmation of Hirschsprung's disease is obtained when biopsy of the mucosa just inside the anal canal shows absence of ganglion cells in the submucous myenteric plexuses and overgrowth of presynaptic neurofibrils in the mucosa and submucosa. (Fig. 21.2). The potential for overgrowth of pathogenic organisms in the dilated and obstructed proximal colon to produce a fulminating enterocolitis, with rapid progression to generalized sepsis and death, makes Hirschsprung's disease an important condition to diagnose early.

Necrotizing enterocolitis

Necrotizing enterocolitis is a serious, acquired abnormality of the bowel which appears to be caused by mucosal hypoxia and ischaemia in association with bacterial invasion of the gut wall by necrotizing and gas-forming organisms (Fig. 21.3). Conditions which produce perinatal stress (e.g. prematurity, obstetric misadventures, sepsis and metabolic disturbances) predispose to its development. The ischaemic mucosa is colonized by certain pathogenic bacteria which include strains of *Clostridium*. These organisms multiply within the layers of the bowel wall and produce large gas bubbles known as 'pneumatosis intestinalis' or 'intramural gas'. Further progression of the infection and ischaemia produces gangrene and perforation of the bowel, which leads rapidly to generalized sepsis and peritonitis.

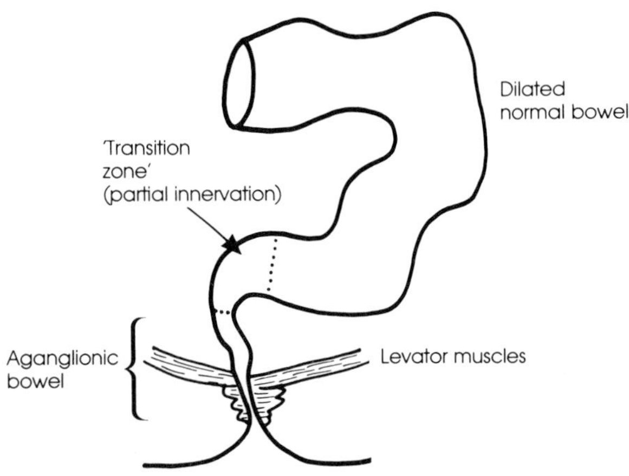

Fig. 21.1: *Hirschsprung's disease.*

Small bowel atresia

In a few patients, ileal or jejunal atresia is caused by an intrinsic abnormality in the development of the bowel, but more frequently it is believed to result from infarction of the bowel *in utero*. It is possible that, in the fetus, the cause of infarction is vascular occlusion of a segmental mesenteric vessel from thrombosis or an embolus.

In addition, mechanical mishaps, such as twisting (volvulus) of the bowel or intussusception, can lead to infarction and subsequent atresia. Vascular or mechanical abnormalities causing perforation also may produce an atresia from scarring at the site of perforation (Fig. 21.4).

Malrotation with volvulus

In the early embryo, the developing mid-gut (which will form the small bowel and the right colon) elongates in the space created by the developing umbilical cord. Progressive narrowing of the umbilical ring accompanies the acquisition of the three-dimensional structure of the embryo

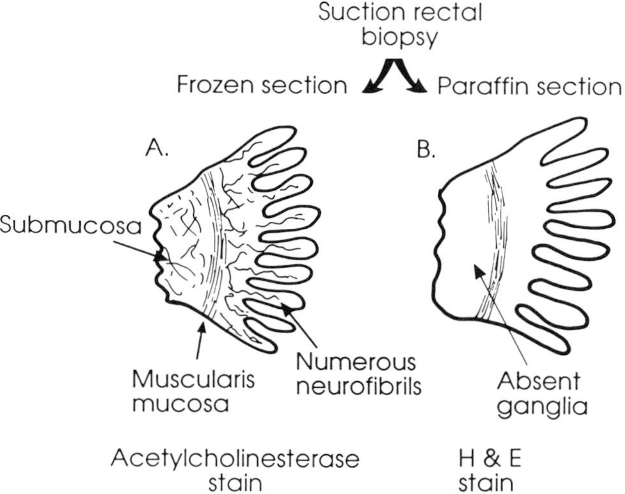

Fig. 21.2: *Pathological diagnosis of Hirschsprung's disease from a suction rectal biopsy stained with acetylcholinesterase* (A) *or* H & E (B). *Acetylcholinesterase staining reveals numerous neurofibrils ramifying in the submucosa and lamina propria.* H & E *shows that ganglion cells are absent from the rectal wall.*

and enlargement of the abdominal cavity: with this process, the right colon and small bowel return to the abdominal cavity at about 10 weeks of gestation. As the bowel continues to elongate on return to the abdomen, it undergoes rotation and fixation to the posterior abdominal wall such that its mesentery, which contains the superior mesenteric vessels, is attached along a wide base from the duodenojejunal flexure to the caecum. The colon is fixed in each flank, and the transverse colon is anchored to the stomach by the great omentum. When rotation is incomplete or ab-

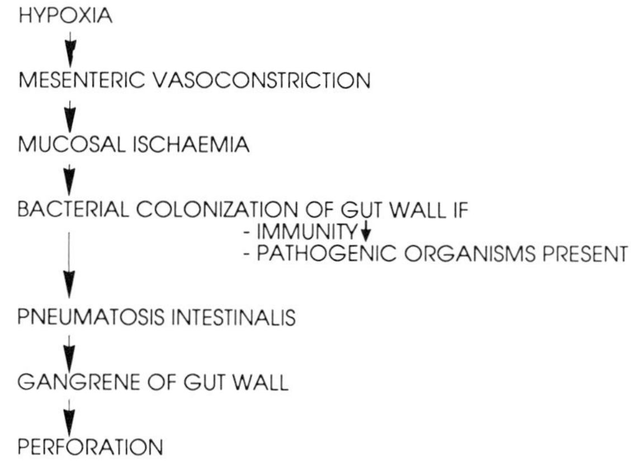

Fig. 21.3: *The pathogenesis of necrotizing enterocolitis.*

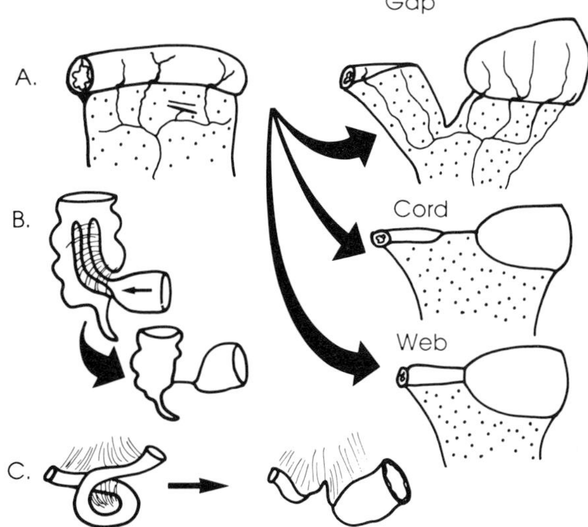

Fig. 21.4: *The pathogenesis of small bowel atresia from vessel occlusion* (A), *fetal intussusception* (B), *or fetal volvulus* (C).

normal, the bowel remains unfixed to the posterior abdominal wall (Fig. 21.5). In the common form of malrotation, the caecum is found just to the left of the midline at the base of the superior mesenteric artery. It has undergone 180° rotation from its original caudal position, but has failed to cross the midline and descend into the right iliac

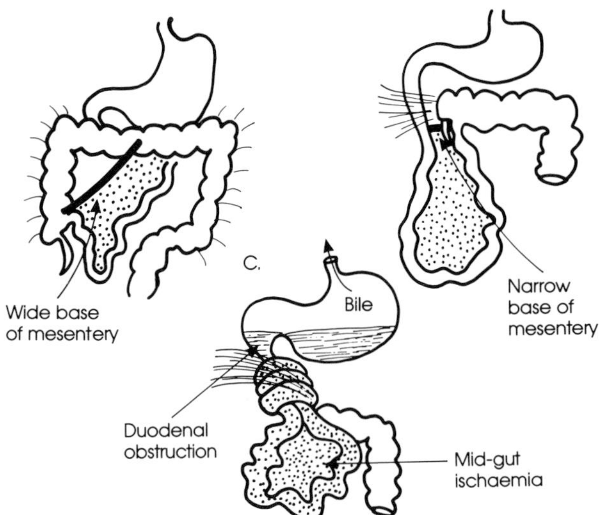

Fig. 21.5: *A comparison of normal gut fixation and rotation (A) with malrotation (B) and malrotation with secondary volvulus (C).*

fossa. In this position, the caecum may be fixed to the right lateral abdominal wall and subhepatic region by fibrous bands of condensed peritoneum which cross the non-rotated duodenum ('Ladd's bands'). This anatomical arrangement predisposes to twisting of the whole of the mid-gut on its narrow mesenteric base to cause duodenal obstruction, with or without mid-gut ischaemia. Bowel malrotation with volvulus is an extremely dangerous condition because it may lead to infarction of the entire mid-gut – a potentially fatal complication.

Duodenal atresia or stenosis

Complete or incomplete intrinsic duodenal obstruction may be caused by failure of recanalization of the duodenal lumen during early development, or by vascular insufficiency. Normally, the fore-gut lumen is transiently occluded by overgrowth of primitive mucosal cells, and subsequently recanalizes. Disturbance of this process produces atresia or stenosis in the second part of the duodenum with abnormalities of the opening of the pancreatic and bile ducts. The clinical importance of intrinsic duodenal obstruction is twofold: first, it is often difficult to distinguish from extrinsic obstruction caused by malrotation with volvulus; and secondly, it is a major abnormality of gut development which is associated with other significant abnormalities, in particular trisomy 21 (Fig. 21.6).

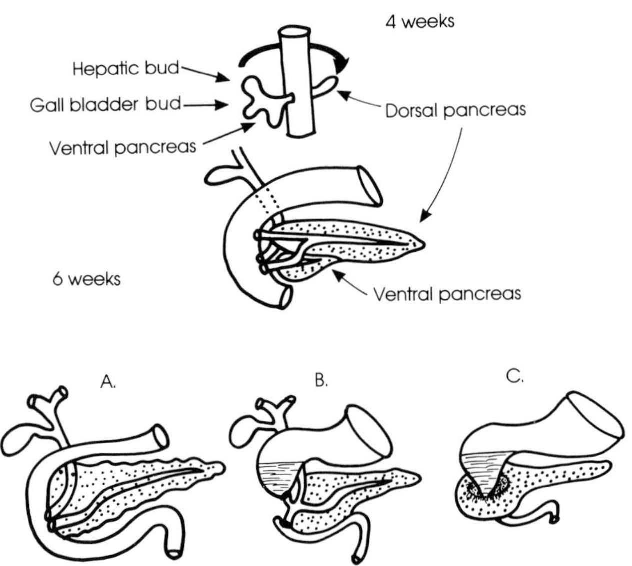

Fig. 21.6: *The pathogenesis of duodenal atresia. Normal development of the duodenum at four and six weeks. After a phase of temporary occlusion with proliferation, the normal duodenum recanalizes (A). Failure to recanalize leads to duodenal atresia (B). Failure of rotation of the ventral pancreas leads to duodenal atresia/stenosis with annular pancreas.*

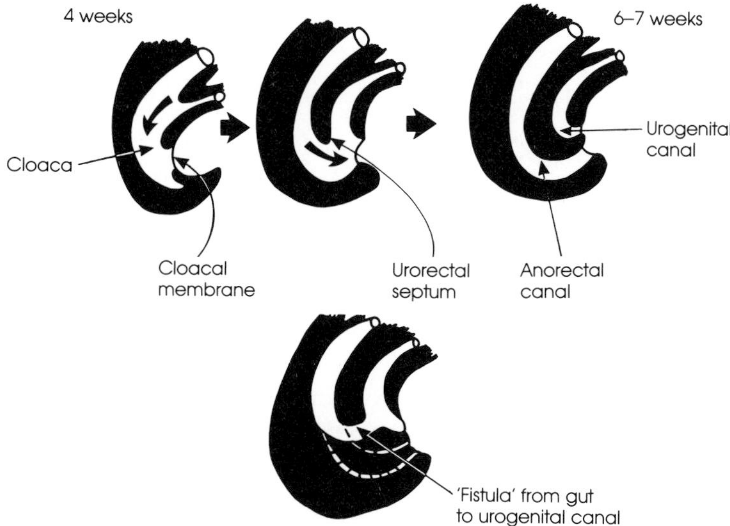

Fig. 21.7: *The normal development of the cloaca into separate anorectal and urogenital canals. Failure of the anal canal to develop is associated with incomplete separation of the gut and urogenital tract, leaving a connecting fistula in many cases.*

Anorectal malformations

Imperforate anus encompasses a complex group of anomalies in which the anal canal or rectum has failed to develop normally. The severity of the abnormality varies, ranging from a simple membranous covering over an otherwise normal anal canal to complete agenesis of the anorectum (Fig. 21.7). In most patients, there is a fistulous connection from the bowel to the perineal skin or urogenital tract, which represents failure of complete separation of the gut from the urogenital tract. The clinical problems in children with imperforate anus include identification of the site of a fistula, if present, and determination of the lowest level of the normal bowel in relation to the pelvic floor muscles and anal sphincter (Fig. 21.8). In addition, patients with imperforate anus commonly manifest multiple anomalies in other parts of the body (e.g. oesophageal atresia, cardiac defects) and significant anomalies in adjacent structures (e.g. urinary tract anomalies and sacral agenesis).

Meconium ileus

Meconium ileus is a functional disorder of the bowel in which the highly viscous meconium becomes impacted and then dehydrated, to obstruct the terminal ileum with dried meconium pellets (Fig. 21.9). It is a manifestation of the common recessive disorder of cystic fibrosis and is its first presentation in 20% of cases. The mucus produced in these patients is tenacious and sticky and makes the meconium sticky, causing obstruction of the distal small bowel lumen. Proximal to the obstruction there is massive dilatation of the proximal ileum, which may undergo secondary volvulus leading to perforation and/or atresia (Fig. 21.9).

Prenatal perforation

Perforation of the bowel *in utero* produces a distinctive form of sterile peritonitis. Leakage of meconium through a perforation initiates a chemical inflammation in the peritoneal cavity and metabolic conditions favourable to calcification. Thus, meconium peritonitis is recognized on abdominal x-ray by irregular calcification in the peritoneal cavity. The underlying abnormality may be any vascular or mechanical event which produces perforation, including (1) meconium ileus with volvulus of heavily laden loops which perforate, or with rupture of the dilated proximal

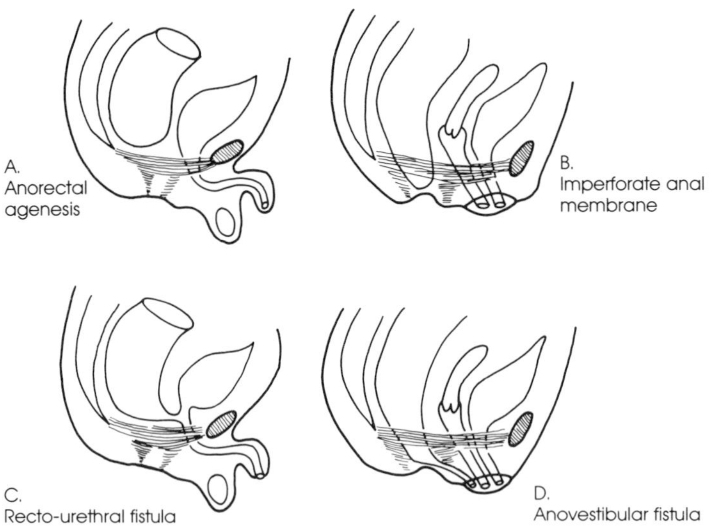

Fig. 21.8: *The four basic anorectal anomalies. In the male, anorectal agenesis occurs* (A), *but commonly is associated with a recto-urethral fistula* (C). *In females, the abnormality usually is less severe, leading to an imperforate anus with persistent cloacal membrane* (B) *or a fistula into the vestibule* (D).

ileum; (2) ischaemia and infarction of the bowel wall secondary to vascular occlusion or fetal hypoxia; and (3) intussusception with gangrene and perforation *in utero*. The timing of the perforation in relation to birth is variable, and occasionally the perforation is secondary to fetal hypoxia which may have occurred within the last few days of pregnancy. When the abnormality has occurred in the fetus at an earlier stage, the perforation seals and healing by scar formation may result in secondary bowel atresia (Fig. 21.10).

THE PRESENTATION OF BOWEL OBSTRUCTION

Three cardinal symptoms herald obstruction of the bowel in the neonate: (1) vomiting, (2) abdominal distension, and (3) failure to pass, or delay in the passage of, meconium

This triad of symptoms is similar to the presentation of bowel obstruction at other times of life. The important principle in management is to assume that, in the neonate, these symptoms represent mechanical obstruction as soon as the three non-surgical causes have been eliminated: (1) local or generalized sepsis, (2) congenital heart disease, and (3) inborn errors of metabolism with vomiting, failure to tolerate oral feeds, and even abdominal distension. Their common characteristic, which is not present in the early stages of mechanical bowel obstruction, is that the baby appears generally unwell or even severely toxic. Once these causes of vomiting have been eliminated by clinical examination, the next priority is to determine whether one of the dangerous causes of mechanical obstruction is present. These include malrotation with volvulus, perforation with meconium peritonitis, necrotizing enterocolitis and Hirschsprung's disease, all of which are potentially life-threatening conditions. Correct management of such a child includes a problem-oriented history and examination to determine the likely site and cause of obstruction, initiation of preliminary treatment or first-aid measures, and early transfer to a paediatric surgical centre. Although the surgical management will be carried out in a specialized unit, general knowledge of the important points to be obtained from the history and examination is essential for the referring clinician who is in the best position to take a full history from the parents regarding the pregnancy and perinatal period, as well as being able to document the timing and type of early symptoms.

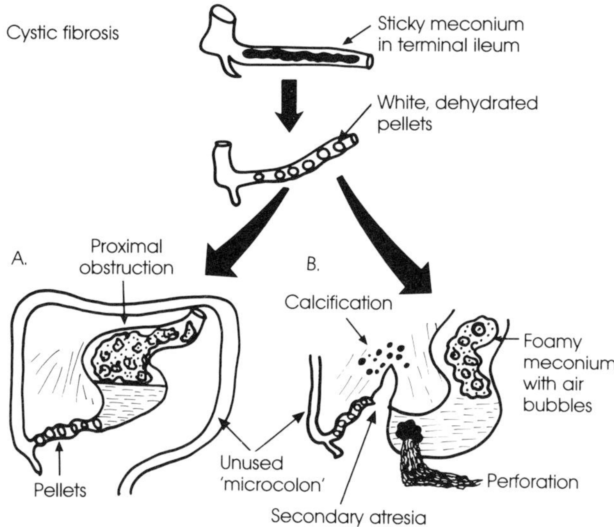

Fig. 21.9: *The aetiology of meconium ileus. The underlying problem is cystic fibrosis in most cases. Pellets of dried meconium obstruct the distal ileum, producing uncomplicated pathology* (A) *or complicated pathology* (B) *at birth. Volvulus and/or perforation is a common sequel to massive distension of the ileum.*

These features help establish the correct diagnosis.

In a neonate with bile-stained vomiting, abdominal distension and failure to pass meconium, the apparent urgency of the clinical situation may lead to the infant's transfer to a surgical centre before proper initial evaluation. However, the clinician should elicit several important points from the obstetric history: (1) details of obstetric problems, including antepartum haemorrhage or pre-eclamptic toxaemia, as these may predispose to fetal hypoxia and secondary gut perforation; (2) details of prenatal screening tests, particularly ultrasound in the second trimester, which may have detected an abnormality; (3) the presence or absence of hydramnios, since swallowed amniotic fluid is absorbed in the distal jejunum. If there is a congenital obstruction in the proximal jejunum, duodenum or oesophagus, there will be significant polyhydramnios. Obstruction distal to the mid-jejunum is unlikely to be associated with polyhydramnios.

A family history of other children with cystic fibrosis, an earlier baby with meconium ileus or a history of Hirschsprung's disease in siblings or parents, is further useful information.

The timing of onset of symptoms provides a clue to the diagnosis since most anatomical obstructions present with symptoms or signs at birth or within the first 48 hours, whereas the functional obstructions, such as Hirschsprung's disease and necrotizing enterocolitis, usually present after the first 48 hours (Fig. 21.11) since they do not cause obstruction *in utero*.

Details of the presenting signs and symptoms may be useful. Vomiting of milk which after a

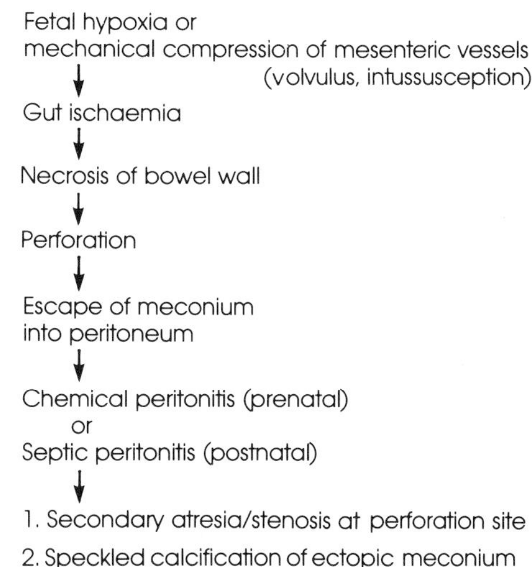

Fig. 21.10: *The pathogenesis of meconium peritonitis (perforation* in utero).

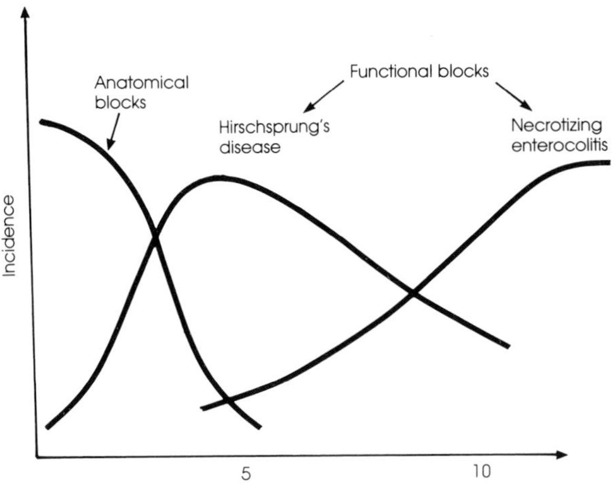

Fig. 21.11: *The incidence of different causes of obstruction compared with the age at presentation. Anatomical causes of obstruction present earlier because they have been present before birth. Functional obstructions cause symptoms and signs after birth.*

period becomes bile-stained, is more likely to be associated with obstruction of the small bowel or colon than when bile-stained vomiting is the initial feature. In this latter situation, the diagnosis favours duodenal obstruction, with the important cause being malrotation with volvulus. In fact, any child who presents with green vomitus as the initial symptom, should be regarded as having malrotation with volvulus until proven otherwise (Fig. 21.12).

Abdominal distension, when present at birth, suggests small bowel obstruction and is typical of meconium ileus. (Fig. 21.13). High obstructions, such as oesophageal atresia, duodenal atresia or malrotation with volvulus and secondary duodenal obstruction, in most instances are not associated with abdominal distension. More distal causes of obstruction, such as imperforate anus, Hirschsprung's disease or necrotizing enterocolitis, do not present with abdominal distension at birth. There are two exceptions to these general principles. First, in oesophageal atresia, marked gaseous abdominal distension may occur from passage of air down a distal tracheo-oesophageal fistula, particularly if the neonate is ventilated for respiratory distress. Positive airway pressure forces gas down the fistula into the stomach and small bowel, and the abdomen rapidly becomes tympanitic and distended. The second exception is malrotation with volvulus, where abdominal distension develops after the volvulus causes obstruction of both the duodenal and colonic ends of the mid-gut. Vascular insufficiency and ischaemia cause fluid to accumulate in the mid-gut lumen, which becomes dramatically distended and exhibits signs of peritoneal irritation.

The first passage of meconium after birth is an important indicator not only of the continuity of

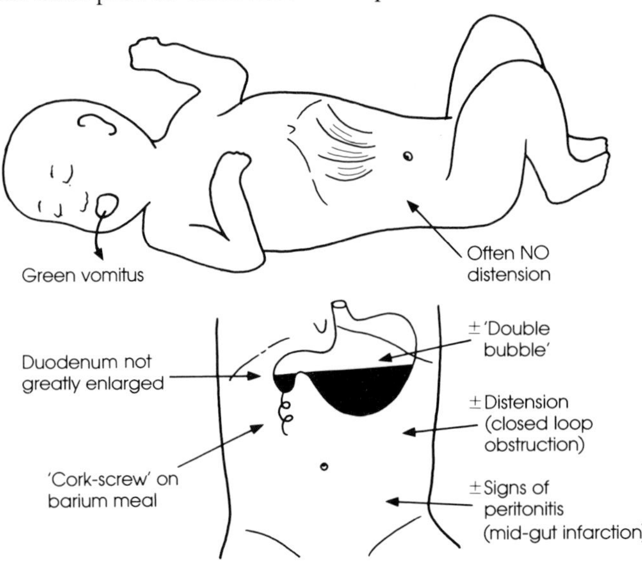

Fig. 21.12: *The clinical picture in malrotation with volvulus.*

the gastro-intestinal tract, but also of its functional competence. One of the cardinal symptoms of Hirschsprung's disease is failure to pass meconium within the first 24 hours of birth. In 90% of normal children, meconium is passed within 12 hours, while in 99%, meconium is passed by 24 hours. In premature or very sick neonates, passage of meconium may be delayed, but even in these the diagnosis of Hirschsprung's disease should be considered.

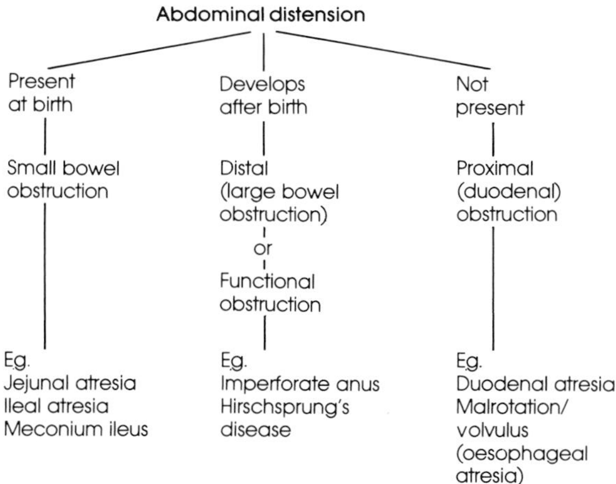

Fig. 21.13: *The relationship of abdominal distension to underlying causes of obstruction.*

PHYSICAL EXAMINATION

When one of the three cardinal signs of bowel obstruction is present, the clinician's first role is to determine whether obstruction is truly present. This is done by collecting all the historical evidence and looking for physical signs of obstruction. Early and extreme abdominal distension, associated with failure to pass meconium, suggests long-standing and complete obstruction. By contrast, moderate or mild distension appearing some days after birth suggests either functional or incomplete obstruction. Where the clinical evidence indicates a bowel obstruction, the next step is to determine the level of obstruction, as this will provide an important clue to the underlying cause.

General examination of the baby should include inspection of the vomitus or nasogastric aspirate to determine whether it contains bile or blood. Acute gastritis caused by accumulation of acid in high obstructions (e.g. duodenal atresia) may present with blood in the vomitus. Observation of the abdomen will determine the degree, extent and location of distension. Duodenal obstruction

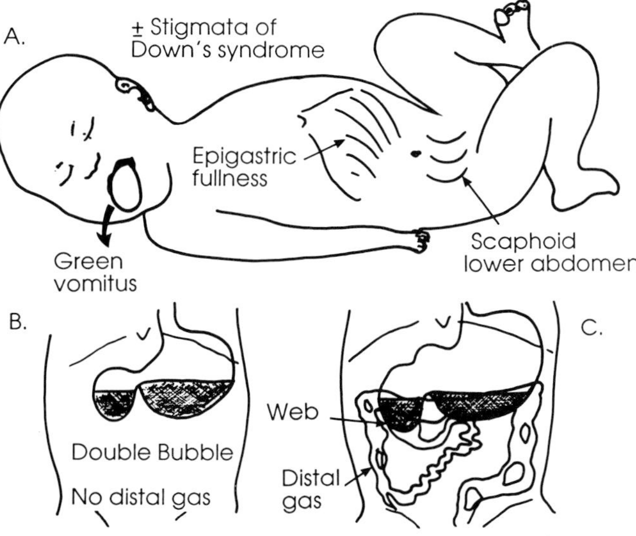

Fig. 21.14: *The clinical picture in duodenal atresia* (A & B) *or duodenal stenosis* (C).

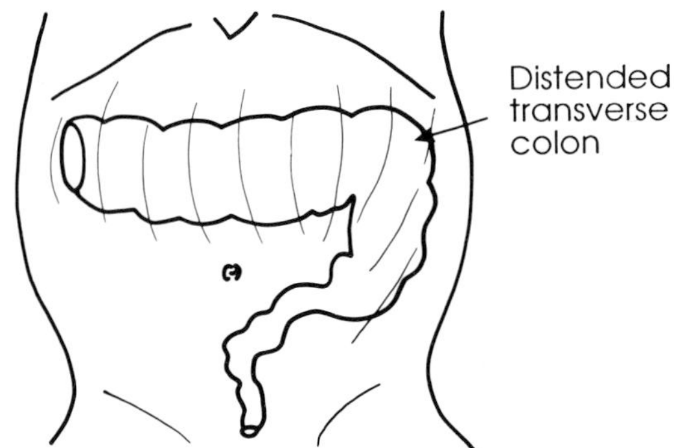

Fig. 21.15: *The first sign in Hirschsprung's disease may be dilatation of the transverse colon, which may be palpated before generalized distension occurs.*

produces epigastric fullness, with a scaphoid lower abdomen (Figs. 21.12 and 21.14). Hirschsprung's disease occasionally presents with dilatation of the colon several days before the small bowel becomes dilated (Fig. 21.15). Volvulus with duodenal obstruction alone presents with a scaphoid abdomen, while distension of the ischaemic small bowel causes generalized distension. Unrelated abnormalities, such as massive hydronephrosis, ovarian cyst or enlargement of a solid organ (e.g. hepatoblastoma), must be considered also, because these may all present with abdominal distension. Percussion of the abdomen determines that the distension is from dilated loops full of air, and should also determine whether the normal area of liver dullness is present, since its absence may be a sign of perforation.

Two important tests should be carried out to exclude oesophageal atresia and imperforate anus. The first involves passage of a 10F catheter through the mouth to test oesophageal patency (see Chapter 20). If oesophageal atresia is present, the tube will be arrested about 10 cm from the gums. The second is to examine the perineum carefully, since even an imperforate anus may appear normal at first glance. Rectal examination should be performed with either the little finger or a thermometer to diagnose anal stenosis or atresia. It might also be useful in the diagnosis of Hirschsprung's disease where dilatation of the anal canal on rectal examination commonly induces reflex evacuation of the colon, even if the tip of the examining finger does not reach the dilated, ganglionated bowel. The sudden gush of air and meconium which follows removal of the examining finger from a child with delayed passage of meconium and abdominal distension, is highly suggestive that the underlying diagnosis is Hirschsprung's disease.

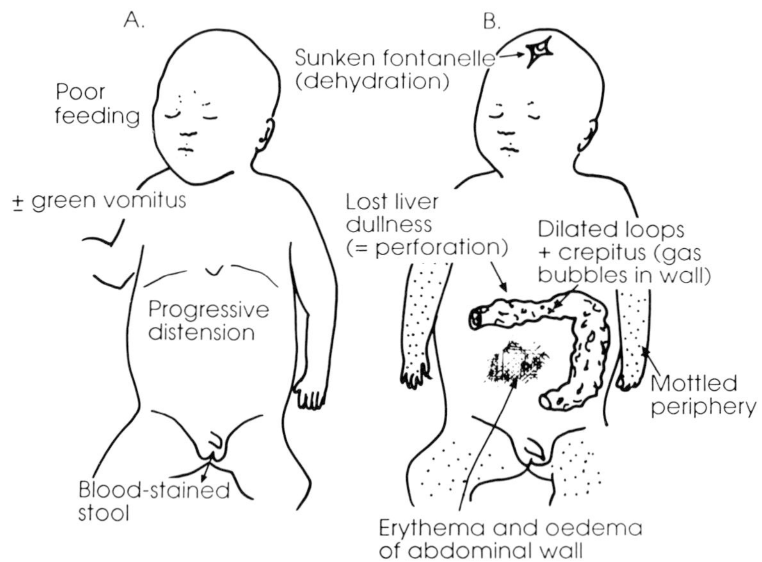

Fig. 21.16: *The clinical picture in early (A) or late (B) necrotizing enterocolitis. At both stages there is abdominal tenderness.*

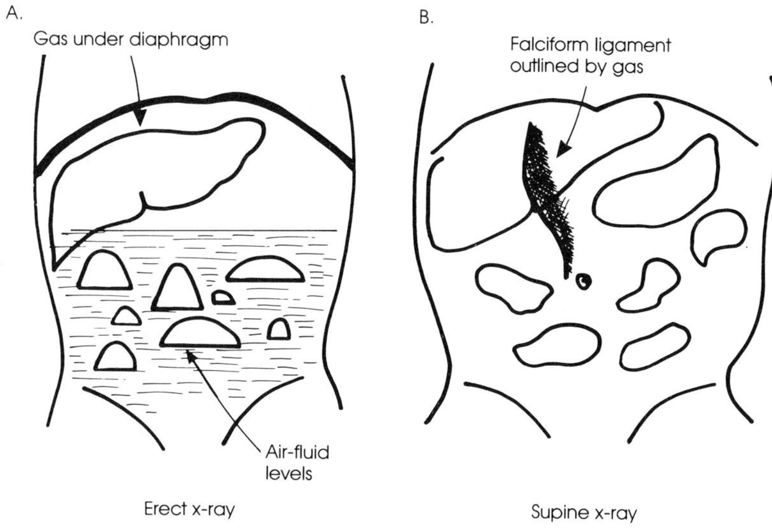

Fig. 21.17: *The features on abdominal x-ray of gut perforation leading to free intraperitoneal gas with or without bowel obstruction.*

Once the presence of a bowel obstruction has been confirmed, two important questions must be answered to determine the urgency of the situation: (1) 'Is there ischaemia of the bowel?'; and (2) 'Is there evidence of perforation?' Gangrene of the gut wall with or without perforation will produce signs of peritonitis. These include abdominal tenderness and guarding, discoloration of the abdominal wall (because it is so thin) and signs of sepsis and shock (Fig. 21.16). The abdomen becomes tight and shiny, with progressive oedema and redness of the abdominal wall. In addition, if there is a persistent perforation, the presence of free gas can be determined by the absence of liver dullness on percussion and by the presence of free gas on the abdominal x-rays. It is important to take an erect or lateral decubitus x-ray, as well as a supine film, to demonstrate free gas in the peritoneal cavity (Fig. 21.17).

What effect does obstruction have on other

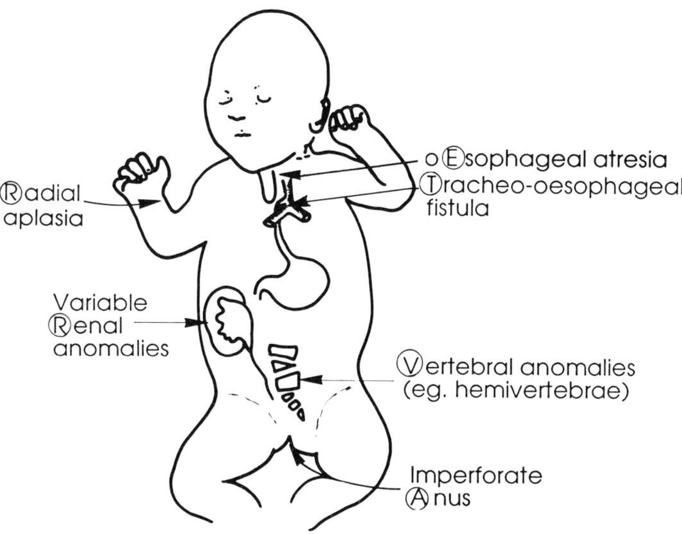

Fig. 21.18: *The clinical features of the* VATER *association.*

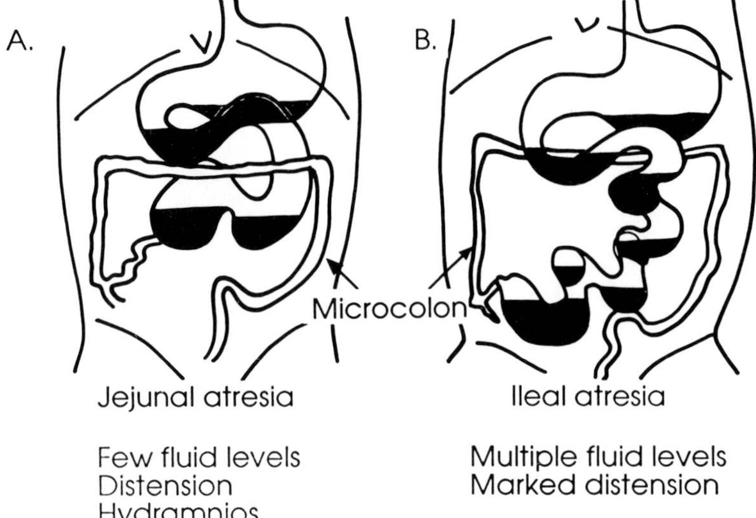

Fig. 21.19: *The clinical and x-ray features of high small bowel (jejunal) atresia (A), compared with low small bowel (ileal) atresia (B).*

areas in the baby? The two systemic effects of neonatal obstruction are respiratory embarrassment from splinting of the diaphragm by the severe abdominal distension, and septicaemia with supervening circulatory collapse secondary to gut gangrene or perforation.

What other abnormalities are present? Some causes of bowel obstruction are associated with important major anomalies elsewhere in the baby. Duodenal atresia is associated commonly with Down's syndrome, and imperforate anus is associated with a range of abnormalities commonly called the 'VATER' association, which includes vertebral, anal, tracheo-oesophageal, cardiac, radial and renal abnormalities (Fig. 21.18).

Abdominal x-rays complement the clinical assessment of the type and level of obstruction, and provide some additional information such as the presence of intraperitoneal calcification in prenatal perforation and intramural gas bubbles in necrotizing enterocolitis. The number and distribution of dilated loops may allow differentiation between high and low bowel obstruction, although the small and large bowel cannot be distinguished readily on x-ray in the neonate (Fig. 21.19). In many instances, the only sure way to determine whether the colon is distended is to perform a barium enema to look for a microcolon. In this situation, the colon is narrow because it has not been stretched by intraluminal contents. Microcolon implies obstruction proximal to the colon rather than an abnormality of the colon itself.

GOLDEN RULES

(1) Green vomitus should be regarded as a potential emergency because of the likelihood of mechanical obstruction and ischaemic damage to the bowel (malrotation with volvulus).
(2) Obstruction of the duodenum should be treated as malrotation with volvulus unless proven otherwise.
(3) Obstruction occurring *after* the evacuation of normal meconium is likely to be (i) malrotation with volvulus, (ii) Hirschsprung's disease, or (iii) necrotizing enterocolitis – all of which are potentially fatal.
(4) Absence of liver dullness in an infant with a distended abdomen indicates perforation.
(5) Hirschsprung's disease should be suspected if a baby fails to pass meconium in the first 24 hours.

22 Ambiguous genitalia: Is it a boy or a girl?

Abnormalities of sexual development present as a wide spectrum of physical appearances ranging from normal female to normal male. This chapter provides a practical approach to the assessment and diagnosis at first presentation rather than emphasizing the pathological classification. The most important intersex abnormality is congenital adrenal hyperplasia because of its frequency and its association with life-threatening vomiting and dehydration shortly after birth.

NORMAL SEXUAL DEVELOPMENT

All embryos are formed with the capacity to differentiate into either a male or a female. At eight weeks of gestation, the urogenital ridge contains a primitive gonad and two ducts. The mesonephric duct (Wolffian duct) forms the vas deferens, and the paramesonephric duct (Müllerian duct) forms the Fallopian tube, uterus and upper vagina.

The two sexes do not form equally: development of the female internal and external genitalia is passive and occurs in the absence of hormones, whereas development of male structures is controlled actively by the hormones secreted by the testes (Fig. 22.1). When a Y chromosome is present, the gonad develops into a testis at eight weeks of gestation and begins to secrete two hormones, an androgen (testosterone) and a glycoprotein (Müllerian inhibiting substance). Testosterone stimulates the Wolffian or 'male' duct to develop into a vas, epididymis and seminal vesicle: in its absence, the Wolffian duct regresses. Müllerian inhibiting substance causes active regression of the Müllerian or 'female' ducts. Without a Y chromosome, the gonad develops into an ovary which secretes low levels of oestrogen during development. In the absence of Müllerian inhibiting substance, the Müllerian ducts form the fallopian tubes, the uterus and upper third of the vagina – the latter two by fusion of the caudal ends of the ducts. In the female embryo, the Wolffian duct undergoes passive regression (Fig. 22.1).

The early development of the external genitalia is the same in both sexes (Fig. 22.2). The cloacal membrane is surrounded by an inner genital fold and a genital tubercle anteriorly. Lateral to the inner genital folds are the outer genital folds, which form either the scrotum or the labia majora. Fusion of the central region of the inner genital folds divides the cloaca into an anterior urogenital membrane and a posterior anal membrane.

Development from eight to 10 weeks' gestation differs between the sexes and is dependent on the presence of testosterone. If testosterone is present (i.e. male or abnormal female), the inner genital folds fuse superficially over the urogenital sinus to form the male urethra, while fusion of the outer genital folds forms the scrotum. Enlargement of the genital tubercle forms the penis. The degree of fusion of inner and outer genital folds is directly related to the level of androgens. In the female,

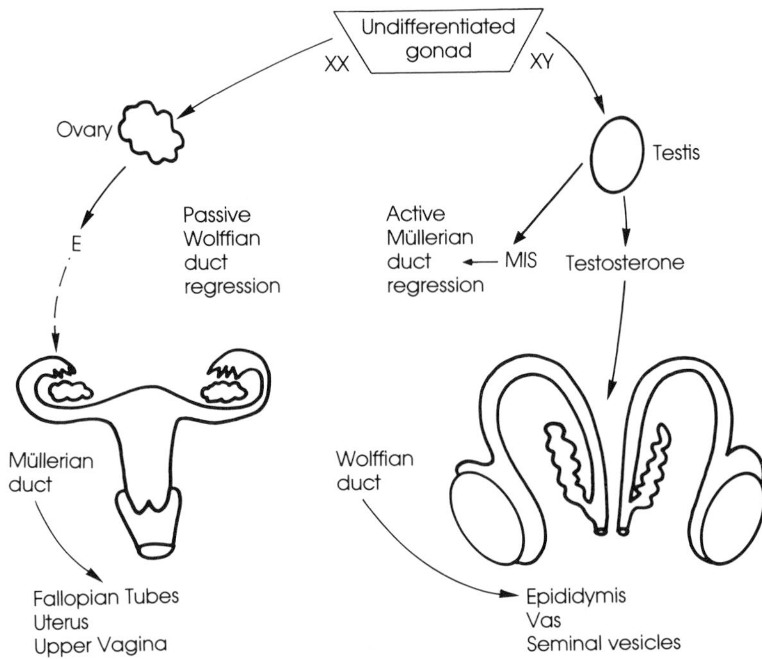

Fig. 22.1: *Sexual differentiation of the internal genital ducts under the influence of oestrogen* (E), *Müllerian inhibiting substance* (MIS) *or testosterone.*

where androgen levels are extremely low, the urogenital membrane breaks down to form the urethral and vaginal openings, and the genital tubercle does not enlarge. The inner genital folds remain separated to form the labia minora, while the outer folds enlarge to form the labia majora. The genital tubercle, which forms the clitoris, remains small and is usually hidden by growth of the genital folds. Although oestrogenic hormones are present in the female embryo, they are not important in the development of the external genitalia. Therefore, if testosterone is absent or unable to function, the external genitalia will have a female appearance even in a genetically male fetus.

Because male development is actively controlled, several important principles useful in clinical practice can be derived.

(1) Any degree of virilization of the external genitalia is proof of androgen secretion, which may be normal or abnormal.
(2) The presence of a vas or epididymis is proof of androgen secretion at an early stage of development, since this implies that the Wolffian duct has been actively stimulated.
(3) Regression of the Müllerian duct is proof of the presence of functional testicular tissue, which has produced Müllerian inhibiting substance.

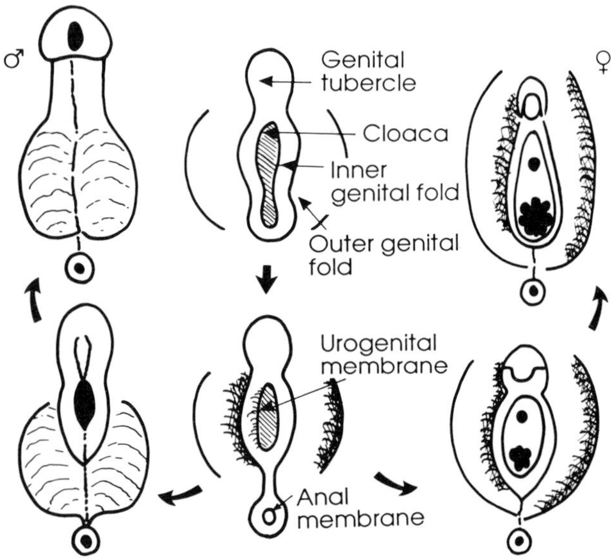

Fig. 22.2: *Sexual differentiation of external genitalia.*

ABNORMAL SEXUAL DEVELOPMENT – AMBIGUOUS GENITALIA

The common conditions which cause ambiguous genitalia are shown in Table 22.1.

Table 22.1 COMMON CAUSES OF ABNORMAL SEXUAL DEVELOPMENT

Congenital adrenal hyperplasia (adrenogenital syndrome)
Dysplastic ovaries (Turner's syndrome)
Dysplastic testes – symmetrical
– asymmetrical (mosaic: mixed gonadal dysgenesis)
Androgen insensitivity (testicular feminization syndrome)
– complete
– incomplete

Congenital adrenal hyperplasia (adrenogenital syndrome)

In congenital adrenal hyperplasia, the most important and common abnormality of intersex, the female embryo is virilized by abnormal androgens. Congenital adrenal hyperplasia does occur as commonly in males, but the excess adrenal androgens do not interfere with sexual development. An enzyme block in the conversion of cholesterol to cortisol and aldosterone causes low levels of cortisol in the blood of the fetus. This reduces the normal feedback inhibition of the hypothalamic secretion of corticotrophin-releasing factor. Consequently, the hypothalamus secretes abnormally high amounts of corticotrophin-releasing factor, thus stimulating the pituitary to produce excessive adrenocorticotrophic hormone (ACTH) and melanin-stimulating hormone. The high levels of ACTH stimulate the enzymes in the pathway for cortisol synthesis, leading to hypertrophy of the fetal adrenals. The usual enzyme deficiency which prevents cortisol from being produced, diverts precursor molecules into side pathways which lead to androgen synthesis. This abnormal androgen synthesis in the presence of excess adrenal function leads to the virilization of female embryos. Lack of aldosterone, which occurs in some enzyme deficiencies, causes loss of sodium chloride from the kidney and leads to severe dehydration. Failure of cortisol secretion produces an infant with low resistance to stress, so that even trivial infections will induce severe vomiting, diarrhoea and dehydration. Occasionally, less usual enzyme deficiencies lead to excess production of deoxycorticosterone and induce hypertension (Fig. 22.3).

Dysplastic ovaries (Turner's syndrome)

The other intersex abnormality common in females is failure of ovarian development caused by Turner's syndrome, but in these children the external genitalia are normal female because external genitalia will develop a female appearance in the absence of any hormone. Babies with Turner's syndrome may be identified clinically by growth retardation and a webbed neck. The fetal lymphatics in Turner's syndrome are abnormal: lymphangiomatous development, which occurs in the cervical lymphatics, leads to the redundant folds of skin of the neck. Lymphangiomatous maldevelopment elsewhere in the fetus with Turner's syndrome may be seen on the dorsum of the hands and feet. Therefore, a baby born with oedematous or puffy feet should be investigated for Turner's

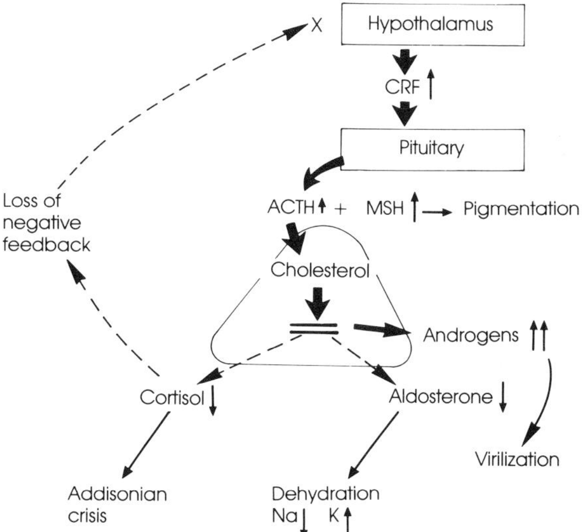

Fig. 22.3: *Biochemical abnormalities in the common forms of congenital adrenal hyperplasia.*

syndrome if the genitalia are normal female in appearance.

Dysplastic testes

Intersex disorders may be produced by dysplastic testes. One or both testes may be affected. When both testes are dysplastic, deficiency of androgen may cause incomplete virilization of the external genitalia, and deficiency of Müllerian inhibiting substance may allow preservation of Müllerian duct structures. Usually, both gonads are undescended because they are unable to secrete the hormone(s) necessary for testicular descent.

Ambiguous asymmetrical genitalia

In the asymmetrical form of dysplastic testes (known as mixed gonadal dysgenesis), one gonad may be a testis which has descended with preservation of the Wolffian duct on that side and local regression of the Müllerian duct. The more dysplastic testis usually remains in the abdomen and is unable to cause regression of the Müllerian duct or preservation of the Wolffian duct. The external genitalia show some virilization with one palpable testis. Children with mixed gonadal dysgenesis may appear to be males with severe hypospadias and one palpable testis. It is an important abnormality to identify, since the dysplastic testes have a significantly increased risk of malignant degeneration. Even though the chromosomes may be male and the gonads are at least partly testicular, these children are almost always best reared as females after gonadal excision.

Androgen insensitivity

Infants with a normal male chromosome pattern but with insensitivity to androgens have a genetic abnormality in the androgen receptor system. This prevents the normal target tissues, such as the Wolffian duct and external genitalia, from responding to androgen stimulation. The abnormality may be partial or complete, and in the complete syndrome (testicular feminization syndrome), the external genitalia are completely female in appearance. Commonly, the clue that the gonads are really testes is their discovery in inguinal herniae. The normal secretion and response to Müllerian inhibiting substance leads to complete regression of the Müllerian duct, while inability to respond to androgens prevents the development of the Wolffian duct into a vas. Thus, there is an absence of internal genital ducts. The failure of the tissues to respond to testosterone prevents complete descent of the testes. Infants with incomplete androgen sensitivity have incomplete virilization of the external genitalia, but the testes are palpable usually in the groin or labioscrotal folds.

THE CLINICAL PRESENTATION OF INTERSEX

Intersex disorders present with three basic types of ambiguous genitalia at birth: female appearance but with an enlarged clitoris; indeterminate genitalia which appear half female/half male; and male appearance, but with hypospadias and impalpable gonads (Table 22.2). Infants with obviously ambiguous genitalia have the LEAST risk of an error being made in the neonatal period, because the attending physician is unable to assign a sex and refers the child for further investigation. The children at greatest risk are those with enlargement of the clitoris where the anatomy appears to be 'female', and those with hypospadias and 'undescended testes' where the anatomy appears to be 'male'. In these two groups, there is strong pressure on the attending physician to assign the sex which is closest to the appearance of the genitalia. This is a serious mistake which may lead to the death of the child, should it be unfortunate enough to have salt-losing congenital adrenal hyperplasia. There is also a risk that the sex chosen for the child is inappropriate once the internal anatomy becomes known.

With clitoral enlargement alone, the genitalia

Table 22.2 CLINICAL PRESENTATIONS OF INTERSEX

'Clitoral enlargement'
Ambiguous genitalia
'Hypospadias with impalpable testes'

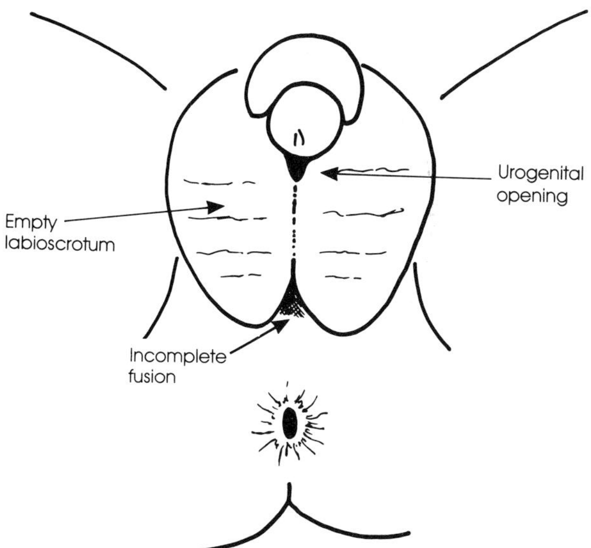

Fig. 22.4: *The appearance of minimally virilized ambiguous genitalia when the phallus is larger than in a normal girl, but no gonads are palpable.*

still look more or less female (Fig. 22.4). Occasionally, the enlarged phallus may not be visible initially, as shown in Figure 22.5. The clitoris is in the normal position but is much larger than normal. From the outside it may not be obvious, but separation of the labia will reveal the enlarged phallus and some degree of urogenital fusion, and the labia may show evidence of androgenic stimulation with wrinkling, reminiscent of the scrotum. Clitoral enlargement is an important physical sign, since the child is likely to have congenital adrenal hyperplasia.

The infant with apparent hypospadias and impalpable testes may appear as in Figure 22.6 or 22.7. When no testes are palpable, it is important to exclude severe virilizing congenital adrenal hyperplasia or one of the causes of dysplastic testes. Since both are best treated by raising the baby as a female, it is extremely important that this appearance is not assumed to be male. Occasionally, the hypospadias is in association with a single palpable gonad. Although this may be a male with a simple undescended testis, it is important to exclude the asymmetrical form of dysplastic testes known as mixed gonadal dysgenesis, since such a child is usually best reared as a female.

CLINICAL EXAMINATION

Ideally, the diagnosis of intersex should be recognized immediately after delivery of the child, and the attending physician should not be tempted to assign the sex most closely representing the anatomy. An antenatal history will exclude the possibility of the mother having ingested drugs which might cause androgenic stimulation. There may be other children in the family with abnormalities of sexual development, such as androgen insensitivity or congenital adrenal hyperplasia

Physical examination of the baby includes an assessment of the general condition, looking for signs of adrenal insufficiency – dehydration, wasting and poor temperature control. The skin should be carefully examined for evidence of excess pigmentation, which is common in congenital adrenal hyperplasia because of the excess melanin-stimulating hormone produced by the pituitary. The pigmentation is commonly in the genital or perianal skin, nipples, palmar creases and knuckles. The body may show a general

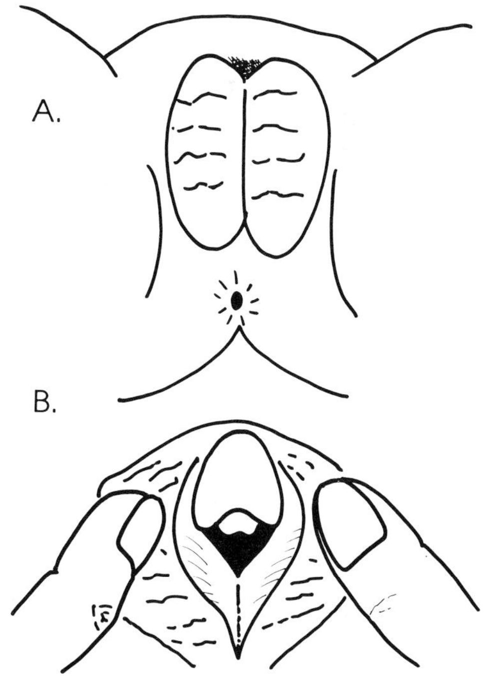

Fig. 22.5: *The genital appearance when the enlarged phallus is concealed by the wrinkled labia* (A). *Separation of the labia reveals the phallus along with partial fusion of the urogenital folds* (B).

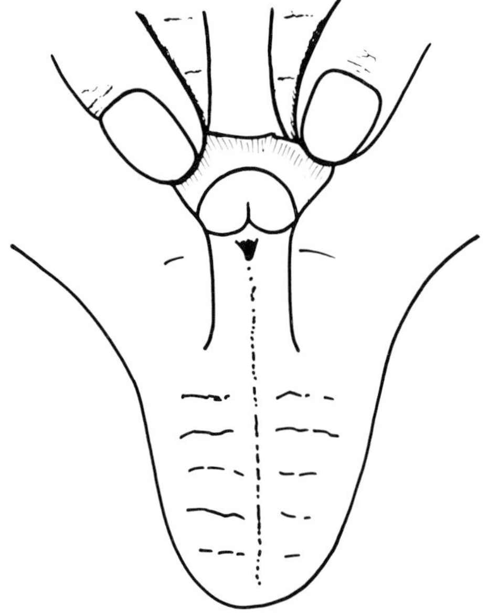

Fig. 22.6: *The appearance of significantly virilized genitalia which mimic 'hypospadias and impalpable testes'.*

increase in melanin pigmentation, including freckles. Darkly pigmented genitalia are especially suggestive of adrenal hyperplasia, allowing for racial characteristics.

The external genitalia should be examined to determine: (1) the size of the phallus; (2) the degree of fusion of the inner genital folds to form a urethra; and (3) the degree of outer genital fold fusion to form a scrotum, with its characteristic-

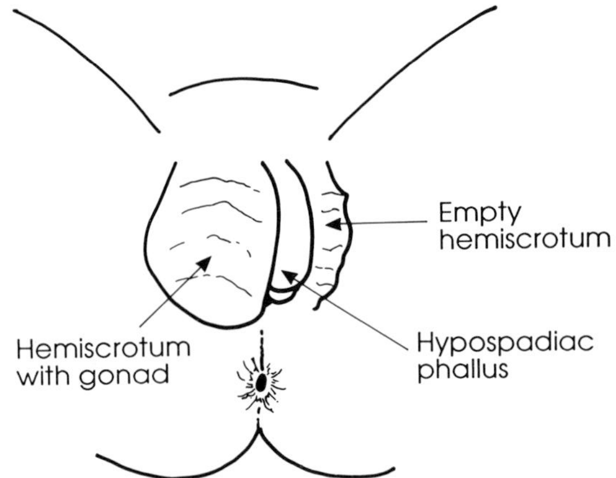

Fig. 22.7: *Asymmetrical dysgenesis of the testes commonly has asymmetrical external genitalia with one descended and one impalpable testis, along with variable deficiency in virilization.*

ally wrinkled skin (Fig. 22.8). Any degree of virilization indicates exposure to androgenic hormones, but does not prove that the child is a genetic male, even if masculinization is extreme. The phallus is lifted up to expose its ventral surface, and the genital folds are spread apart with the fingers: the position of the urethral orifice can be identified and the degree of urogenital fusion estimated (Fig. 22.9).

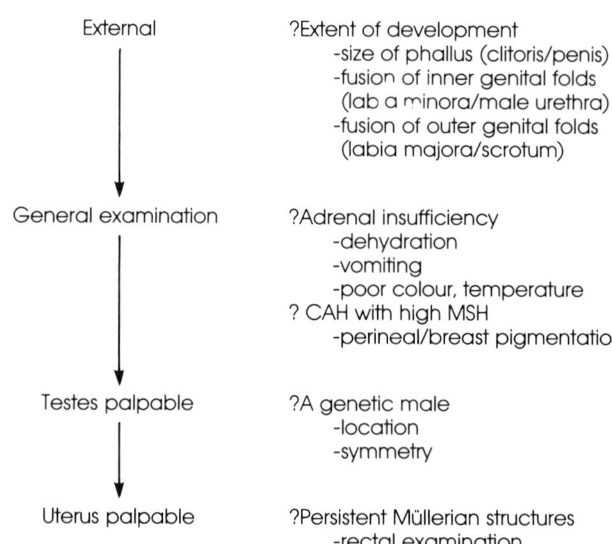

Fig. 22.8: *The clinical examination of a child with ambiguous genitalia.* (CAH = *Congenital adrenal hyperplasia*)

The next step is to determine whether there are palpable gonads. The labioscrotal folds need to be palpated carefully for the presence of testes, as do the regions around the external inguinal ring. The presence of two palpable testes in the scrotum indicates that not only is the underlying sex of the child male, but also there has been sufficient androgen stimulation to cause testicular descent. In such cases, the sex of rearing is appropriately male with later surgical reconstruction (hypospadias repair).

If there are no testes palpable in the groins or labioscrotal folds, the next step in the clinical examination is to determine the presence of a uterus. A cervix may be palpable on rectal exam-

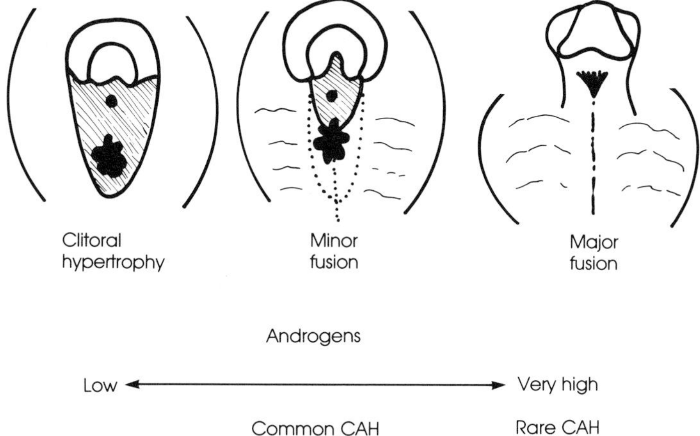

Fig. 22.9: *The degree of virilization is proportional to the amount of urogenital fusion (and phallus size). Increasing amounts of androgens stimulate development of a penile urethra. Severe virilization can occur, but is rare in congenital adrenal hyperplasia (CAH).*

ination with the little finger (Fig. 22.10). The presence of a uterus implies that there has been either absent or insufficient Müllerian inhibiting substance – as may occur in a female with androgen-stimulated virilization, or where there are very dysplastic testes. The presence of a uterus means that female reconstruction is likely to be successful. This is an important surgical consideration, since it is much easier to reduce the phallus and separate the labioscrotal folds to form female genitals, than it is to augment the phallus to make a penis. The presence of a uterus and vagina allows normal female sexual function, which is preferable to male reconstruction if the result is a penis too small for normal sexual function.

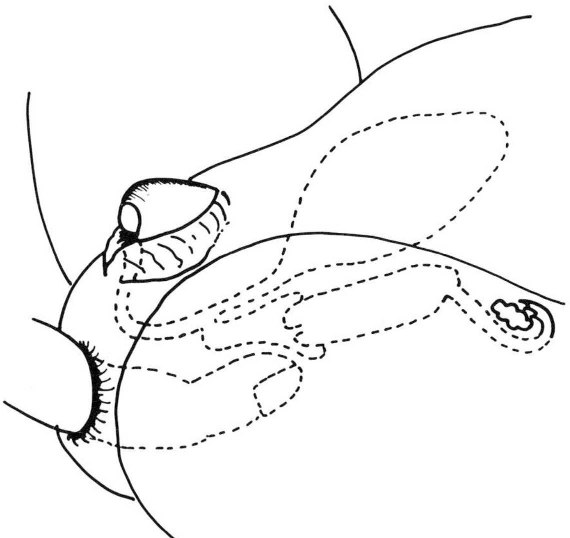

Fig. 22.10: *Rectal examination in babies with ambiguous genitalia: is a uterus palpable?*

A child with congenital adrenal hyperplasia usually will demonstrate a recognizable pattern of clinical signs (Fig. 22.11). There is vomiting which may suggest gastro-enteritis. The child is thin and dehydrated, depending on the degree of salt loss and whether the diagnosis has been made immediately after birth or has been delayed. The nipples, skin creases and genitalia may be pigmented. The melanin pigmentation gives the appearance of a suntan to the affected areas. Virilization of the external genitalia is proportional to the degree of urogenital fusion (Fig. 22.9): the concentrations and potency of androgens present in the fetus determine the size of the phallus and the development of a male type of urethra. Low levels of androgens occurring late in gestation will lead only to clitoral hypertrophy, since this is the last part of the external genitalia to develop. Higher levels of androgens produced earlier in gestation cause fusion of the urogenital folds which cover the introitus. In rare forms of adrenogenital syndrome in which very high levels of androgens are produced at the time of sexual differentiation, the external genitalia may be completely masculinized, producing a very large phal-

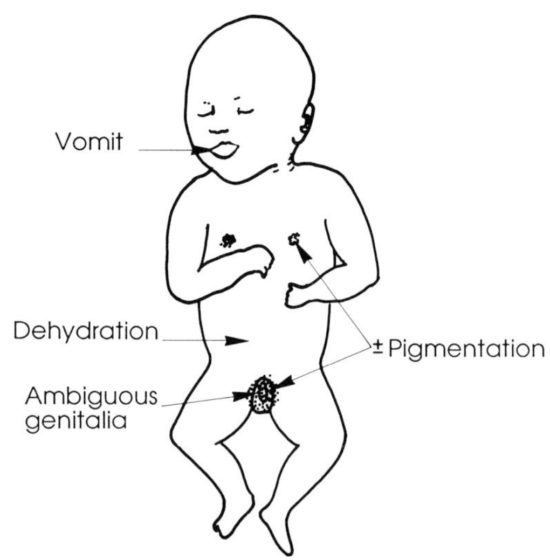

Fig. 22.11: *The child with congenital adrenal hyperplasia presents with ambiguous genitalia and signs and symptoms of adrenal insufficiency or excess melanin-stimulating hormone.*

lus identical to a penis (and containing a penile urethra) and a short upper vagina which opens into the posterior urethra. The only clue to the true sex of the child is the absence of the testes. The common form of anatomy in children with congenital adrenal hyperplasia is shown in Figure 22.12. The urogenital fusion causes partial covering of the introitus beneath which there is a normal uterus and vagina.

INVESTIGATION

Any child born with ambiguous genitalia should be referred for immediate investigation, including chromosome analysis, electrolyte estimation (for evidence of low sodium and high potassium concentrations in the serum), blood glucose concentrations (hypoglycaemia is commonly associated with adrenal hyperplasia), and 17-hydroxyprogesterone concentrations in order positively to identify children with the common form of adrenal hyperplasia. Urinary gas-liquid chromatography may show some of the less common forms of abnormal steroid production. In addition, an urgent urogenital sinugram, with or without endoscopy, needs to be performed to delineate the anatomy of the urethra and possible vagina, while a pelvic ultrasound confirms the presence of a uterus. Occasionally, laparoscopy or even laparotomy and gonadal biopsy, may be required. The sex of the child needs to be determined as quickly as possible, but this can be done only after consultation and proper investigation.

ABSENT VAGINA

This is a frequent concern of mothers of normally feminized infants: during washing or a change of nappy, the mother notices that the introitus cannot be seen. She assumes that the girl has an absent vagina, and seeks immediate medical opinion. The usual diagnosis in this circumstance is labial adhesion, although true atresia of the vagina does occur.

Labial adhesion is thought to be secondary to inflammation and ulceration of the labia minora in an infant with ammoniacal dermatitis. When the labia re-epithelialize, the two sides of the introitus become stuck together by bridging of the new epithelium. Although some authors have suggested that this could be a congenital abnormality, it is seen in infancy or early childhood but not at birth. Moreover, the fusion of the labia is quite different from the fusion seen in females exposed to virilizing androgens. The labia can be separated by simple traction or by pushing a thermometer posteriorly between them.

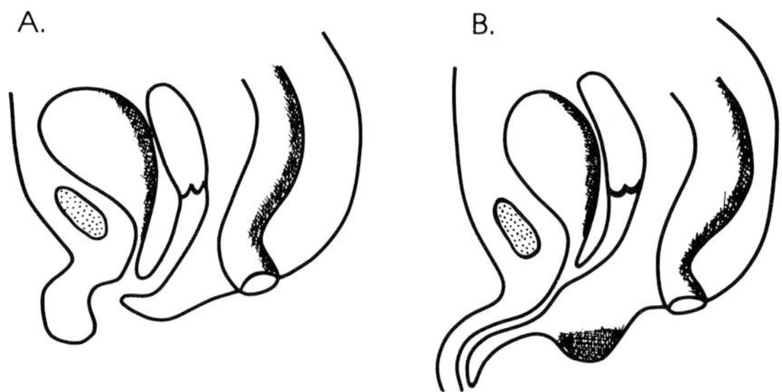

Fig. 22.12: *The interal anatomy of a genetic female with congenital adrenal hyperplasia. A. In the common situation, the introitus is partly covered by urogenital folds and the clitoris is enlarged. B. Rarely, when the androgen levels are very high, the phallus looks like a penis and the urogenital fusion has reduced the lower vagina, which opens in the posterior urethra.*

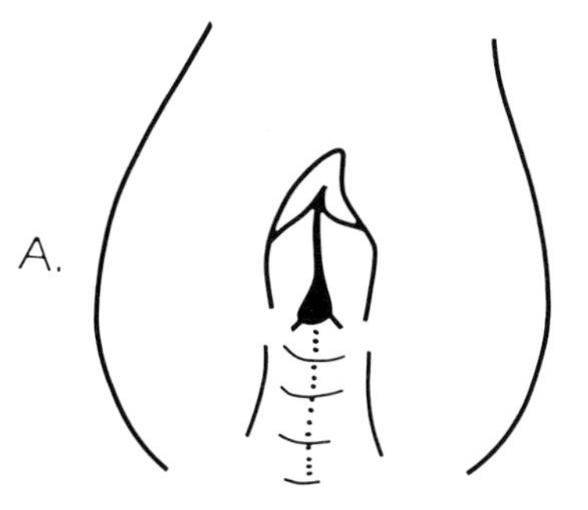

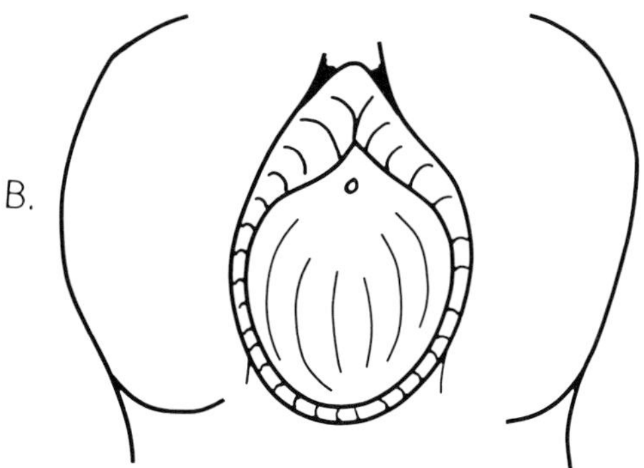

Fig. 22.13: *The different appearance of the vulva in labial adhesions in infancy (A), and vaginal atresia of a neonate (B).*

There are several points which enable the common adhesion of the labia to be distinguished from vaginal or hymenal atresia (Fig. 22.13). In labial adhesions, the labia cover the posterior half of the introitus like a curtain. The posterior rim of the labia is absent around the site of the fourchette. In vaginal atresia (Fig. 22.13B), the condition presents at birth or puberty (times of exposure to hormone stimulation) rather than in infancy. The hymen bulges out between an obvious rim of the labia minora, which is continuous posteriorly around the fourchette.

GOLDEN RULES

(1) The diagnosis and sex of rearing need to be determined *as soon as possible after birth*, to avoid the salt-losing crisis of adrenal hyperplasia and to prevent undue psychological and social stress on parents, relatives or the child.

(2) Do *not* assign the sex of a child born with ambiguous genitalia. Perform complete physical examination, investigations and urgent referral to an expert. Referral *must* be on the *first day of life*.

(3) Virilization of the external genitalia is proof of androgen secretion (normal or abnormal): the clitoris enlarges, the labia minora fuse to create a male urethra and the labia majora unite as a scrotum and become wrinkled.

(4) The presence of a vas/epididymis is proof of androgen secretion at an early stage of development.

(5) Any regression of the Müllerian duct indicates functional testicular tissue producing Müllerian inhibiting substance.

(6) Congenital adrenal hyperplasia must be diagnosed as soon as possible (even if there is no salt-losing) because *virilization progresses with age* and, if correctly treated, a girl with congenital adrenal hyperplasia may be fertile.

(7) Vomiting, diarrhoea and dehydration in the neonatal period in a phenotypic 'male' may indicate a girl with congenital adrenal hyperplasia.

(8) Perineal pigmentation is suggestive of congenital adrenal hyperplasia when high amounts of melanin-stimulating hormone have been produced by the pituitary gland.

(9) The presence of Müllerian structures can be determined clinically on rectal examination by palpation of the cervix and uterus.

(10) The presence of two testes indicates a genetic male, even if the external genitalia are feminized; it does *not* indicate the correct sex of rearing. This is determined after referral and complete investigation.

(11) A baby with hypospadias should not be assumed to be male unless *both testes are palpable in the scrotum*: the baby may have testicular dysgenesis and be better raised as female after gonadal excision and perineal reconstruction.

(12) In discussion with parents, avoid the use of emotionally disturbing terms, such as 'hermaphrodite', 'pseudohermaphrodite', or even 'intersex'. 'Genital abnormality' is an acceptable label while awaiting definitive diagnosis and deciding the sex of rearing.

Index